Birthing Outside the System

This book investigates why women choose to 'birth outside the system' and makes connections between women's right to choose where they birth and violations of human rights within maternity care systems.

Choosing to birth at home can force women out of mainstream maternity care, despite research supporting the safety of this option for low-risk women attended by midwives. When homebirth is not supported as a birthplace option, women will defy mainstream medical advice and, if a midwife is not available, choose either an unregulated careprovider or birth without assistance. This book examines the circumstances and drivers behind why women nevertheless choose homebirth by bringing legal and ethical perspectives together with the latest research on high-risk homebirth (breech and twin births), freebirth, birth with unregulated careproviders and the oppression of midwives who support unorthodox choices. Stories from women who have pursued alternatives in Australia, Europe, Russia, the UK, the US, Canada, the Middle East and India are woven through the research.

Insights and practical strategies are shared by doctors, midwives, lawyers, anthropologists, sociologists and psychologists on how to manage the tension between professional obligations and women's right to bodily autonomy. This book, the first of its kind, is an important contribution to considerations of place of birth and human rights in childbirth.

Hannah Dahlen is the Professor of Midwifery and Higher Degree Research Director in the School of Nursing and Midwifery at Western Sydney University in Australia. Hannah is also a privately practising midwife with a group practice called Midwives @ Sydney and Beyond. Hannah has been the Doctoral/Master's/Honours supervisor for seven of the contributors to this book. In 2012 Hannah was named in the *Sydney Morning Herald's* list of top 100 leading 'science and knowledge thinkers'. In 2019 she was made a Member in the General Division of the Order of Australia for her services to Midwifery, Nursing and Medical Education and Research.

Bashi Kumar-Hazard is an Australian trained competition and consumer rights lawyer, and the upcoming Chair of Human Rights in Childbirth. Bashi has represented families in coronial inquests and hospital midwives pursued by the healthcare regulator. Internationally, she has prepared Amicus briefs and UN human rights submissions on mistreatment in childbirth and women's reproductive rights. Bashi is currently working on a doctorate in Competition Law and Human Rights at the University of Sydney, examining anti-competitive practices in the provision of maternity healthcare in Australia.

Virginia Schmied is Professor of Midwifery and Deputy Dean, Research and Engagement in the School of Nursing and Midwifery, Western Sydney University. Her research focuses on transition to motherhood and perinatal mental health with a strong focus on the organisation of healthcare, workplace culture and the facilitators and barriers to the delivery of high-quality, compassionate maternity and child healthcare. Most recently, Virginia and her colleagues have been studying the experiences of women and men from diverse cultural backgrounds living in western Sydney.

Routledge Research in Nursing and Midwifery

Pragmatic Children's Nursing
A Theory for Children and their Childhoods
Duncan C. Randall

A Theory of Cancer Care in Healthcare Settings
Edited by Carol Cox and Maya Zumstein-Shaha

Motherhood, Spirituality and Culture
Noelia Molina

Joy at Birth
An Interpretive, Hermeneutic, Phenomenological Inquiry
Susan Crowther

The Shadow Side of Nursing
Paradox, Image and Identity
Margaret McAllister and Donna Lee Brien

Birthing Outside the System
The Canary in the Coal Mine
Edited by Hannah Dahlen, Bashi Kumar-Hazard and Virginia Schmied

For more information about this series, please visit: www.routledge.com/Routledge-Research-in-Nursing/book-series/RRIN

Birthing Outside the System

The Canary in the Coal Mine

Edited by
Hannah Dahlen, Bashi Kumar-Hazard and Virginia Schmied

Routledge
Taylor & Francis Group
LONDON AND NEW YORK

HUMAN RIGHTS in CHILDBIRTH

First published 2020 by Routledge
2 Park Square, Milton Park, Abingdon, Oxon OX14 4RN

and by Routledge
605 Third Avenue, New York, NY 10017

Routledge is an imprint of the Taylor & Francis Group, an informa business

British Library Cataloguing-in-Publication Data
A catalogue record for this book is available from the British Library

Library of Congress Cataloging-in-Publication Data
Names: Dahlen, Hannah G., editor. | Kumar-Hazard, Bashi, editor. | Schmied, Virginia, editor.
Title: Birthing outside the system: the canary in the coal mine / edited by Hannah Dahlen, Bashi Kumar-Hazard and Virginia Schmied.
Description: Milton Park, Abingdon, Oxon; New York, NY: Routledge, 2020. | Includes bibliographical references and index. |
Identifiers: LCCN 2019051068 (print) | LCCN 2019051069 (ebook) | ISBN 9781138592704 (hardback) | ISBN 9780429489853 (ebook)
Subjects: LCSH: Natural childbirth. | Childbirth at home. | Maternal health services. Classification: LCC RG661 .B575 2020 (print) | LCC RG661 (ebook) | DDC 618.4/5–dc23
LC record available at https://lccn.loc.gov/2019051068
LC ebook record available at https://lccn.loc.gov/2019051069

ISBN: 978-1-138-59270-4 (hbk)

DOI: 10.4324/9780429489853

Typeset in Times New Roman
by Newgen Publishing UK

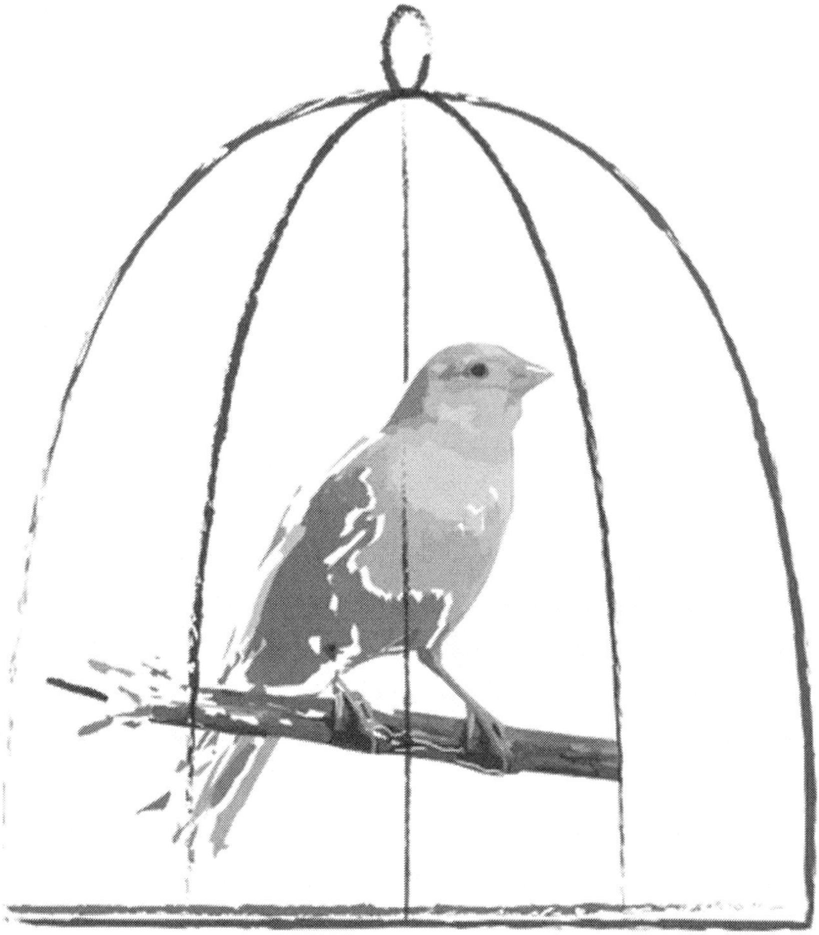

Artwork by Lydia Dahlen.

Contents

Acknowledgements

We would like to acknowledge the women who told their stories and trusted us to make changes through our research. We take this remit very seriously. It is hard to truly quantify the pain and enduring impact of trauma discussed in these pages or the extreme measures some women took and currently take to avoid mainstream care. We hear, and have felt, the fear and frustration you felt when you were backed into a corner of the system's making. We hope that this book triggers a revolution in the thinking and listening that is so desperately needed to the voices of women and their choices. This is the beginning and we must not let it be the end.

ENOUGH

ENOUGH to the lies women are told about their 'incapable' bodies
ENOUGH to the bullying and coercion they experience when they say 'No'
ENOUGH to the trauma that scars them and those who love them for life
ENOUGH to ignoring the scientific evidence AGAIN and AGAIN and AGAIN
ENOUGH to the power middle class men hold when it comes to women
ENOUGH to the PTSD that is rising in childbirth and the rising rates of suicide
ENOUGH to the horror stories that strip women of their hopes and dreams
ENOUGH to the impersonalised care we give, knowing we can do better
ENOUGH to a system focused on itself, not women, despite the mission statements
ENOUGH to anxious babies looking for love in their haunted mother's eyes
ENOUGH to our money spent on causing harm in health care, not preventing it
ENOUGH to weak leaders and politically correct tiptoeing around the issue
ENOUGH when we know better
ENOUGH when we know how
ENOUGH when we know why
ENOUGH when it can change now
ENOUGH!
ENOUGH!
ENOUGH!

Hannah Dahlen, 25 July 2015

Figures

Tables

Notes on contributors

Alison Barrett is a Canadian-trained consultant obstetrician and gynaecologist. She lives in New Zealand, where she continues to practise medicine while finishing a law degree at the University of Waikato. Before she went to medical school, she studied ecology at the University of Toronto.

Andrew Bisits is the Medical Co Director of Maternity at the Royal Hospital for Women in Randwick. He is an active obstetrician whose professional practice has always been in the public sector. Dr Bisits has worked closely with midwives to promote midwifery models of care. He has a conjoint Associate Professorial Appointment with UNSW. He is active in teaching and research.

Melanie Briggs is an Aboriginal woman and a descendant of the Dharawal and Gumbangirr peoples and lives on Wandandian country in the Yuin nation. She is a midwife with ten years' experience working with Aboriginal families in the community. She is the Co-Chair of the National Strategic Birthing on Country Committee and works as the Project Officer at Waminda in Nowra for the Executive Shoalhaven Birthing on Country Strategic Committee.

Cherisse Buzzacott is an Arrernte woman and midwife from Alice Springs, NT, Australia and the Project Officer for the Australian college of Midwives Birthing on Country Project. She is also the Chair of the Rhodanthe Lipsett Indigenous Midwifery Charitable Fund. Her work focuses on supporting national objectives through consultation, with a goal of improving maternity care outcomes for Aboriginal and Torres Strait Islander women and families.

Agy Cater was working as an Assistant Accountant for the Commonwealth Games, Australia before becoming pregnant. She is currently still on maternity leave, advocating for positive birth experiences and sharing her birth story by working as a Consumer Representative for Maternity Choices Australia.

Melissa Cheyney is Associate Professor of Clinical Medical Anthropology at Oregon State University with additional appointments in Global Health and Women Gender and Sexuality Studies. She is also a Licensed Midwife in active homebirth practice and the Chair of the Division of Research for the Midwives Alliance of North America.

Sue-anne Cutmore identifies as a Wandi Wandi woman from Gomeroi country. Sue-anne is committed to working with communities, families and individuals around equity in all areas of life. She has a mediation background and is moving into Family Group Conferencing. She is currently completing a Bachelor of Social Work after working in the field for 30-plus years.

Dea Delaney-Thiele is a very proud Dunghutti, Kamilaroi and Yuin Aboriginal woman and is the National Executive Director of *Dhiiyaan Mirri*, Bridging Cultures Unit at OzChild. Dea also worked in the ACCHO network for over 26 years at all levels. Dea strongly advocates for Aboriginal People's right to self-determination and Child Safety.

Farah Diaz-Tello is a US human rights attorney focusing on the full spectrum of pregnancy outcomes. She is Senior Counsel for If/When/How: Lawyering for Reproductive Justice, where she works to ensure everyone can make reproductive decisions with dignity. Her publications address obstetric violence, economic coercion during birth and criminalisation of pregnancy.

Daniela Drandić is the Head of the Reproductive Rights Program, Roda – Parents in Action (Croatia). She is a student undertaking her MSc in Maternal and Infant Health (University of Dundee). Daniela is also the Reproductive Rights Program Lead, Roda – Parents in Action (Croatia).

Claire Feeley is a recent Doctoral student at the University of Central Lancashire in Preston, UK. Claire is practising as a midwife at the Royal Free NHS Trust in London, UK. Claire also works as an Associate Lecturer at three universities.

Deborah Fox is a Lecturer in Midwifery at the Centre for Midwifery, Child and Family Health at the University of Technology Sydney, Australia. Her qualifications include a Doctorate, Master of Science (Midwifery and Women's Health) and Bachelor of Midwifery. With obstetric colleagues in 2011, she implemented the first midwifery continuity of care model to be established in Singapore. Her research is focused on optimising birth experiences for women who experience complications and unexpected outcomes in childbearing.

Rixa Freeze is a Visiting Assistant Professor at Wabash College in Indiana, USA. Her doctoral studies focused on maternity care and childbirth. She is the mother of four children, all born at home. In 2018 she founded Breech Without Borders, a non-profit organisation dedicated to breech training and education.

Kathryn Gutteridge was a consultant midwife since the role first developed. She has worked all of her midwifery career within the NHS in the UK developing and supporting midwifery-only facilities. She is a well-renowned author/presenter and founder of Sanctum Midwives, set up to provide maternity workers with advice about caring for survivors of sexual abuse. Although Kathryn has undertaken research and completed academic studies, she is first and foremost devoted to being with 'woman'.

Donna Hartz identifies as a member of the Kamilaroi nation. She is midwife and nurse with 34 years' experience as a clinician, educator, lecturer, manager, consultant and researcher, and has worked in variety of settings including homebirth. She is currently an Associate Professor in Midwifery at Charles Darwin University, Sydney.

Martine Hollander is an obstetrician and staff member at the Radboud University in Nijmegen, the Netherlands. She wrote her doctoral thesis on women who go against medical advice in their choices surrounding (place of) birth and birth attendant, and on traumatic childbirth experiences. Martine was a community midwife in the early 2000s and attended many homebirths.

Jo Hunter is a privately practising midwife in Sydney supporting women who choose to give birth at home. She completed her Honours research in 2019 through Western Sydney University under the supervision of Hannah Dahlen. Jo is also a film-maker and has spent 3 years co-creating a documentary called *Birth Time*.

Suha Hussein is a Higher Degree Research student in the School of Nursing and Midwifery at Western Sydney University in New South Wales, Australia. Her research focuses on changing non-evidence birthing practices in Jordan and the Middle East. Most recently, Suha has been studying childbirth experiences of Jordanian women living in Jordan or Australia. Suha has been supervised for her Master's and doctorate by Virginia Schmied and Hannah Dahlen.

Svetlana Illarionova is a new graduate midwife who completed her Bachelor of Midwifery as a second degree at Monash University, Melbourne, Australia in 2017. Svetlana now lives in Ufa, Russia. Svetlana is in the process of getting registration as a midwife and currently supports women in their childbirth journey as a doula.

Melanie Jackson is a research midwife with a focus on birth outside the system and also works as a private midwife in New South Wales, Australia with her private group practice Midwives @ Sydney and Beyond. Melanie has also worked as a Midwifery lecturer at Western Sydney University and done consultancy work with The Australian College of Midwives. Melanie undertook her doctoral research under the supervision of Hannah Dahlen and Virginia Schmied.

Bec Jenkinson is a maternity consumer activist and researcher. Bec completed her doctorate in 2017, examining women's, midwives' and obstetricians' experiences of situations where pregnant women decline recommended care. She is currently co-leading the development of Queensland Department of Health guideline for partnering with women who decline recommended maternity care.

Hazel Keedle is a Lecturer of Midwifery and doctoral candidate at the School of Nursing and Midwifery at Western Sydney University in New South Wales, Australia. Hazel's Master's Honours thesis focused on homebirth after caesarean and her doctoral work is exploring women's experiences of planning a VBAC in Australia. Hazel's Higher Degree Research studies have been supervised by Hannah Dahlen and Virginia Schmied.

Andrew Kotaska is an Obstetrician/Gynaecologist at Stanton Territorial Hospital in Yellowknife, Canada. He is president of the Northwest Territories Medical Association and has academic appointments as Adjunct Professor with the School of Population and Public Health at the University of British Columbia and Lecturer at the Universities of Manitoba and Toronto.

Kaveri Mayra is an Indian midwifery and nursing researcher. She has over 12 years' research experience in nursing and midwifery workforce policies and care provision, mainly in India. Having seen mistreatment during childbirth early on as a student midwife and experienced lack of leadership and decision-making power, Kaveri started researching and advocating about this. Kaveri is a global speaker on disrespect and abuse during childbirth. She is trained in nursing, midwifery and public health in India and is currently pursuing a doctorate at the University of Southampton, UK.

Sarah O'Connor is a mother of four, living in Victoria, Australia. Sarah recently resigned from her Dental Assistant occupation to focus on raising her children and studying to become a Midwife. Sarah is a Bachelor of Nursing student at Charles Darwin University, intending to transfer into their Bachelor of Midwifery programme.

Elizabeth Rigg is a Senior Midwifery lecturer in the School of Nursing and Midwifery at the University of Southern Queensland in Queensland, Australia. Elizabeth is also a registered midwife with over 30 years' experience working in clinical practice and undertook her Doctoral studies under the supervision of Hannah Dahlen and Virginia Schmied.

Nicholas Rubashkin is Associate Professor of Obstetrics, Gynecology, and Reproductive Sciences at the University of California San Francisco (UCSF) where he serves as an inpatient obstetric hospitalist. He is also a doctoral candidate in Global Health Sciences (also at UCSF). His research concerns respectful, evidence-based maternity care and uses methods that integrate the perspective of women's advocacy groups. His dissertation research will examine the role of race and racism in access to VBAC in the United States. He is a board director with Human Rights in Childbirth in which capacity he has given testimony in court cases around the world where women's rights have been violated in pregnancy and childbirth.

Tamara Sadovaya is a founder and the Director for Development in the Centre of Traditional Midwifery and Family Medicine in Moscow, Russia. Tamara is a practising midwife since 1995, an educator and initiator of the project 'Gentle Birth' in several maternity hospitals in big cities across the country.

Heather Sassine was a Traditional Chinese Medicine practitioner and a midwife in private practice. She is currently devoting her time to raising her two beautiful boys. Heather did her Honours research under the supervision of Hannah Dahlen and presents some of the results in her book chapter.

Maddy Simpson is a doctoral candidate at Western Sydney University, supervised by Hannah Dahlen and Virginia Schmied. Her main research area is understanding the experiences of women who have experienced traumatic births and the development of post-traumatic stress disorder after childbirth. Maddy is a registered midwife and nurse, currently working in a nursing and midwifery management role.

Laura Tanner is a doctoral candidate in Feminist Studies with an emphasis on productive and reproductive labours at the University of California, Santa Barbara, USA. Her dissertation research examines the motivations and experiences of women who plan freebirths.

Gill Thomson is a Reader (Associate Professor) in Perinatal Health in the Maternal and Infant Nutrition & Nurture research unit at the University of Central Lancashire, UK. Gill has a psychology background, and has a long history of undertaking research and evaluation-type projects within community, private and academic sectors.

Foreword

Every chapter of this book reminds us of the profound and far-reaching importance of humanising birth: for women,[1] their families, societies and humanity, whatever the context. The authors have shared their research and experiences about a wide range of issues for women who choose to give birth at home when their pregnancies are considered to be 'high risk', including those who decide to 'freebirth' (give birth unattended by health professionals). The imperative to understand, respect and support women who make these choices is illuminated by quotations, stories and the authors' own searing accounts of experiences that have motivated them to speak and write of the unacceptable face of institutionalised childbirth in the twenty-first century.

The stories in this book also speak, though, of resilience and courage, giving examples of situations and actions that promote a sense of agency for women who give birth. In reading and re-reading this book, I am reminded of the power of stories to open our minds to the situations and feelings of others, particularly those who do not necessarily share the same ideologies or culture as us: those who we might consider as 'other'.

For many of us, the accounts in this book will trigger memories of women we have known throughout the years who have chosen to give birth at home 'against medical advice'. The language may have shifted so that women now bear the label of having a 'high-risk pregnancy', but stories of the animosity they encountered echo throughout this book.

Reading this book transported me back to a time in the 1980s when I worked as an 'independent' (privately practising) midwife in London. I was invited to speak at a Royal College of Midwives' Professional Day. My talk, 'Filling the gaps and picking up the pieces', was published in 1991 in the RCM journal, at that time still called *Midwives Chronicle and Nursing Notes*. Like the many examples in this book, this article described how women were turning to independent midwives after encountering negativity and hostility in their interactions with NHS staff. These included midwives, obstetricians, GPs, or a combination of maternity care professionals who were hostile and intent on convincing women of the 'selfish' risks they were inflicting on their babies. The women most likely to describe feeling powerless and humiliated were those who had had previous traumatic experiences of giving birth. Then, as now, these women were the ones who were most likely to turn to independent (privately practising) midwives, digging their heels in: 'I am *not* going back into that system. I feel safer staying at home to give birth'. Importantly, the paper also provided descriptions of independent midwives who were effectively liaising with supportive obstetricians and senior midwives, who listened to women and trusted them to make informed decisions, even when these were not the decisions they would make themselves.

Throughout this book there are messages about the importance of ensuring that structures are in place to promote respectful consultation and transfer if needed. We need to work on the concept of going to hospital if 'help is needed' rather than 'the failed homebirth'. This approach involves hospital staff trusting and supporting midwives who attend births at home, especially where women have made choices that evoke disapproval and fear.

When I first heard about women 'freebirthing' I found it very challenging. And then I remembered … I remembered stories over the years of women who may have left it too late to call the midwife or go to hospital … I remembered my own story of doing this and offer it here in the spirit of this book, not as an example of someone making a conscious informed decision to bypass giving birth in hospital, but to raise awareness of more passive, intuitive resistance that we may encounter from time to time.

It is 1970. I am 22 years old and pregnant with my second child. We are living in a semi-detached farm cottage in rural Somerset, surrounded by fields, at the end of a mile-long, narrow, unsurfaced lane. I want to give birth at home but I'm told I must go to hospital to have this baby – the lane is seen as an access problem for an ambulance.

At antenatal visits I repeatedly ask if I can give birth at home. My mother had babies at home (including undiagnosed twins) and as the eldest of five children, I have wonderful memories of greeting my siblings in my parents' bedroom. In this second pregnancy, I am haunted by memories of giving birth to my first baby in hospital. The seven days' routine 'confinement' in hospital makes me shudder and I don't want to leave my first child, who is 22 months old. No one tells me that I have any rights to question or challenge anything I am told. I am anxious to be seen as a good mother and feel powerless in the face of authority.

Fretful about going to hospital, I am not sleeping well. In the antenatal clinic they hand out a new benzodiazepine sleeping pill – 'Temazepam' – to help pregnant women with their restless legs and difficulties getting to sleep.

As with my first baby, I am still pregnant three weeks past the official due date, healthy with a well-grown baby. My contractions start in the evening. Memories of my last birth swirl around my head: the routine shave and 'high, hot and a helluva lot' enema; not being believed when I was in strong labour; the pethidine that was given without consent and which took away my voice; the policy of not allowing my husband to be present; the slapping of my hands when I reached down during the crowning of her head; the lining up of new mothers in the postnatal ward at a trough-like sink, made to scrub our nipples with a nail brush before each feed; perineal swabbing while lying in bed over a bedpan four-hourly; the nightmare tuition and exam in 'bathing baby'; and worst of all, the separation: the routine removal of my baby to the nursery, starting with the long night after I gave birth, lying awake aching for her – babies lived in the nursery and were ceremonially brought to us for a breastfeed every four hours. I cannot face going in. I take two Temazepam in the hope that sleep will delay the night-mare prospect.

I wake in the night with fierce contractions; barely a break in between them – there is no way I can go to hospital. Our next-door neighbours click into action – Mick cycles to the telephone box at the pub at the end of the lane and phones the village midwives; Jo slices up empty plastic fertiliser sacks to protect the mattress. I am in my own birthing world, no longer even thinking about going to hospital.

Sister Jones arrives in the upstairs bedroom and wags a finger at me – 'You should have gone to hospital earlier'. I respond with: 'I want to PUSH'. She stops looking stern and we smile at each other. Two pushes later, I stop wondering whether an enema is a crucial part of having a baby and gently, I breathe her out, this perfect, beautiful baby. I gather her to me and weep with love and exhilar-ation. No one is going to take this baby from me or dictate when I can feed her.

There is much celebration going on. The GP is downstairs (Sister Jones must have called him). He's drinking brandy and recovering from getting lost and falling into the rose bushes by the garden path. He comes upstairs, pokes his head round the door, says 'Congratulations' and goes downstairs for a top-up.

This was the start of me wanting to spread the word about how birth can be. I entered the world of birth activism.

Nine years later – and in different circumstances – I gave birth to my third child at home. Significantly, in the intervening years, the Western world had also changed. The Women's Liberation Movement was promoting a culture of coming together to demystify and take control of our health away from medical hegemony. The concept of 'woman-centred care' – placing the individual woman at the centre of her care – was articulated as the way health services for women should be developed. These ideas were first promulgated in the book produced by the Boston Women's Health Collective (1971): *Our Bodies, Ourselves*. Suzanne Arms' (1975) *Immaculate Deception* and Ina May Gaskin's (1976) *Spiritual Midwifery* were two of the influential books challenging what Robbie Davis-Floyd would later call 'technocratic birth'. The notion of 'the personal is political' became a unifying feminist slogan for reflecting on women's experiences, including childbirth, in terms of power dynamics. In all of this heady reappraisal of our lives, coming together in groups involved consciousness-raising, practising assertiveness, writing articles and planning collective action – features of the Association of Radical Midwives meetings in the UK for over 40 years.

Moving into the twenty-first century, as this book describes, birth activism has a new, different face and a far greater global reach than ever before. The proliferation of communication technology sees the linking of woman-centred care during childbirth to human rights and the need to address issues such as racism, misogyny, 'obstetric violence' and the persecution of midwives. The websites of organisations such as 'Human Rights in Childbirth' and 'White Ribbon Alliance' continue to identify the urgency to act in ways that place individual women at the centre of maternity care in people-led movements. Examples in this book offer hope by identifying where these actions have made a difference.

Many people have suggested that our efforts to create a more humane world start with promoting a positive experience for each individual woman giving birth. This goes way beyond promoting 'normal birth' to creating cultures in which all women are treated with respect and dignity. Increasingly, this is seen as a global human rights issue. In *The prevention and elimination of disrespect and abuse during facility-based childbirth* (WHO, 2015), the World Health Organisation has identified that women experience disrespectful and abusive treatment during childbirth in facilities worldwide and that this is a major factor in women avoiding contact with health professionals. The statement calls for 'greater action, dialogue, research and advocacy'. This book makes an important contribution to all of those recommendations.

If ever you had any doubts about the reasons why women choose to give birth outside of the system or in ways that do not fall within maternity service guidelines, these will fall away as you read this book. For many of us this will trigger memories that may be both painful and uplifting. There is no doubt that the book has the potential to heighten our awareness about our own role in perpetuating or challenging power dynamics in childbirth. After reading it, I felt compelled to talk to friends about the issues it raises and the impact it had on me.

The overwhelming message here is simple. We need to listen to women, respecting that safety for many of them cannot be reduced to decision-making based on a series of 'evidence-based facts'. As I write, I catch an interview on the BBC news with Tracey Neville, retired English netball player and ex-head coach of the English national netball team. She is talking about her pregnancy and her desire to change the conversations around 'older' pregnant women:

> We know the stats ... We know that I'm 42 and the risks are higher, but it creates a fearful environment ... If only there was just a bit more positivity around health and well-being. [With our athletes] we don't sit down and quote stats at them, and quote how many times we've lost. We sit down and look at how we can win. [The doctors] go down the route of: 'Well, we're preparing you for the fail.' I don't prepare my team for the fail. Why is pregnancy not targeted like that? Why is it not given that positivity? I'd come out of a miscarriage and another consultant was giving me these stats again. No, tell me what can I do.

In our conversations with pregnant women, the potential positive and negative impact we have at both a conscious and a subconscious level cannot be underestimated. 'Safety' for pregnant women includes making sure that they feel respected in all aspects of their identity when making choices. Being a mother (or parent) will involve a lifetime of grappling with uncertainty as we make decisions to protect and enhance the health and well-being of our children. A key challenge for birth workers is, therefore, to consider how we engage with pregnant women around uncertainty. This involves far more than focusing on the fraught notion of 'informed choice'.

This book provides the imperative for us to join with others – users and providers of maternity services – in exploring local and global efforts to humanise birth. This will inevitably include looking at the discrimination and power imbalances that pervade institutionalised birth environments. The stories, research findings and suggestions for the way forward presented here will help to both inform and challenge us in those discussions. The authors have offered us evidence and valuable resources that will enhance our efforts to engage with pregnant women in whichever way they see fit on their unique journey through childbirth.

Nicky Leap
Adjunct Professor of Midwifery, University of Technology Sydney, Australia

Note

1 I have used the words woman and women in this foreword. This is not meant to exclude those who give birth and do not identify as women, for whom the honouring principles of respectful maternity care described here are equally important.

References

Arms, S. (1975). *Immaculate deception: A new look at women and childbirth*. Boston, MA: Houghton Mifflin.

Boston Women's Health Book Collective. (1971). *Our bodies, ourselves*. Boston, MA: New England Free Press.

Gaskin, I. M. (1976). *Spiritual midwifery*. Summertown, TN: Book Publishing Company.

Part 1

Understanding the problem

Introduction

Hannah Dahlen, Bashi Kumar-Hazard and Virginia Schmied

> The question should not be why do women not accept the service that we offer, but why do we not offer a service that women will accept?
>
> (Fathalla, 1988)

Introduction

This book has had a very long gestation. It was conceived many years ago, even though we did not realise it at the time. As you will see below, your editors (Hannah, Bashi and Virginia) came together by chance, three very different women with different expertise and backgrounds, who connected through a common focus and a powerful synergy in our research, work and personal experiences.

This book is about women who choose to birth 'outside the system'. We defined birthing outside the system as either 'freebirth' – where women plan a birth at home with no registered health provider in attendance (also known as unassisted birth or unhindered birth) – or 'high-risk homebirth' – where the presence of significant risk factors cause most health providers and guidelines to recommend hospital birth as the safest option (for example, breech and twin birth). Essentially, women who birth 'outside the system' are making a choice of birth place (usually home) or provider (such as unregulated birth workers), or both, in circumstances that would not be recommended by the majority of health professionals and fall outside health service guidelines. Note that we refrained from saying 'evidence-based guidelines' because it will become apparent, as you read this book, that the guidelines commonly used within the system are not necessarily evidence-based or woman-centred.

This book is a political opus, and we make no apologies for that. If you think you can sit back and be entertained, think again. We intend to upend thinking and disturb assumptions. We intend to shock, at times distress and most certainly to exasperate. Finally, we hope to inspire you to be a part of the change we so desperately need. We guarantee that you will think differently after reading this book and hope you will join a revolution to humanise childbirth for every woman, everywhere. We have a challenge on our hands in maternity care today, but we also hold the answer to that challenge.

The state of childbirth in the world

Women are not choosing birth outside the system because they are spoilt for choice; far from it. They choose to birth outside the system because what we offer is hurting them and we are simply not listening to their concerns. The world authorities are now taking this issue very seriously, in the face of mounting scientific evidence of harm.

Recent world reports

Medical intervention in childbirth has reached unprecedented levels. While it is sometimes necessary to save lives, it is apparent we have gone too far with little consideration given to short- and long-term consequences on health (Dahlen et al., 2013; FIGO, 2018; WHO, 2018). The 2018 Lancet Series on Caesarean Section warned against excessive use – now reaching epidemic proportions – of obstetric interventions like caesarean section (Boerma et al., 2018). The authors called for a reduction in overuse of interventions causing avoidable harm and leading to a cascade of interventions that cause even further harms that are not being adequately monitored. The authors also found, based on data from 169 countries that included 98.4% of the world's births, that nearly 30 million caesarean sections had occurred in 2015 (21%) – almost double the rate since 2000 (12%) (Boerma et al., 2018). Many countries reported caesarean section rates significantly higher than the World Health Organisation (WHO)-recommended rates of 10–15% (Betran et al., 2015; WHO, 2015). For example, caesarean section was up to 10 times more frequent in Latin America and the Caribbean region (44.3%) when compared with the west and central African region (4.1%) (Boerma et al., 2018). By contrast, the rate in Africa is too low. There was significant variation between countries with similar socio-demographics; for example, Cyprus has a rate of 55% while the Netherlands was at 16% in 2016 (OECD, 2018). The Nordic countries not only have the lowest caesarean section rates in the developed world, they also have some of the best maternal and perinatal outcomes. Caesarean section use is almost five times higher in the richest countries when compared to the poorest (Boerma et al., 2018). High caesarean section use was also seen among low-risk births, especially among women who are more educated (Brazil and China). Caesarean section use was at least 1·6 times more frequent in private facilities than in public facilities (Boerma et al., 2018). Similar findings were reported in Australia (Dahlen et al., 2014).

Caesarean section is not without significant consequences. The Lancet Series on Caesarean Section (CS) states:

> The prevalence of maternal mortality and maternal morbidity is higher after CS than after vaginal birth. CS is associated with an increased risk of uterine rupture, abnormal placentation, ectopic pregnancy, stillbirth, and preterm birth, and these risks increase in a dose–response manner. There

> is emerging evidence that babies born by CS have different hormonal, physical, bacterial, and medical exposures, and that these exposures can subtly alter neonatal physiology. Short-term risks of CS include altered immune development, an increased likelihood of allergy, atopy, and asthma, and reduced intestinal gut microbiome diversity. The persistence of these risks into later life is less well investigated, although an association between CS use and greater incidence of late childhood obesity and asthma are frequently reported.
>
> (Sandall et al., 2018, p. 1349)

Related obstetric intervention rates are also rising across the globe. In 2016, the Lancet Series on Maternal Health reported high rates of induction of labour, described as care that is 'too much, too soon' (Miller et al., 2016). The Lancet Series on Midwifery (Renfrew et al., 2014) and the *WHO recommendations: intrapartum care for a positive childbirth experience* (WHO, 2018) also call for a reduction in unnecessary birth intervention. These major reports offer a simple solution: a move towards relationship-based models of care, the gold standard being continuity of midwifery care for all women, regardless of risk. In the Lancet Series on Midwifery, the authors found over 50 outcomes were improved with midwifery care, including reductions in maternal and neonatal mortality and morbidity, stillbirth, preterm birth and unnecessary interventions, and improved psychosocial outcomes. Homer and colleagues (2014) showed that the effect of scaling up midwifery to 95%, in countries with the highest incidence of adverse maternal and newborn outcomes, could avert 61% of maternal and perinatal deaths. The Quality Maternal and Newborn Care framework (Renfrew et al., 2014) emphasised the importance of care that is respectful and tailored to a woman's individual needs within her context in her community.

A global network of researchers recently published a research priorities paper calling for the need to recognise the importance of positive experiences for women during pregnancy, birth and the postpartum period alongside the reduction of adverse events. This is leading to a critical change in the conversation and prioritisation of research in this space (Kennedy et al., 2018). The paper called for three inter-related research themes: (1) examination and implementation of models of care that enhance both well-being and safety; (2) investigating and optimising physiological, psychological and social processes in pregnancy, childbirth and the postnatal period; and (3) development and validation of outcome measures that capture short- and longer-term well-being (Kennedy et al., 2018). These first steps may well herald a new era in childbirth research and policy that will actually improve care for women, babies and their families.

Birth trauma and mental health

In the first study on freebirth and high-risk homebirth in Australia undertaken by our (Hannah and Virginia) PhD student Melanie Jackson (see

Chapter 2), 85% of the women interviewed had given birth previously, most in hospital. Many reported highly negative previous birth experiences involving interventions without informed consent. For some, the treatment they received was emotionally and physically devastating (Jackson, Dahlen, & Schmied, 2012). It was clear that these women wanted what was the best and safest for their baby and were highly educated (70% had university degrees). They perceived the intervention and interference they had previously experienced in hospital as a greater risk. They also understood that the health system would not respect or support their choices, so they chose to disengage from, and birth outside, the system (Jackson et al., 2012).

Once we add the complexities around mental health concerns to mistreatment in childbirth, the vulnerabilities women with mental health issues face in birth are compounded and exacerbated. Worldwide, maternal mental health problems are considered one of the most significant public health issues, with several developed nations, including Australia, now reporting maternal suicide as the leading single cause of maternal death (Ellwood and Dahlen, 2019). One in five women experience high levels of anxiety in pregnancy and this appears to be increasing (Kingsbury et al., 2017; Dahlen et al., 2018), with significant and enduring impacts on women and their babies (Austin et al., 2017). The American Psychiatric Association (2018) found that anxiety had increased in the population by five points in just one year on a 0–100 scale, to reach an average of 51 points. In Australia, the 2018 Women's Health Survey reported that 66.9% of the 15,000 women interviewed felt nervous, anxious or on edge during several or more days over a four-week period (Women's Health Survey, 2018).

Risk factors for perinatal anxiety and depression include: (a) previous history of depression or anxiety (Clavarino et al., 2010; Rubertsson, Hellström, Cross, & Sydsjö, 2014; Dennis, Brown, Falah-Hassani, Marini, & Vigod, 2017); (b) birth interventions associated with post-traumatic stress disorder (PTSD) in the mother (Rubertsson et al., 2014; Dennis et al., 2017; Simpson, Schmied, Dickson, & Dahlen, 2018); (c) difficult socio-economic circumstances, with low-level social support, or migrant and refugee backgrounds (Rubertsson et al., 2014); and (d) women who report perfectionist characteristics (i.e. striving to meet the 'good mother' ideal) (Hays, 1996; Liamputtong, 2006; Maher and Saugeres, 2007; Goodwin and Huppatz, 2010; Pedersen, 2012). In this book, you will read that a past traumatic birth and/or PTSD is a major reason motivating women to leave our maternity system (see Chapter 12).

When military personnel return from war with PTSD, we do not send them back to the same battlegrounds where the trauma was first triggered. By contrast, with childbirth trauma, we not only require women's exposure to the same trauma, we bully and coerce them into accepting it, again and again. When traumatised women seek to avoid further trauma (in hospital), care providers accuse them of being selfish, journalists portray them as bad or stupid mothers and laws are proposed to 'criminalise' their efforts to protect themselves. Demonising and criminalising women to control and herd them back into an abusive environment is coercion and, in itself, a form of violence against women. It serves as an easy, duplicitous distraction for health professionals who want to ignore their contribution to the mistreatment of women.

Recent evidence demonstrates that respectful care has an impact on physical and psychological health. A Cochrane review of routine uptake of antenatal services across 41 countries (high-, medium- and low-income) found women were more likely to access antenatal care if they saw care as individualised, positive, reflecting their cultural values and beliefs, accessible, affordable and flexible. Women in the review valued good information and advice, and wanted to feel safe, respected, and be treated with kindness (Downe, Finlayson, Tuncalp, & Gulmezoglu, 2019).

Obstetric violence

A review on 'obstetric violence' reported that publications about this topic have increased substantially since 2015 (Barbosa Jardim and Modena, 2018). The authors found, from reviewing 24 papers, that obstetric violence constitutes a violation of human rights and is a serious, global public health problem. It manifests in the negligent, reckless, omissive, discriminatory and disrespectful acts of health professionals and is legitimised by 'the symbolic relations of power that [both] naturalize and trivialize their occurrence' (Barbosa Jardim and Modena, 2018). Despite the reporting, research and complaints, we know that governments don't like to talk about or acknowledge obstetric violence. Recently in Brazil, where the term was first officially recognised, the new conservative-led government announced that the term will now be avoided and, if possible, banned from use in government public policy documents (Ignacio, 2019). The Ministry of Health later softened its position somewhat in response to a backlash from medical specialists, activists and human and women's rights groups. When the truth offends, the offended can either change themselves or change the truth. Their reaction is often as revealing as the truth.

Racism in maternity care

The latest research has quantified a further, disturbing dimension to mistreatment in pregnancy and childbirth – the negative effects of racism in facility-based care on health outcomes. Racism is not a new phenomenon in itself. Ethnic minority groups across the globe face a complex set of adverse social and psychological challenges linked to their minority status, all of which often imbued with racial discrimination. Racism in healthcare, however, is only now being subjected to the scrutiny it deserves. The behaviours that take place in hospitals are merely a reflection of these all too common social dynamics occurring within a society. As you will read in this book, systemic racism is a comfortably settled component of hospital maternity care in every country in which dominant ethnic groups have learnt to apply skin colour, or external physical characteristics, as a defining criteria for exclusion, domination and/ or dehumanisation.

Further, a growing body of literature is recognising the relationship between racial discrimination and poor health outcomes (Berger & Sarnyai, 2015). When it comes to pregnancy and childbirth, we know that racism can have a significant impact on mothers and babies. The much-publicised case of a pregnant woman in Ireland who ruptured her membranes at a pre-viable gestation and died of sepsis captured the attention of the world. As Savita Hallapanavar suffered a slow and agonising death from maternal sepsis, a nurse told her that she couldn't have an abortion 'because Ireland is a Catholic Country' (Bowers, 2013). In the USA and the UK, significant disparities in mortality and morbidity for women and babies of colour can no longer be dismissed as being due to socio-economic or other external factors (Knight et al., 2018; National Partnership, 2018). The numbers speak for themselves: in the richest countries around the world, women of colour and their babies are significantly more likely to die from pregnancy-related causes than their white counterparts. Most recently, Vedam et al. (2019) reported a cross-sectional survey of maternity experiences among women from diverse backgrounds in the United States. She found that 17.3% of the 2138 women surveyed reported experiencing some type of mistreatment, including loss of autonomy, being shouted at, scolded or threatened, or simply ignored. Women who birthed in hospital reported higher rates of mistreatment (28.1%) compared to women birthing at home (5.1%). Significantly, women who were white, older (> age 30), multiparous, had a vaginal birth, a home or birth centre birth and had midwifery care were less likely to report mistreatment (Vedam et al., 2019).

The genesis of this book

I (Hannah) commenced my Honours thesis in 1995. It was a grounded theory study looking at the experiences of women giving birth to their first babies at home and in hospital. Looking back, I think I was researching my own birth options as I had not yet become a mother. The study profoundly influenced my thinking about homebirth as I listened to the different stories from women who had a homebirth as compared to women who had a hospital birth. They could not have been more different, despite the fact they were all experiencing a similar phenomenon as first-time mothers birthing and navigating the unknown (Dahlen, Barclay, & Homer, 2008a, 2008b, 2010). I realised that homebirth was less about the 'bricks and mortar' and more about the philosophy of care and the power a woman reclaims in her own space.

Later, I (Hannah) would go on to analyse 832 publicly available consumer submissions to the 2009 Australian National Maternity Services Review. I published two papers on what the submissions said about homebirth (Dahlen et al., 2011b) and birth centres (Dahlen, Jackson, Schmied, Tracy, & Priddis,

2011a), with Virginia Schmied (co-editor) and Melanie Jackson, who worked as my research assistant before undertaking her dissertation on freebirth and high-risk homebirth. This was the first study on the subject of freebirth in Australia at the time. Melanie Jackson, Elizabeth Rigg, Heather Sassine, Hazel Keedle, Suha Hussein, Jo Hunter and Maddy Simpson commenced Honours/Master's/PhDs under the supervision of Hannah and Virginia at Western Sydney University, and each contributed a chapter on their research to this book.

We (Hannah and Virginia) began to see a pattern emerging as these further studies were being undertaken. Birth trauma, lack of choice and inability to access midwifery continuity of care seemed to be recurring, emerging themes. Meanwhile, in 2010, Melanie and I (Hannah), along with two other midwives (Robyn Dempsey and Jane Palmer) formed a private midwifery group practice called *Midwives at Sydney and Beyond*. Our practice 'catches' around half the homebirth babies in NSW. This was where Hannah met Bashi.

Bashi is a lawyer who came to our midwifery group practice after two traumatic caesarean sections with her first two babies. She came into our care with a steely determination, born out of betrayal and birth trauma, not to repeat her first births with her third baby. Bashi went on to give birth to Connor vaginally after two caesareans, and the fire in her belly grew (Bashi's story comes later in this chapter and in Chapter 9). Bashi and Hannah spent many hours talking about human rights in childbirth, meeting in coffee shops and each other's homes where we slowly but surely hatched an idea for a book about a bird that was not actually about a bird – but more on that later!

Bashi started representing women who had been treated poorly in the system and midwives who had been reported. In 2015, she was invited to join the Board of Human Rights in Childbirth (HRiC) Board, and directed the inaugural Human Rights in Childbirth Mumbai Conference, with the support of the Lancet Maternal Health Series, the WHO, International Confederation of Midwives, White Ribbon Alliance and Birth India. Bashi is transitioning to the head of the organisation in 2019. Through HRiC, she continues to fight for women's human rights in childbirth on a global scale.

Virginia was working with Hannah and co-supervising many of the same students. Her own work focused on postnatal care and maternal attachment. It wasn't long before she began to see the effects of trauma and mental health consequences on the mother/baby bond and the developing family.

Perched on a slippery slope

In 2012, I (Hannah) wrote a blog entitled '*Are Australia women's birthing rights perched on a slippery slope?*' (Dahlen, 2012). I was inspired to write the blog after my time as an expert witness in a coroner's inquest in South Australia, investigating the deaths of three infants who died under the care of a (voluntarily deregistered) midwife working as an unregulated birth worker attending homebirths (see Chapters 5 and 14). The adverse outcomes were all associated with high-risk women who chose homebirth (contrary to medical advice) after their efforts to obtain flexible care options within the system were dogmatically resisted. The coroner had the perfect opportunity during the inquest to examine the drivers that led three women to choose a high-risk birth outside the system (see Chapter 14). Instead, the coroner pointed the finger at the women and the ex-midwife. I wrote the following:

> The coroner identified some serious system and legislative problems that contributed to these incidents and made some potentially important recommendations, along with some potentially concerning ones. The potentially positive recommendations are that the practice of midwifery should be permissible only in the case of registered midwives under National Law as this ensures accountability and the meeting of standards that protect the safety of the public … However, what is most concerning is the recommendation that legislation be introduced that would 'impose a duty on any person providing a health service, including midwifery services to report to the South Australian Department of Health and Ageing the intention of any person under his or her care to undergo a homebirth in respect of deliveries that are attended by enhanced risk of complications.' The concern with this is twofold. Firstly, it may in fact push some women further underground and lead to them not seeking any engagement with health services at all and this will be a significant disincentive to safety and secondly, it could lead to a serious intrusion into the rights of women to determine what happens to their bodies during pregnancy and birth … the question we seem unable to ask once again is why would women take the 'risk' of having a baby at home when they have significant risk factors? Do these women love their babies less or do they fear our health system more? … For the vast majority of women their baby is their number one priority. When they make choices that are not always in the best interests of themselves and their baby, one should ask why? … If women are avoiding our system isn't it incumbent upon us health professionals to work together with women to fix the problems? … In 2005, the WHO challenged health practitioners not to ask, 'Why women do not accept the service that we offer?' but to question, 'Why do we not offer a service that women will accept?' Let's stop calling for 'legislating' against women's choice or bullying them into submission and let's start trying to understand why that choice is made and put in place responsive sensitive maternity care systems that cater for the individual and see birth as more than a medical event. If we can do this we won't have to erode women's rights and we can pull ourselves back from the top of this slippery slope we are currently perched on in this country.
>
> (Dahlen, 2012)

In response to my post, a woman commented:

> The instincts of a pregnant woman are highly attuned to safeguarding the interests of her unborn child – if she has reason to believe harm may be done, she will naturally avoid that at all costs. In Stone Age times, we would have applauded the same mother for finding herself a safe, secluded cave to birth in, tucked away from potential predators who might be roaming outside. Let us see the freebirthers and the increasing number of women choosing midwife attended homebirth here in Australia as the 'canaries in the mine' of the birthing industry here. Obviously, something is amiss and women are voting with their feet as a sign of where they feel most safe in birth.

And so, the title for our book was born. It is a culmination of seven years of work, during which time the evidence mounted and we grew in our separate, and shared, wisdom and insight.

An international effort for an international problem

You could say this book was destined to be. While half the chapters come from us (Hannah, Virginia and Bashi) and are informed by our research students and experiences, we soon realised that many other researchers were examining these issues around the word. So, we share not just our research and experience but those of authors from ten countries, four continents and 12 disciplines, each with a unique perspective on the canary in the coal mine. Consumers collaborate with researchers in this book. Their shared stories form the intricate, delicately woven web which binds the chapters of stark, formal research and analysis. That silver-threaded web is the connection we all share in our quest to humanise birth. Their hearts and voices make this book accessible to all, and this is essential reading for midwives, obstetricians, lawyers, government, health departments and, most important of all, consumers of maternity services.

This book is not a manifesto

This book is not a manifesto on freebirth, it does not promote the use of unregulated birth workers and it does not advocate birth at home for women with significant risk factors. Rather, we point a finger directly at mainstream maternity care (the coal mine) and those registered healthcare providers/managers (the miners) who, with their lack of evidence-based practice and inflexible and disrespectful attitudes, drive women to birth outside the system. In this book, we claim these women as the 'canary in the coal mine'. We call on everyone engaged in this space (consumers, midwives, obstetricians, family doctors, doulas, service managers, government, regulators, world health bodies, lawyers and coroners) to recognise this important subset of violence against women and energise all of us to find a solution.

The history of the canary and the coal mine

Canaries were used in English coal mines to protect miners between 1911 and 1986 until alternatives were introduced. The canary is a bird known for its sweet, steady stream of song and sensitivity to dangerous gases like carbon monoxide. Canaries need large quantities of oxygen to enable them to fly to great heights. Their anatomy allows them to get one dose of oxygen when they inhale, and another as they exhale, as they hold air in extra sacs. They also breathe rapidly and get affected quickly. Canaries therefore get a double dose of air and any poisons the air might contain, giving miners an earlier warning. John Scott Haldane, 'the father of oxygen therapy', recommended the first canary for the coal mine. In his research on carbon monoxide, he realised that canaries were more sensitive to colourless, odourless carbon monoxide and other gases also poisonous to humans. Miners used them as a warning to evacuate. Most people would be familiar with the famous black and white images of miners holding the canary in small cages (Eschner, 2016). These valued birds were housed in a special type of birdcage with specially placed ventilation holes. If the canary fell off its perch in the cage, miners closed an airtight door over the ventilation holes and used oxygen to revive the bird. Some miners apparently even carried small vials of oxygen so they could revive a poisoned bird (Alberta Culture and Tourism, 2019). Miners knew their survival depended on the canary.

The miners loved and cared for the canary because they knew they would perish without it. In this book, childbearing women are the canary and the mine is the mainstream maternity system. Around the world, many of our maternity systems are broken, with poisonous gases oozing steadily from the fissures caused by human rights abuses, lack of evidence-based practice, inflexible services and lack of choice. The canary is getting sick, and becoming more desperate in its attempts to flee. So too the women who find other options, such as freebirth, unregistered birth workers and high-risk homebirth. We respond to these powerful survival instincts by blaming the canary for lacking resilience, for not singing in accordance with norms, for not pleasing her carers. We prod and poke the canary in her cage while making disparaging comments about her age, her weight, her ethnicity, her appearance and her sexual behaviours. We ignore her distress – or worse, we portray her pain as weakness or disadvantage, and we laugh at or taunt her. In our frustration with her seemingly incessant fretting, we rattle the cage or hit the canary. We are in denial – to detriment of all of us.

When the canary stops singing, it should be time to immediately evacuate the mine and clear the gas. Mainstream maternity care is highly resistant to change. If anything, systems are doubling down on efforts to lock the entrance and trap the canary, without realising that these same toxic structures are slowly destroying our healthcare providers, fathers and babies who go home with a broken mother. This book sounds the emergency alarm, shares a vial of oxygen and hopefully, the chance to re-examine the structures of the coal mine.

About the Editors

You will notice, in every chapter, we asked the author(s) to tell us a little bit about themselves and what drew them to their work. We wanted to share this fascinating insight into our authors who themselves have been shaped, so profoundly, by their own experiences in and around maternity healthcare systems. It is important that we also share our experiences and what motivated us to produce this book.

Hannah Dahlen

I am a mother, a midwife, a researcher and a political activist in the birth world. I came to the realisation, at a young age, that birth was not just a feminist issue but perhaps *the* feminist issue left unaddressed by the feminists of our, and earlier, times. I was born and grew up in the Middle Eastern country of Yemen and observed daily the way that women and girls were treated and their lack of worth in society, simply because they were born female. At 11 years of age, I attended a birth that changed my life forever. The pregnant woman was the 16-year-old sister-in-law of my best childhood friend. I had walked with her to the nearby community clinic with her young girls to get iron injections as she was seriously anaemic. When I asked her husband to drive them, to avoid the hot one-hour walk to the clinic, he said he did not want to waste his petrol. I was awakened to women's rights and the invisibility of women in countries like Yemen. I went on to witness the woman give birth to a beautiful baby girl (named Hannah after me) and was deeply affected by her reaction when she learned her baby was not the boy she hoped for and asked me to take it away. The mother knew her value as woman and wife was tied to her ability to produce sons, not daughters. It was that moment that both my love for and admiration of women's capacity and my deep anger at the injustice women experience was born. That was the moment I realised midwives had to be feminists, and I have not lost this certainty. I also knew then that midwifery was a way to change the world and that women's rights were key to achieving this. I returned to Australia from Yemen at the age of 15, finished school and trained to be a nurse before taking off to the UK to study midwifery. Brought up on the intoxicating stories of life as a midwife in the Docklands of London – told to me by my mother, who was also a midwife – I pursued the dream and began a midwifery career which, nearly 30 years ago, captivated me for life.

At 34 years of age, much to my surprise, as this was not planned, I became pregnant. I contacted two women who were to be my midwives through four births over the next seven years (Shea Caplice and Sheryl Sidery). The care I received, the dignity I retained and the respect I was privileged to experience buffered me through the most harrowing of journeys. I have written my story elsewhere, so will share a brief version here.

Being pregnant shook me to the core. I had not planned this, but the microscopic cells deep in my belly let me know, in no uncertain terms, my life would never be the same. I finally understood that fear that snakes around the heart of a parent. The fear I saw in my own mother's eyes when she lost not one but two of her children. I experienced the slow and subtle stripping away of my protective chest wall, and the exposure of my vulnerable heart to the possible, terrible, loss of my child. I have never loved so terrifyingly, yet completely.

Lydia, my firstborn, was perfect. She was strong and she was given to us first so we could bear what was to come. During my labour with her, I was transferred from my planned homebirth to hospital due to thick meconium (probably due to being 42 weeks and taking far too much castor oil to avoid an induction), but I had my very familiar midwives at my side every step of the way. I was woman and I heard myself roar. That powerful birth changed me forever.

Four years later, in 2002, my son Luke was born after a 23-hour labour, another transfer from home, a further 12 hours labouring in hospital, and finally, an emergency caesarean at 8 cm. He arrived and he did not breathe. Two days later, we held him in our arms and switched off the ventilator. I finally 'knew there was no celestial tally; there was no justice when it comes to loss, and all the impossibilities so logically dismissed were now possible' (Dahlen, 2017). The autopsy produced no answers, so we embarked on another pregnancy, three short months later. I heard the experts roll out their theories: It was 'definitely an infection' said one, it was 'definitely a missed hypoxia' said another, and on it went. My midwives were my rock even though I knew people were judging them as homebirth midwives, and judging me for making such a 'selfish choice' – for putting my needs above those of my baby. I know, first-hand, the almost impossible burden of grief and guilt women feel when they give birth outside the system and lose their babies (see Chapter 17). So, with my next pregnancy, I handed myself over to the medical experts for ultrasounds and investigations – all were perfect – while still clinging to my midwives and harbouring secret desires of birthing at home again. I even dreamed of birthing alone, under cover of night, with no one near me. I finally understood that desire to freebirth that I have since heard women describing in interviews. However, when the rubber really hit the road, I wanted my midwives by my side.

A year to the day after we buried Luke, at almost the exact same time, I birthed our second son, Ethan. I again went to 42 weeks. With an oblique lie and the same dread that told me something was wrong in the latter weeks of my pregnancy with Luke, I surrendered and had a caesarean section. This time, I was sacrificing myself for my baby. This was the bargain I struck to get myself a live baby. Ethan was born and, just like his brother, he did not breathe.

For 11 days, my perfect-looking full-term baby was ventilated while my husband and I were tested for every possible condition. Finally, we discovered that my instincts (that something was wrong) were right, and the judgement and blame towards my choice to birth at home were wrong. My boys had a rare X-linked disorder, one that a thorough and appropriately trained perinatologist should have picked up when performing an autopsy on Luke. My homebirth choice was never the issue; perhaps jumping to conclusions based on beliefs and judgements was.

This story has a happy ending. I gave birth to Bronte in 2005. Once again, I wanted a homebirth. This time, with a history of two previous caesareans and two previous neonatal deaths, I made everyone nervous, but my midwives never showed it. Destined to go overdue, I went to 42 weeks again, attempted an induction which did not succeed, and finally, had another caesarean.

This I can honestly say – I was not traumatised. I was heartbroken and I was grieving, but in all the four births we experienced, my midwives were at my side and my care was respectful and loving. Had it not been, I can't imagine who I would be today – this book may never have been written! I wish for every woman the care I experienced in my births. Despite a journey that was beyond my control, we were offered every choice imaginable along the way. I gave birth surrounded by love and respect, and for that, I will always be grateful. Sadness we can cope with, scarring our souls with trauma is much less easy to deal with.

Birthing the canary in the coal mine

After a 20-year career working in fragmented care in hospitals, in 2008, I became an academic. By now, I had a PhD and a rising fire in my belly about human rights in childbirth. I met Melanie Jackson, then a newly qualified midwife, who worked as my research assistant while she apprenticed with private midwife Robyn Dempsey. Together, we analysed and wrote papers on the submissions to the National Maternity Services Review in 2009. We were blown away by how many women requested greater access to homebirth and who disclosed they had freebirthed due to lack of respectful options. Melanie decided to pursue a doctorate, the first Australian study on freebirth and high-risk homebirth, nominating Virginia and me as her supervisors (see Chapter 2). At that time, Rixa Freeze from the US (see Chapter 1) was the only other researcher examining the practice of freebirth. The stories from women we interviewed for Melanie's study fired my passion even more. More PhD students came to research topics related to '*birthing outside the system*' – the title of Melanie's thesis. Hazel Keedle did her Master's on women who choose to VBAC at home and is now pursuing a PhD on VBAC (see Chapter 7). Elizabeth Rigg did her PhD on unregulated birth workers in Australia and the women who use their services (see Chapter 5). Heather Sassine undertook the largest Australian survey on why women choose homebirth for her Honours thesis (see Chapter 6), Jo Hunter (Chapter 11) examined the reporting of homebirth midwives in Australia to the Australian Health Practitioner Regulation Authority (AHPRA), Suha Hussein (Chapter 8) examined birth care in Jordan and showed the treatment women experienced in hospitals there, and finally, Maddy Simpson (Chapter 12) investigated the impact of birth trauma and post-traumatic stress on women postnatally. It was only a matter of time before this book needed to be written as a matter of urgency. Working with Virginia, and meeting Bashi, made this possible.

Bashi Kumar-Hazard

I began my journey into parenthood as innocently as any new mother. I was a corporate lawyer specialising in consumer and competition law. From my ivory corporate tower, I assumed that consumer laws applied to medical maternity practice and that, like me, medical professionals understood my rights as a woman. My GP, who knew I was privately insured, gave me a list of private obstetricians to contact. I was young, fit and healthy, didn't drink or smoke and enjoyed an uneventful pregnancy, but none of that mattered to my chosen obstetrician. The 15-minute antenatal appointments fuelled an unnecessary anxiety about whether I would even make it through the pregnancy. Having come from a family of women who birthed naturally during the Great War and after, I just could not understand why it was such a drama. I had an ultrasound at every visit. I had every possible test, none of which were presented as a choice. When tests revealed nothing, my obstetrician started complaining about the large size of the baby and my small stature and pelvis.

My effort to raise childbirth options were charmingly deflected until the last antenatal appointment. Suddenly, the charm was replaced with panic. We were in imminent danger, the baby was huge, I was small and she had the solution: an induction at 38 weeks to greatly increase my chances of delivering naturally. When I resisted, she booked me in 'just in case'. Over the next week, I received phone calls every day from a hospital midwife telling me I was due for an induction. The induction was put to us as a matter of convenience – to speed up labour and ensure a natural delivery. I didn't know that, if the induction failed, I would have a caesarean. I didn't know how many inductions generally failed, let alone in a private hospital, but the odds were very much against me. On the day, my waters were broken and a drip administered, I was put on a monitor, and left alone for 11 or so hours. At 5 p.m., a midwife came tearing into the room to check on the drip and she hurriedly raised the dose; my pain became excruciating. The midwife said, 'Oh! She can't take the pain' to my husband. She offered me gas, which made me throw up. She left us to clean up and we didn't see her again.

I then heard someone sing out 'Last chance for an epidural before I go home.' As soon as I accepted the epidural, I was strapped down in bed and put on a monitor. My obstetrician marched in shortly after to announce an emergency: the monitor was showing signs of foetal distress and I needed a caesarean. What just happened? Can we just stop all this? 'No, not really' she said before turning to my husband and saying, *in front of me*, 'If this was my baby, I would not be letting her do this.'

Fathers are the latest weapon of coercion in modern obstetrics. They have been raised on a diet of Hollywood-style dramatic births and are blissfully unaware of the disembodiment of pregnant women in obstetric practice. My husband panicked and appealed to me to think about our baby. He, without knowing it, had succumbed to the fear in the room at my expense. I gave in, signing that form like a guilty criminal expressing contrition. Unbeknownst to both of us at the time, he was going to pay a very high price for it.

As soon as I signed that form, the atmosphere in the room lifted. The urgency and concerns simply evaporated. Staff chatted over my body like I was a table. Midwives joked about the 6 p.m. 'queue' into theatre as I lay exposed, shivering and vomiting. I was a cow on the conveyor belt; only I was being trollied into the operating theatre of a very expensive private hospital in Sydney's lower north shore. I was cut open and my baby removed. Inside, I was screaming – I don't want this, why is this happening to me? I desperately wanted to run away. I kept telling myself that I was saving my baby, but then I learned he was just 3.1 kg, with an APGAR score of 9:10. If that wasn't bad enough, staff took him away from me. When we finally met, hours later, he was rudely awoken and shoved against my breast. He screamed in protest, but I couldn't hold or soothe him. I was helpless, and useless – not fit to be a mother.

The obstetrician convinced my husband that I had had a 'straightforward procedure', easily managed with sensible pain relief. Looking back, it concerns me that we trusted someone who so wilfully disregarded the impact of major surgery. The pain was difficult enough to manage on its own, let alone with a newborn and my shattered emotional state. The next few days were a nightmare – noisy, disruptive and arguing over mismanaged pain medication. I tried to talk to the hospital lactation consultant. Why did I feel like I was dead? 'Oh, you'll be fine', she said breezily, 'Think how lucky you are that your baby is alive and well.' She lectures me on poor feeding habits instead. At 6 weeks, the obstetrician added to my litany of deficiencies: my body grew a baby too big, was not fit to labour, failed to respond to standard treatments and had to be saved. It was a wonder that this and other such typically faulty female bodies had ever withstood the test of time.

At home, I began to imagine terrible things happening to me and my baby. I relived those birth events, again and again, wondering what I could have done to change my fortunes. This got worse over time, not better. I told myself every day that this was part and parcel of having a baby, that I was no different to anyone else, that I should be grateful. Sometimes, I tried to so hard, whole days would slip by while I simply sat motionless, caught up in vivid 'daymares'. The GP claimed I was having trouble adjusting to motherhood. The psychiatrist, who seemed to run a thriving practice treating a roomful of women like me, heard my story, shrugged her shoulders and offered me medication.

Three years later, we heard about VBACs, so we decided to have another child. To my surprise, when I contacted the obstetrician to get my records, she offered to help. She seemed to favour it, until we got to the end of another uneventful pregnancy. Then, she started again, saying she didn't think I was capable of labouring or achieving a VBAC.

I went into labour on my due date. I enjoyed a few hours of labour at home. To this day, I regret walking into that hospital. I was the 'trial of scar'; no one asked for my name. I continuously battled staff about ridiculous matters, like whether I could stand up during contractions. At some point, the obstetrician arrived with an entourage. The lights went on, a group of people wandered in, chatting and joking loudly, as I was pulled out of the shower. The obstetrician said, 'Bashi, labouring all by yourself – amazing!' As I was being examined, my waters broke and the labour ground to a halt. No one knew what to do next. My obstetrician accused the midwife of wasting her time. It never occurred to her that her behaviours or the structure she put around me may have been the problem. I was soon tied down with drips and monitors, and left alone to contemplate that looming caesarean. As I lay there sobbing and shaking, midwives would storm in, check the monitor and glare at me accusingly before storming off again. As I conceded to a caesarean, I felt that familiar sensation of the energy draining out of my body. I didn't see my baby for hours. I didn't try to feed or hold her. I lay next to her all night, unable to move or even see her. I called for a drink of water but no one came. Finally, just before sunrise, a midwife came, snapped at me and went to fetch water. She never came back.

Some time later, a trainee nurse tried to get me out of bed. I pulled the covers over my head. After a few hours, my obstetrician came in. She feigned surprise at my physical and mental state and left. Staff actively avoided me after that. The hospital's social worker couldn't even manage to see me before I was discharged. I sat, like an eyesore, in the foyer of this very expensive hospital, numb, staring into the distance with a crying newborn next to me, waiting alone for hours, as wealthy, white people sauntered past. Some stared, the receptionist glared and the rest just averted their eyes. When she finally arrived, the social worker took a photo of my baby and gave me a phone number for the local health service. This was supposedly the gold standard of expensive, private hospital care – where babies are pulled out as quickly as possible, and healthy, happy mothers are sliced open, emotionally shattered and sent packing with a sweet smile and a hefty bill.

My compliance and good behaviour made no difference to how I was perceived: I was dehumanised until it caused me suffering, and then punished for expressing my suffering. Out came the growing army of health professionals propped up to treat the harms regularly and knowingly perpetrated on mothers and babies in pregnancy and childbirth: psychologists, psychiatrists, physiotherapists, neonatologists, paediatricians and social workers. Their ineffectual treatments were deliberately focused on piecemeal symptoms; like putting expensive Band-Aids over bullet wounds. Did the health service counsellor care that I had PTSD? No, she just warned me that accessing publicly funded mental health services could trigger a child protection alert. Did the psychiatrist know how many women had the same complaint as me? Yes, but it wasn't her problem. Did the GP listen? No, she changed the subject – every, single, time. The neonatologist who saw my sick baby? He shouted at me for refusing to formula-feed her. The paediatrician? He said he knew, but didn't want to get involved. These providers, when faced with questions from women like me, engaged state enforcement services to blindly pursue their ends. My complaints made things worse for me – the local health nurse inspected my home, including where my baby slept, and looked for evidence of alcohol or drug consumption. When I questioned her right to invade my privacy, she threatened to report me to child protection services, and she did. In the months that followed, I survived PTSD, managed a child protection officer, cared for a seriously ill baby and a distressed toddler, contemplated suicide and separated from my husband for some time. I gave up my job. But through all that, I knew better than to seek help from a system that is so openly hostile to women of colour.

We tried to get as far away from all this as we could, but then came Baby Connor, whose birth was a watershed moment in my life. This pregnancy proved a real challenge. I lost 10 kilos from hyperemesis and became chronically iron-deficient. I also knew that I would jump off a cliff before repeating my hospital experiences, but I couldn't find a doctor to help me. After a lot of research, I found a private midwifery practice, which is where I met Hannah. This was my first step towards a journey of learning, empowerment and healing. Everything changed when my midwife and I started talking. I realised, as she gently nurtured me and my children through this pregnancy, she was slowly nurturing me back to life. My confidence grew, alongside my well-being. THIS is the gold standard in maternity care that should be offered to all women in this country.

I also saw, through my lawyer lens, that she was working in an openly hostile and unsupported environment. My previous obstetrician wouldn't release my records directly to her. The next obstetrician wouldn't take her calls. The hospital wouldn't give her visiting rights. My GP wouldn't share information with her, even at my request. I couldn't get insurance coverage or rebates for her care, but I had no trouble getting rebates for the useless ultrasounds at the obstetrician's surgery every 6 weeks. When, during my precipitous labour, I called an ambulance (see Chapter 9), the ambulance officer refused my midwife's debrief and instead misreported my circumstances to the hospital. The final knife twist, for me, was watching an arrogant, incompetent obstetrician bully and berate her for doing her job exceptionally well, while ignoring the job he was paid to do.

Finally, I understood. I had unwittingly entered a world where my mind, wishes and rights were irrelevant and pregnancy an excuse to dismantle my physical and mental well-being. This was the raw end of a journey through systemic discrimination and dehumanisation, where prejudice and pregnancy collide. It is so endemic and so acceptable, anyone even mildly associated with me, whether my white Australian husband or my midwife, was destined for the maternity gulag.

I knew we were dealing with more than just someone's bad day, one bad egg or one system outlier – whatever excuse our governments throw up when adverse events take place in hospital maternity wards. In the months that followed, with Connor in arms, I began cornering poor Hannah at her practice's monthly gatherings to pick her brains about midwifery practice, regulations and the health system. The rest, as they say, is history.

Virginia Schmied

I (Virginia) studied midwifery in the UK in 1981 and loved it, particularly working in the community and with women in their homes. On returning to Australia, I moved into nursing education for a range of reasons, and studied sociology and women's studies in undergraduate and postgraduate degrees. From here, my commitment grew to ensuring that all women have access to the sexual and reproductive healthcare they need, particularly the right to be treated with dignity and respect in all healthcare encounters no matter her age, cultural background, class, etc. Bringing feminist thought to my teaching in the mid-1980s often attracted surprisingly negative reactions from students who had trained as nurses and midwives in an apprenticeship system.

In the early 1990s, I had my two lovely sons, now adults. Both were born in a birth centre, 10 minutes' walk from home. During my pregnancies I was cared for by midwives, many of whom I knew. My births were both normal births – 8 hours long – and I was then visited at home by a midwife I taught as a student nurse. While I did not have continuity of carer, I had continuity of care and philosophy. Breastfeeding went well and I was thrilled with the amount of weight I shed until I found out I was thyrotoxic. The endocrinologist, a very personable man, informed me that I would have to give up breastfeeding to take eight tablets of propathyuracil a day. My response was very emotional, breastfeeding was central to my identity as a mother. Not knowing what to do with me, he suggested I could take three tablets a day and continue to feed. So I did some rapid research overnight and continued to feed for two years. When I read the stories of women in this book and women who have participated in our research over the years, I realise how empowering it is to be treated with dignity and respect in care encounters. All women deserve that.

Roughly coinciding with becoming a 'breastfeeding' mother, I landed an exciting new job in a research centre, working alongside Professor Lesley Barclay, the first clinical chair in nursing in Australia, and simultaneously commenced my PhD which, you may guess, was on breastfeeding, entitled '*Breastfeeding as discursive construction and embodied experience*'.

In 2004, I took a senior management role in a research centre in the NSW Department of Community Services, the state government's child protection department. This position brought into sharp focus the impact of abuse and neglect on children, but also importantly the role of intergenerational trauma and violence on the mothers and fathers who were now struggling to parent their children. In Australia, First Nations children are disproportionally represented in our child protection system. This is as a direct result of systemic mistreatment and abuse of generations of Aboriginal people.

I came to understand the enormous challenges of building parenting capacity in women and men to ensure infants and children develop secure attachments. When you consider that the parents themselves have not had the same opportunity and are vulnerable because of mental health problems, drug and alcohol misuse and/or are experiencing intimate partner or family violence, the costs of addressing these issues downstream are very high. I also learnt that the opportunity to address these issues upstream through prevention is crucial and yet, there is limited use of, indeed limited recognition of, the role of our universal maternal and child health services in Australia. Specifically, there is little or no discussion of the holistic role midwives can play in providing care to all women in the public health system and their ability to support women who are vulnerable, particularly in the context of midwifery-led models of care.

When I moved back to an academic and research role, I made a commitment to ensuring that the universal maternal and child health services would become recognised and involved in designing services for vulnerable families. One of my first projects at Western Sydney University (where I work with Hannah) was entitled '*Towards seamless services: Improving the response of universal health services to the needs of disadvantaged and vulnerable Australian children and families*'. This work formed the basis of ongoing research consultancy and eduation related to women, children and families experiencing complex psychosocial issues and a commitment to interdisciplinary efforts to buid a support network of services, to ensure that no woman would fall through the gap.

But, what I had not fully realised at the time, and what our onging research and this book demonstrates, is that the system itself is often the root of the problem.

A book in two parts

This book is divided into two sections: Part 1 defines and describes the systemic problems we face in maternity healthcare around the globe, through the eyes of women increasingly seeking to birth outside this system; and Part 2 examines strategies and solutions. You will see, as we did, that the women who birth outside the system are not mad or bad or selfish, as is often the claim, they are the 'canary in the coal mine'.

Part 1 – Listening to the canary

In Part 1, the first five chapters examine freebirth and high-risk homebirth in the USA, Australia, the UK and the Netherlands. Chapters 6–10 examine what women are seeking, and fleeing from, when they choose to give birth at home against medical advice or avoid the system. We focus on homebirth generally (Chapter 6), vaginal birth after caesarean section (VBAC) (Chapter 7) and birth in the Middle East (Chapter 8), South Asia (Chapter 9), Eastern Europe and Russia (Chapter 10). In Chapter 11, we explore the modern-day witch hunt against midwives who support women who choose to birth outside the system. We end this section by focusing on birth trauma, which has appeared as a major underpinning theme in every chapter in Part 1 (Chapter 12). We describe birth trauma as the poisonous gas anaesthetising and eventually destroying the canary.

By the end of the first part of this book, you will be well-briefed on multiple perspectives about birthing outside the system, and will have grasped some of the distressingly common and recurring themes emerging throughout the research.

Part 2 – Fixing the system

In Part 2, we look at ways we can fix the system so women re-engage with mainstream care. We begin with two chapters (Chapters 13 and 14) which discuss the legal framework that underpins and, to some extent, protects the faulty maternity healthcare system which is alienating women around the globe. Legal practitioners need to come to terms with the disconnect around human rights and choice on the one hand, and medico-legal principles and coronial investigations on the other hand. These authors, both experienced lawyers in defending women's reproductive rights, discuss accessing legal processes to assert and protect women's rights, as well as advocacy to challenge legal principles and interpretations driven by misogyny, prejudice and care providers' interests, in violation of women's human rights. In Chapter 15, we detail examples of how to keep women within our system through the use of maternity care plans and supporting respectful homebirth transfer when required. Five Aboriginal women write, in Chapter 16, about Australia's '*Birthing on Country*' initiatives and how to engage and care for Aboriginal and Torres Strait Islander women with respect and cultural dignity. Chapters 17 and 18 explore initiatives by amazing midwives who offer safe, within-system, options for women who make 'off-menu' choices in childbirth, together with details on counselling responsibilities when doing this. In Chapters 19 and 20, obstetricians share refreshing and valuable insights on the system's sustainability and coercion in childbirth, and how to talk meaningfully with women about risk, breech birth and VBAC.

Finally, in the concluding chapter, we editors examine the recommendations the authors put forward at the end of each chapter, to discuss the immediate issues we need to address, right now, to keep the canary singing and women birthing in the system. We share our thoughts on a global solution and way forward.

Conclusion

As we were writing this Introduction, several events happened around us. Midwives contacted us about the plight of childbirth in Russia, so we made room for their story and interviewed four additional people for the book. A *Lancet* paper found that facility birth does not necessarily convey a survival benefit for women or babies (Gabrysch et al., 2019). Why? is a question we have heard so often over the past decade from mystified, well-meaning, head-shaking, often privileged middle-class people – but do we really want to hear the answer? Do we want to hear that the problem at hand may largely be to do with us the health provider and what we don't offer women in mainstream maternity system? It is an uncomfortable realisation. It is much easier to demonise and compartmentalise this as a problem with THOSE women. But what if those women are our canary in the coal mine and not listening to them is not only harmful to them, but to us?

We hope you find this book motivates you to improve care for women. Reading each chapter has been like watching a fog slowly lift from a complex and at times hard to understand issue. We hope you find the same when you read this book. We echo the quote that we began this chapter with: *The question should not be why do women not accept the service that we offer, but why do we not offer a service that women will accept?* (Fathalla, 1988)

References

Alberta Culture and Tourism. (2019). Canaries in the coal mine. Alberta Culture and Tourism. Retrieved from http://history.alberta.ca/energyheritage/coal/the-early-development-of-the-coal-industry-1874-1914/early-methods-and-technology/canaries-in-the-coal-mine.aspx

American Psychiatric Association. (2018). Americans they are more anxious than a year ago; Baby Boome report greatest increase in anxiety. Retrieved from www.psychiatry.org/newsroom/news-releases/americans-say-they-are-more-anxious-than-a-year-ago-baby-boomers-report-greatest-increase-in-anxiety

Austin, M.-P., Highet, N., & The Expert Working Group. (2017). Mental health care in the perinatal period: Australian clinical practice guideline. *COPE perinatal mental health guideline*. Retrieved from http://cope.\org.au/wp-content/uploads/2017/10/Final-COPE-Perinatal-Mental-Health-Guideline.pdf

Barbosa Jardim, D., & Modena, C. (2018). Obstetric violence in the daily routine of care and its characteristics. *Revisto Latino-Americana de Enfermagem*, *26*, e3069.

Berger, M., & Sarnyai, Z. (2015). 'More than skin deep': Stress neurobiology and mental health consequences of racial discrimination. *Stress*, *18*, 1–10.

Betran, A. P., Torloni, M. R., Zhang, J., Ye, J., Mikolajczyk, R., Deneux-Tharaux, C., … Gülmezoglu, A. M. (2015). What is the optimal rate of caesarean section at population level? A systematic review of ecologic studies. *Reproductive Health*, *2015*, 57.

Boerma, T., Ronsmans, C., Melesse, D., Barros, A., Barros, F., Juan, L., … Temmerman, M. (2018). Optimising caesarean section use 1 Global epidemiology of use of and disparities in caesarean sections. *The Lancet*, *392*, 1341–1348.

Bowers, F. (2013). Midwife confirms she told Savita Halappanavar Ireland is a 'Catholic country'. *Raidió Teilifís Éireann*. 11 April. Retrieved from www.rte.ie/news/health/2013/0410/380613-savita-halappanavar-inquest/

Clavarino, A., Mamun, A. A., O'Callaghan, M., Aird, R., Bor, W., O'Callaghan, F., … Alati, R. (2010). Maternal anxiety and attention problems in children at 5 and 14 years. *Journal of Attention Disorders, 13*, 658–667.

Dahlen, H. (2003). Personal diaries.

Dahlen, H. (2012). Are Australian women's birthing rights now perched on a slippery slope? *Crikey*. Retrieved from https://blogs.crikey.com.au/croakey/2012/06/08/are-australian-women%E2%80%99s-birthing-rights-now-perched-on-a-slippery-slope/

Dahlen, H. (2017). Reproductive loss and grief. In G. Thomson & V. Schmied (Eds.), *Psychosocial resilience and risk in the perinatal period: Implications and guidance for professionals*. Abingdon: Routledge.

Dahlen, H., Barclay, L., & Homer, C. (2008a). The novice birthing: Theorising first time mothers' experiences of birth at home and in hospital in Australia. *Midwifery, 26*, 53–63.

Dahlen, H., Barclay, L., & Homer, C. (2008b). Preparing for the first birth: Mothers' experiences at home and in hospital in Australia. *Journal of Perinatal Education, 17*, 21–32.

Dahlen, H. G., Barclay, L., & Homer, C. S. E. (2010). Processing the first birth: Journeying into 'motherland'. *Journal of Clinical Nursing, 19*, 1977–1985.

Dahlen, H., Jackson, M., Schmied, V., Tracy, S., & Priddis, H. (2011a). Birth centres and the National Maternity Services Review: Response to consumer demand or compromise? *Women and Birth, 24*, 165–172.

Dahlen, H., Schmied, V., Tracy, S., Jackson, M., Cummings, J., & Priddis, H. (2011b). Home birth and the National Australian Maternity Services Review: Too hot to handle? *Women and Birth, 24*, 148–155.

Dahlen, H. G., Kennedy, H. P., Anderson, C. M., Bell, A. F., Clark, A., Foureur, M., … Downe, S. (2013). The EPIIC hypothesis: Intrapartum effects on the neonatal epigenome and consequent health outcomes. *Medical Hypothesis, 8*, 656–662.

Dahlen, H., Tracy, S., Tracy, M. B., Bisits, A., Brown, C., & Thornton, C. (2014). Rates of obstetric intervention and associated perinatal mortality and morbidity among low-risk women giving birth in private and public hospitals in NSW (2000–2008): A linked data population-based cohort study. *BMJ Open, 2014*(4), e004551. doi:10.1136/bmjopen-2013–004551.

Dahlen, H. G., Foster, J. P., Psaila, K., Badawi, N., Fowler, C., Schmied, V., & Thornton, C. (2018). Gastro-oesophageal reflux: A mixed methods study of infants admitted to hospital in the first 12 months following birth in NSW (2000–2011). *BMC Pediatrics, 18*. doi:10.1186/s12887–018–0999–9.

Dennis, C. L., Brown, H. K., Falah-Hassani, K., Marini, F. C., & Vigod, S. N. (2017). Identifying women at risk for sustained postpartum anxiety. *Journal of Affective Disorders, 213*, 131–137.

Downe, S., Finlayson, K., Tuncalp, O., & Gulmezoglu, A. M. (2019). Provision and uptake of routine antenatal services: a qualitative evidence synthesis. *Cochrane Database of Systematic Reviews, 2019*(6), CD012392.

Ellwood, D., & Dahlen, H. (2019). FactCheck: Is suicide one of the leading causes of maternal death in Australia? *The Conversation*. Retrieved from

https://theconversation.com/factcheck-is-suicide-one-of-the-leading-causes-of-maternal-death-in-australia-65336
Eschner, K. (2016). The story of the real canary in the coal mine. Smithsonian.com. 30 December. Retrieved from www.smithsonianmag.com/smart-news/story-real-canary-coal-mine-180961570/
Fathalla, M. (1988). Preface. *Paediatric and Perinatal Epidemiology*, 12 (Suppl. 2), vii–viii.
FIGO. (2018). FIGO position paper: How to stop the caesarean section epidemic. *Lancet*, *392*, 1286–1287.
Gabrysch, S., Nesbitt, R. C., Schoeps, A., Hurt, L., Soremekun, S., Edmond, K., … Campbell, O. M. R. (2019). Does facility birth reduce maternal and perinatal mortality in Brong Ahafo, Ghana? A secondary analysis using data on 119 244 pregnancies from two cluster-randomised controlled trials. *The Lancet*, *7*, e1074–e1087.
Goodwin, S., & Huppatz, K. (2010). *The good mother: Contemporary motherhoods in Australia*. Sydney: Sydney University Press.
Hays, S. (1996). *The cultural contradictions of motherhood*. New Haven, CT: Yale University Press.
Homer, C., Friberg, I., Bastos Dias, M., Hoope-Bender, P., Sandall, J., Speciale, A. M., & Bartlett, L. A. (2014). The projected effect of scaling up midwifery. *The Lancet*, *384*, 1146–1157.
Ignacio, A. (2019). Brazil's debate over 'obstetric violence' shines light on abuse during childbirth. *HuffPost Brazil*. Retrieved from www.huffpost.com/entry/obstetric-violence-brazil-childbirth_n_5d4c4c29e4b09e72974304c2.
Jackson, M., Dahlen, H., & Schmied, V. (2012). Birthing outside the system: Perspectives of risk amongst Australian women who have high risk homebirths. *Midwifery*, *28*, 561–567.
Kennedy, H. P., Cheyney, M., Dahlen, H. G., Downe, S., Foureur, M., Homer, C. S. E., … Renfrew, M. J. (2018). Asking different questions: A call to action for research to improve the quality of care for every woman, every child. *Birth*, *45*, 222–231. DOI: 10.1111/birt.12361.
Kingsbury, A. M., Gibbons, K., McIntyre, D., Tremellen, A., Flenady, V., Wilkinson, S., & Najman, J. M. (2017). How have the lives of pregnant women changed in the last 30 years? *Women and Birth*, *30*, 342–349.
Knight, M., Bunch, K., Tuffnell, D., Jayakody, H., Shakespeare, J., Kotnis, R., … Kurinczuk, J. J. (Eds.) (2018). *On behalf of MBRRACE-UK, Saving lives, improving mothers' care – Lessons learned to inform maternity care from the UK and Ireland Confidential Enquiries into Maternal Deaths and Morbidity 2014–16*. Oxford: National Perinatal Epidemiology Unit, University of Oxford.
Liamputtong, P. (2006). Motherhood and 'moral career': Discourses of good motherhood among Southeast Asian immigrant women in Australia. *Qualitative Sociology*, *29*, 25–53.
Maher, J., & Saugeres, L. (2007). To be or not to be a mother? Women negotiating cultural representations of mothering. *Journal of Sociology*, *42*, 5–21.
Miller, S., Abalos, E., Chamillard, M., Ciapponi, A., Colaci, D., Comande, D., … Althabe, F. (2016). Beyond too little, too late and too much, too soon: A pathway towards evidence-based, respectful maternity care worldwide. *Lancet*, *388*, 2176–2192.
National Partnership for Women and Families. (2018). Black women's maternal health: A multifaceted approach to addressing persistent and dire health disparities.

Issue Brief, April. Retrieved from www.nationalpartnership.org/our-work/health/reports/black-womens-maternal-health.html
OECD. (2018). Health at a glance: Europe. OECD. Retrieved from www.oecd.org/about/publishing/Corrigendum_Health_at_a_Glance_Europe_2018.pdf
Pedersen, D. E. (2012). The good mother, the good father, and the good parent: Gendered definitions of parenting. *Journal of Feminist Family Therapy*, *24*, 230–246.
Renfrew, M., McFadden, A., Bastos, M., Campbell, J., Channon, A. A., Cheung, N. F., … Declercq, E. (2014). Midwifery and quality care: Findings from a new evidence-informed framework for maternal and newborn care. *Lancet*, *384*, 1129–1145.
Rubertsson, C., Hellström, J., Cross, M., & Sydsjö, G. (2014). Anxiety in early pregnancy: Prevalence and contributing factors. *Archives of Women's Mental Health*, *17*, 221–228. doi:10.1007/s00737-013-0409-0.
Sandall, J., Tribe, R., Avery, L., Mola, G., Visser, G., Homer, C., … Temmerman, M. (2018). Short-term and long-term effects of caesarean section on the health of women and children. *The Lancet*, *392*, 1349–1357.
Simpson, M., Schmied, V., Dickson, C., & Dahlen, H. G. (2018). Postnatal post-traumatic stress: An integrative review. *Women and Birth*, *31*, 367–379.
Vedam, S., Stoll, K., Taiwo, T., Rubashkin, N., Cheyney, M., Strauss, N., … The GVTM-US Steering Council. (2019). The Giving Voice to Mothers study: Inequity and mistreatment during pregnancy and childbirth in the United States. *MBMC Reproductive Health*, *16*. Retrieved from https://reproductive-health-journal.biomedcentral.com/articles/10.1186/s12978-019-0729-2
WHO. (2015). *WHO Statement on Caesarean Section Rates*. World Health Organisation Department of Reproductive Health and Research.
WHO. (2018). *WHO recommendations: Intrapartum care for a positive childbirth experience*. Geneva: WHO.
Women's Health Survey. (2018). Women's Health Survey 2018: Understanding health information needs and health behaviour of women in Australia. Jean Hailes For Women. Retrieved from https://jeanhailes.org.au/contents/documents/News/Womens-Health-Survey-Report-web.pdf

1 Freebirth in the United States

Rixa Freeze and Laura Tanner

> My first birth resulted in a traumatic episiotomy without my consent and horrible PTSD from previous sexual assault. My second birth resulted in me being discharged from care by my homebirth midwife for being postdates. I ended up having a completely unnecessary caesarean without any labour, listed in my medical records as an 'elective primary caesarean'. I was/am outraged. That is what led me to freebirth.
>
> (Tanner, 2019)

About the authors

This chapter brings together the research and experiences of Rixa Freeze and Laura Tanner, two scholars who have researched freebirth and who have themselves freebirthed children.

Rixa

I (Rixa Freeze) am a mother to four children and I hold a PhD in American Studies. I completed my dissertation, *Born free: unassisted childbirth in North America*, in 2008 and I have since maintained a pregnancy, birth and mothering blog called *Stand and Deliver*. I have published several articles about birthing at home, and recently co-authored an article on planned vaginal breech home and birth-centre birth.

I am one of the unusual cases. I chose to freebirth my first baby, despite not having experienced any previous obstetrical, sexual trauma or disappointing hospital experiences. I knew I would give birth at home and already had a midwife picked out. I knew my chosen midwife well, having worked as her assistant during my doctoral studies. However, I moved away from my chosen midwife to Illinois before I was able to get pregnant. I started assisting another midwife while working on my dissertation and got pregnant after several years of trying and one unsuccessful IVF cycle. Direct-entry midwifery was, and still is, illegal in Illinois. While I greatly admired the midwife I was now assisting, I didn't want her at my own birth. At 80 miles away, that midwife was also the closest available option. As I spent my days immersed in freebirth message boards and discussion forums, I became more convinced that I wanted to give birth unassisted.

In the USA, some women who freebirth belong to religious groups that eschew obstetric care. My religion of origin (Mormonism) did not dictate the place or manner of birth. When I needed that final drop of certainty, however, I drew from my spiritual traditions. As Mormons do with big life decisions, I sought to know if my choice to freebirth was right. That final assurance came through prayer, reflection, and blessings from my husband. My belief in Mormonism has since dissolved. I sometimes wonder if I would have had the courage to freebirth without that thread of religious certainty.

When I was pregnant with my second baby, I did not feel drawn towards freebirth like I did the first time around, so I sought midwifery care. I had three more children at home, all with the same midwife, although baby number three was born unassisted, by accident, as the midwife was still en route. I have no regrets about my freebirth. It taught me about how I give birth and what I needed during labour. It helped me find the perfect hands-off nurse-midwife, Penny Lane, who was happy to let me do it all myself and only step in if (a) asked to or (b) an emergency arose warranting assistance.

Laura

I (Laura Tanner) am a mother to three children and I am currently completing my PhD in Feminist Studies at the University of California, Santa Barbara. I have been involved in both homebirth and freebirth communities for 24 years and I am a radical supporter of women's birthing autonomy. My dissertation, tentatively titled *Birthing against the grain: women's autonomy in birth*, is in progress as of 2019.

I freebirthed my third, and last, baby. I would have freebirthed my first, but lacked the language needed to express that I wanted to birth, on my own, in total privacy. All I knew, at the time, was that I was mortified by the idea of having anyone near me and ashamed to be so modest and inhibited. I had two midwife-assisted births within 14 months of each other. Both were quick and straightforward, but I was left dissatisfied. I wasn't traumatised, but felt that, each time, some things the midwives said or did had diminished my experience. I felt I needed to be entirely alone in labour to go deep inside myself and to be completely uninhibited.

Over the next six years, I learned about freebirth and became involved in freebirth online communities, before becoming pregnant with my third child. I became involved with the freebirth community and obsessively educated myself about it.

My third birth was quick, almost too quick to enjoy properly – two hours. This time, I laboured alone in the bathroom while my husband slept. I feel this labour was exactly as it was meant to be. One of the things I was unhappy with, in my first two births, was how quickly my midwives had moved to deliver the placentas with cord traction within minutes of the baby being born. At the time, I knew just enough to think this was an unnecessary intervention (and it usually is), but not enough to really understand the physiology of it. I did not anticipate that my efficient uterus would clamp down so quickly after my freebirth, with the placenta becoming partially lodged in my cervix minutes after the birth. No amount of pushing could dislodge it. I called a local midwife for help, but was refused because I was not a client. Seven hours after the birth, I told my husband to take me to hospital. I spent one hour in the maternity ward where a doctor pulled out the placenta and tried to convince me to have a transfusion which, in retrospect, I feel I should have taken. I then discharged myself against medical advice.

My freebirth experience fell into that grey area where something happened which required assistance but which was not (at least initially) an emergency. With a bit more knowledge, I could have guided my husband on how to help me. Or, if the midwife I called had agreed to help, I could have stayed home and potentially had a much easier recovery. Hiring a midwife in the first place would have prevented these problems as, by the time I went to the hospital, it was a life-threatening emergency. This emergency was created solely by lack of support and the isolation that comes from birthing outside of the system. This experience gave me a rich perspective on the pros and cons of freebirth.

Introduction

The US spends more money on health care – per-capita and as a percentage of gross domestic product (GDP) – than any other country in the world (World Bank, 2019). The US also has the worst maternal and infant mortality rates of any other high-income country. It is the only developed country with a rising maternal mortality rate, where black women are 3.5 times more likely to die in childbirth than white women (MacDorman et al., 2016; Martin & Montagne, 2017; World Bank 2019). Clearly, something has gone terribly wrong in US maternity care. In addition to high costs and poor health outcomes, paternalistic control, dehumanisation, emotional abuse and physical violence have become normalised features of US maternity care. Medical intervention is so widespread, simply emerging from birth without a surgical delivery constitutes a lucky win (Declercq, Sakala, Corry, & Applebaum, 2007; Diaz-Tello, 2016; Exposing the Silence Project, 2019; Maternal Safety Foundation, 2019).

Fertility, pregnancy and birth in America are the battleground of a complex struggle between women's knowledge and autonomy on the one hand and the medico-legal control of their bodies on the other. Women have advocated to improve childbirth through reforming hospital policies and obstetrical practices as well as by championing midwifery care and birth at home (Mathews & Zadak, 1991; Daviss, 2002; Kline, 2019). A small percentage of women have chosen to opt out of maternity care completely, to give birth either on their own or with close family and friends, in what is variously termed unassisted childbirth (UC), undisturbed birth, unattended birth and freebirth (Freeze, 2008). These women are canaries in the proverbial coal mine: their stories, choices and experiences provide insights into what has gone wrong in maternity care and how we can better support women in childbirth.

Genealogy of freebirth in the US

If we were to write a genealogy of freebirth in the US, Patricia Cloyd Carter would be named the quirky, eccentric grandmother. Born in 1916, she gave birth to ten children. Her first two births were traumatic. She experienced extreme pain, discomfort and mortification from what were, at that time, typical hospital births. She then had a pain-free birth with her third baby when she unknowingly went into labour while in the hospital for an unrelated condition and rejected the hospital system altogether. Her remaining seven babies were born at home in Titusville, Florida, with no medical assistance during the 1940s and 1950s.[1]

Pat Carter might have remained the solitary neighbourhood 'crazy lady', had she not been friends with reporter Mary Lou Culbertson of the *Daytona Beach News-Journal*. Culbertson photographed and wrote about Carter's births, and her articles were published on national and international newswires (Associated Press and United Press) in 1955 and 1956 (Shanley, 2018). Women began writing to Carter, describing traumatic births and asking how they could improve their experiences. This correspondence later turned into a self-published book *Come Gently, Sweet Lucina* (1957), a newsletter *The Wellborn Wag*, and the organisation *League of Liberated Women*, a group founded in 1960 to advocate for Carter's ideas about birth. Author Pamela Klassen describes *Come Gently* as 'the first how-to text for home birth in a culture of medicalized birth … a quirky assortment of physiology, literary quotations, autobiography, and jeremiads against the medical approach to childbirth' (Klassen, 2001, p. 29).

If Pat Carter was grandmother, then British obstetrician Grantly Dick-Read was great uncle to the freebirth movement. Carter was heavily influenced by Dick-Read's theory of the fear–tension–pain cycle. His books, *Natural Childbirth* in 1933 and *Childbirth Without Fear* in 1943, were bestsellers. Dick-Read lecture-toured the US in 1947. He inspired the natural childbirth movements that, in turn, informed the Lamaze and Bradley methods and the creation of the National Childbirth Trust (NCT) in the UK, household names today. Dick-Read surmised that fear during labour creates tension which creates pain. Eliminate fear and tension during childbirth, and you can eliminate pain (Dick-Read, 1943).

Carter argued that while Dick-Read was on the right track, his births were still disturbed, especially during the pushing stage. In Carter's view, birth was instinctual, undisturbed, easy and nearly painless. If it isn't, she argued that women should take anaesthesia early on – none of this 'half and half business that is the fashion now, with obstetricians allowing their patients to be fully conscious during their *unnatural* births while attendants are doing *unnatural* things to them'. Proper mental and physical preparation were key, such that the presence (or not) of an attendant was of minor concern. If women achieved a 'brainless, will-less birth', the benefits were not only no pain or suffering but also enhanced bonding with baby and husband, as well as a sense of achievement and empowerment (1957, pp. 217, 338).

A midwife for every woman, or every woman her own midwife?

The natural childbirth and feminist women's health movements of the 1960s and 1970s were another strong influence in developing freebirth philosophy. Women were reclaiming knowledge and trust in their bodies and demanding freedom from male-dominated medical care (Craven, 2010). Without available midwives, however, some were having 'do it yourself' (DIY) homebirths with friends. Some women continued attending births in what had become a newly created grassroots direct-entry midwifery practice (Reid, 1989). For these birthing-women-turned-midwives, freebirth was the bridge to professional midwifery. Their heritage looms large in some well-known midwifery (and their partners') names, such as Ina May Gaskin (*Spiritual Midwifery*, 1977) and other farm midwives Peggy O'Mara and Marion Sousa (*Childbirth At Home*, 1976), and David and Lee Stewart of InterNational Association of Parents & Professionals for Safe Alternatives in Childbirth (NAPSAC International) and the authors of *Five Standards For Safe Childbearing* (1981).

Conversely, other freebirth advocates envisioned midwifery as a bridge leading to a (desired) professional self-extinction. Midwife Jeanine Parvati Baker freebirthed the last three of her six children in the 1980s. She wrote *Prenatal Yoga & Natural Birth* in 1974, and included her freebirth experiences in the 2001 edition. She saw freebirth as an outgrowth of lay midwifery. Her ideal was that every woman would become her own midwife and that couples would reclaim responsibility for their own births.

Genital love gifts

In the 1980s, a new strain of freebirth thinking emerged which was a curious blend of sexuality and religion. Marilyn Moran described birth as a 'dialogue of love' between married couples. A devout Catholic and mother of ten children, Moran argued that birth is the penultimate sexual act and belongs *only* between husband and wife. During intercourse, the man gifts his sperm to the woman. Nine months later, the woman gifts the baby back to the man. Midwives or doctors can interrupt the completion of the human sexual cycle by receiving the baby or 'genital love gift' meant *only* for the husband. In addition, Moran argued, sexual play during labour – kissing, cuddling, nipple stimulation and orgasm – not only cements marital bonds, it also enhances the birth process naturally, making it safer and more efficient (1981).

Moran wrote two books which described her freebirth views, including *Birth and the Dialogue of Love* (1981) and *Pleasurable Husband/Wife Childbirth*

(1997). She also edited a collection of freebirth stories, *Happy Birth Days* (1986), many of which are about Christian couples' births. Lynn Griesemer's 1998 book, *Unassisted Homebirth*, agreed with many of Moran's ideas. This book was less theoretical and more practical, providing advice to women on managing common complications. Griesemer, a mother of six, was heavily influenced by Moran's ideas of sexual 'complementarity' (the reciprocity of sexual gift-giving) and by her Catholic theological interpretations of birth. Griesemer was a bit looser with her restrictions on who could be present. In her view, children were also welcome to see the process, rather than just husband and wife.

Midwifery as inherently interventive

In the United States, there are two basic types of midwives. The first, *certified nurse midwives* (CNMs), are university-trained nurses who take an advanced degree in midwifery and who practise primarily in hospitals. The second, *direct-entry midwives* (DEMs), are trained through apprenticeship or by attending a midwifery programme. They are called 'direct-entry' because they do not obtain a nursing degree before opting to become midwives. The most commonly used credential to describe direct-entry practice is the *certified professional midwife* (CPM). Regardless of whether they are licensed, certified or unregulated, direct-entry midwives practise primarily in the home and sometimes in birth centres. Unlike midwives in many other countries, direct-entry midwives are generally not allowed to practise in hospitals. The only direct-entry midwifery allowed in hospitals is the one that holds the CM (Certified Midwife) credential, which is recognised in only five states (ACNM, 2017).

In the 1980s and 1990s, homebirth advocates, scholars and mothers began to critique what they saw as the growing medicalisation of direct-entry midwifery. They argued that professionalisation, legalisation and regulation of direct-entry midwifery had shifted homebirth towards an undesirable model in which midwives could not necessarily be trusted to provide non-medicalised care (Weitz & Sullivan, 1985). Women started using the term 'midwifery' to distinguish between midwives who were committed to a non-medical orientation of childbirth and those who supported the obstetric viewpoint (Morgan, 2002; Cameron, 2014). Jeannine Parvati Baker is often credited with coining and popularising this term in her critiques of professionalised midwifery (Baker, 2002). She commented:

> Too many midwives have identified with the oppressor, learned to speak the conquerers [sic] language, and otherwise been vanquished to emerge as obstetrically-trained 'Medwives'. In other words, many midwives have given up being guardians and keepers of natural birth at home, in order to survive as professionals.
>
> (Green, 2019)

Laurie Annis Morgan took this critique further, arguing that even midwives committed to non-medicalised care could impose unnecessary and potentially dangerous interventions in women's birthing spaces. Morgan had her first baby in 1995 with midwives in a freestanding birth centre. She later articulated that the care she received was abusive and violating. She subsequently freebirthed her last three children. Alongside other freebirth writers, Morgan specifically wrote about the downsides of homebirth midwifery in *The Power of Pleasurable Childbirth* in 2002. 'Even the holistic, loving tradition of midwifery (not "med" wifery)' she claimed, 'is interventive to its very core'. Based on her belief that normal birth is inherently private and sexual, she argued that any outsider presence would interfere with the process, no matter how 'hands-off' they promised to be.

Coming full circle: from Pat Carter to Laura Shanley

Laura Shanley, arguably the best-known freebirth advocate today, reinvented Pat Carter's wheel without knowing it. She gave birth to five children, unassisted, in the 1970s and 1980s. Her approach to giving birth was remarkably similar to Carter's, even though she did not discover either Carter or that other women were having freebirths until after she finished having children. Shanley described her feeling of isolation in choosing freebirth:

> When I gave birth to my first child unassisted in 1978, I assumed I was one of the few women in the Western world who had actually *chosen* to give birth this way. In fact, fourteen years would pass before I would realize that the unassisted childbirth movement was alive and well in this country and had been since the 1950's.
>
> (Shanley, 2018)

Shanley read and supported Dick-Read's fear–tension–pain cycle before her first pregnancy. Her overarching thesis in *Unassisted Childbirth* (1994) is that the way birth unfolds depends on our attitudes and beliefs. If we believe that birth is inherently safe and painless, then the need for intervention and assistance will diminish. Fear, shame and guilt will hinder the birth process. On the other hand, qualities such as love, patience, forgiveness and persistence will enhance a woman's labour. As with Carter's book, the presence or absence of a birth attendant was of minor concern to Shanley. In fact, it was Shanley's editor at Bergin & Garvey who suggested the title 'unassisted birth'. It became the first book about freebirth to be released by a major publishing house (Shanley, 2005).

Within a decade of Shanley's book release, the freebirth movement lost its geographic tethers, thanks to the Internet. From early discussion forums on Yahoo! or Mothering.com platforms, the bulk of online communication about freebirth grew into social media sites, particularly on Facebook. Today, a person interested in freebirthing is as likely to connect with someone in

Australia or the UK as she is with someone in her own hometown or region. Freebirth communities may still have linguistic boundaries, but location no longer impedes the flow of thoughts, ideas and information. This, in part, explains the rise of freebirth in western countries.

Entering academia

While the popular literature on freebirth comes from mothers and midwives in the USA, a small body of academics have produced quality literature on the issue, some of whom have contributed to this book. US scholars have published works on the following:

- Understanding freebirth and women who freebirth (Freeze, 2008; Brown, 2009; Miller, 2009) (see Chapter 1)
- How freebirthers conceptualise risk (Cameron, 2014; Plested & Kirkham, 2016)
- The stigma of freebirth choices (Miller & Shriver, 2012)
- Freebirth as a quest for well-being (Plested, 2014)
- Freebirth in the law (Hickman, 2010)

Much of the academic research about freebirth, however, comes from outside the USA:

- Australia (Dahlen, Jackson, & Stevens, 2011; Jackson, Dahlen, & Schmied, 2012; Dannaway & Dietz, 2014; Rigg, Schmied, Peters, & Dahlen, 2018) (see Chapters 2, 5 and 7)
- The Netherlands (Holten & de Miranda, 2016; Hollander et al., 2017; Hollander, Holten, Leusink, van Dillen, & de Miranda, 2018) (see Chapter 4)
- The United Kingdom (Feeley, Burns, Adams, & Thomson, 2015; Feeley & Thomson, 2016a, 2016b; Feeley, 2016a, 2016b) (see Chapter 3)
- Sweden (Lundgren, 2010; Lindgren, Nässén, & Lundgren, 2017)
- Ireland (OBoyle, 2016)

Why do women freebirth in the USA?

Women rarely freebirth for one reason alone. Their decisions come from a combination of factors that *push* them away from maternity care and factors that *pull* them towards freebirth.

Push factors include trauma or dissatisfaction experienced in a previous birth, knowing about trauma that someone else has experienced, avoiding medical practices or policies that are seen as harmful or demeaning, a lack of resources for accessing care and policies or regulations that disqualify access to normal birth. Even women who want the support of an experienced birth worker may end up freebirthing because they are unable to find or access the kind of care and birth environment they need.

Pull factors include belief in the non-medical normalcy of childbirth, belief that freebirth is safer, more pleasurable or more satisfying than medicalised birth and a desire for privacy and intimacy (Morgan, 2002; Buckley, 2009; Feeley et al., 2015; Holten & de Miranda, 2016). Some women embrace freebirth primarily as an outreach of deeply held beliefs. They prefer to give birth either alone or with close family members or friends. These women would rather give birth on their own, even if a supportive midwife was available.

A common scenario is where push factors create the impetus to look for alternatives to standard hospital or midwife-attended birth care. Once women learn about freebirth, however, their reasons become equally as much or more about the benefits of freebirthing.

This section below focuses on two broad categories of push factors: (1) a lack of acceptable options within the maternity care system (called *push-O*) and (2) previous birth trauma (called *push-T*). These factors make freebirth a woman's best, and sometimes only, viable option. We then discuss pull factors that draw women to freebirth and how freebirth fulfils their needs.

In Rixa's dissertation research a decade ago, she compiled themes from 60 open-ended essay responses to the question 'why did you choose a freebirth?' (see Table 1.1).

Ten years later, Laura's survey research shows similar trends for both push factors. When asked to rate motivational factors for planning a freebirth, a large majority of respondents (n = 233) highlighted trauma avoidance as a significant factor (Table 1.2).

Table 1.1 Reasons for freebirthing (Freeze)

Frequency	*Reason(s)*	*Theme*
19	push-O&T	Dangers of hospitals and unnecessary interventions
18	pull	Trust and confidence in birth and in their bodies
16	pull, push-O	Privacy
13	pull, push-O&T	Autonomy and control
12	push-O	Lack of midwives/midwives were a bad fit
11	pull, push-O	Safety
10	pull, push-O	Comfort and peace of home environment
8	pull	Birth as a family event
5	pull	Always wanted a homebirth/freebirth
5	pull	Belief in instinct/intuition
5	push-T	Birth trauma: want to avoid, or previous traumatic birth
5	pull	Just felt right
4	pull	Do-it-yourself ethic
3	pull	Desire to take responsibility for the birth

Table 1.2 Push factors for choosing freebirth (Tanner) (n = 233, rounded)

Reason	*N/A*	*Not really*	*Slightly*	*Fairly*	*Very*
Avoiding something negative experienced in her own previous birth (*trauma*)	60 (26%)	15 (6%)	13 (6%)	24 (10%)	121 (52%)
Avoiding a negative experience she knows that someone else has had in birth (*trauma*)	43 (18%)	43 (18%)	30 (13%)	39 (17%)	78 (34%)
'Risked out' of a natural vaginal hospital birth due to hospital policy (*options*)	89 (38%)	25 (11%)	12 (5%)	26 (11%)	81 (35%)
'Risked out' of midwife-attended homebirth due to midwifery regulations (*options*)	107 (46%)	32 (14%)	18 (8%)	24 (10%)	52 (22%)

Policies and regulations that restrict options (*push-O*)

In some situations, women are actually *barred* from attempting vaginal birth in hospitals. This is due to a combination of hospital policies and provider practices that mandate surgical delivery. The most common reasons given by doctors for refusing women the option to give birth vaginally include (a) previous surgical delivery, (b) twin or multiple births or (c) breech birth. Vaginal birth bans are not evidence-based and do not conform to medical ethics (Wendland, 2007; Dodd, Crowther, Huertas, Guise, & Horey, 2013; ACOG, 2019), yet they are deeply entrenched in US maternity care.

In such cases, out-of-hospital birth may be a woman's only chance for a normal birth. As midwifery has increasingly found legitimation through state licensure, however, similar restrictions have been built into state practice regulations so that midwives may not be legally permitted to attend births labelled as 'higher-risk'. These restrictive regulations extend medical models of risk into the home and constrain women's choices, particularly in the case of vaginal birth after caesarean (VBAC), breech, and multiple births.

Vaginal birth after caesarean (VBAC)

Unlike other parts of the human body that are expected to fully heal and resume normal functioning after surgery, the uterus is forever suspect after a caesarean. This suspicion follows a historical precedent of pathologising women's bodies in medical research, literature and practice (Morgan, 1998; Davis-Floyd, 2004; Owens, 2017). While the incidence of certain complications – most notably abnormal placental attachment and uterine rupture – are increased after caesarean section, this increased risk is relatively small, and repeat caesareans carry a different set of risks to both mother and baby.

While Chapter 7 discusses VBAC more fully, it is instructive to take a brief look at the statistics associated with the VBAC debate from the US perspective. The risk of mortality from a planned VBAC is low, with an overall perinatal mortality rate of 1.3/1000 compared to 0.5/1000 for elective repeat caesarean section (ERCS) (Guise et al., 2010). Approximately 0.5% of women attempting a VBAC will experience a uterine rupture. Among women *with* uterine ruptures, there may be an estimated zero maternal deaths and between 0% and 2.8% foetal deaths (Metz, Berghella, & Barss, 2019). Meanwhile, maternal mortality is 3.6–3.9 times greater for a first-time caesarean delivery than for vaginal birth, and the risk of both maternal mortality and morbidity increases with each additional caesarean (Harper et al., 2003; Deneux-Tharaux, Carmona, Bouvier-Colle, & Bréart, 2006; Silver et al., 2006; Childbirth Connection, 2012). Maternal morbidity is increased with planned caesarean delivery, with higher rates of haemorrhage requiring blood transfusion or hysterectomy, infection, admission to the intensive care unit and extended hospital stay (Liu et al., 2007; Curtin, Gregory, Korst, & Uddin, 2015). In addition to these risks, women must take into account the effect of mode of birth on recovery time, the ability to care for other children or return to work, breastfeeding and bonding after birth, future health risks for both mother and baby and the impact on subsequent births. In all of these areas, vaginal birth is undeniably better for the well-being of mother and infant.

Despite the known downsides to repeated caesareans, the risks of VBAC generally and of uterine rupture in particular are emphasised over those of ERCS. Why? The American maternity care system favours medical management, by treating pregnancy and childbirth as inherently pathological and preferencing surgical solutions over non-intervention. Thus, as researchers have noted, 'the "exploding uterus card" receives such a disproportionate amount of attention that VBAC is considered categorically worse for the foetus – and sometimes the mother – than a repeat C-section' (Torio, 2010; Hallgrimsdottir, Shumka, Althaus, & Benoit, 2017). As many US hospitals impose 'VBAC bans', the hospital policy is in fact mandating ERCS. In 2013, only 20% of women who had one previous caesarean even attempted a subsequent vaginal delivery. That rate dropped to 7% for women with two or more previous caesareans (Metz et al., 2019).

In 2009, the International Caesarean Awareness Network (ICAN) conducted a telephone survey of every US hospital offering maternity services to determine if they supported VBAC. Forty-nine percent of US hospitals banned VBAC with either an express policy ban (28%) or a ban by default (no providers willing to support VBAC, 21%) (Paul, 2009; Birth Monopoly, 2019b). VBAC bans continue to this day, despite the low risk of uterine rupture and the higher success rate for planned VBAC. Hospital VBAC success rates (i.e. how many planned VBACs actually *end* in a vaginal birth) range from 47% to 87% (Guise et al., 2010). VBAC success rates in planned home or birth centre births are consistently around 87% (Lieberman, Ernst, Rooks, Stapleton, & Flamm, 2004; Cox, Bovbjerg, Cheyney, & Leeman, 2015; Rowe,

Knight, Brocklehurst, & Hollowell, 2016).[2] One study estimated that the repeat caesarean rate would drop to 25.5% if all women who screened as 'good candidates' actually attempted a VBAC (Metz et al., 2019). In other words, the low national VBAC attempt rate comes largely because hospital and provider policies ban it, not because of an inherently high failure rate.

The American VBAC situation leaves many women with no hospital options for VBAC. At the same time, access to midwife-attended VBAC at home or in birth centres is also restricted. There are currently no laws prohibiting women from giving birth at home, regardless of their perceived risks status. States indirectly restrict women's homebirthing choices by restricting who a midwife can serve. (The effect of this regulation on midwives is explored further in Chapter 11.)

Regulation of midwifery in the US is complex because laws and regulations vary from state to state and may be different depending on whether a birth worker is a nurse or direct-entry midwife, and whether direct-entry midwives are certified and/or licensed or not. While CNMs can attend homebirths in 49 states (with or without various restrictions such as the requirement for physician supervision), only 3% actually attend homebirths (Hamilton, Martin, Osterman, Curtin, & Matthews, 2015). CPMs are currently licensed or authorised in 33 states, which leaves direct-entry midwifery in illegal, a-legal or unregulated spaces in the remaining states (The Big Push for Midwives, 2019).

Saraswathi Vedam and her research team recently released data on VBAC restrictions in all 50 US states and the District of Columbia (Vedam et al., 2018). The current status of access to VBAC with licensed midwives is:

27 states: VBAC prohibited, or DEMs are unregulated
Five states: VBAC allowed only by restrictive conditions (e.g. physician approval)
14 states: VBAC allowed by meeting certain conditions and with informed consent
Five states: VBAC unrestricted

Notably, VBAC with licensed direct-entry midwives is only freely or reasonably available in 19 states. In unregulated states, women can VBAC at home with an unlicensed 'underground' midwife, if they can find someone willing to serve. That said, access to home VBAC is not guaranteed even in states that currently permit it. For example, proposed regulation changes in Oregon could limit access to VBAC after multiple caesareans (Oregon Health Authority, 2019).

Breech and multiple births

Vaginal birth of multiples and breech-presenting babies are considered by the medical community to be high-risk births. As with VBAC, the assumed risks of vaginal birth are emphasised while the negative consequences of caesarean

Table 1.3 Restrictions on breech and multiples for licensed homebirth midwives

Restrictions on breech and multiples for licensed homebirth midwives	*Breech*	*Multiples*
Prohibited at home	13*	12*
With restrictive conditions	3	3
With certain conditions	4	5
No restrictions	4	4

*In Utah, licensure is optional and unlicensed midwives have no restrictions on supporting VBAC, breech, or multiple pregnancies.

are minimised. Since the 1960s, caesarean rates for breech presentation have been rising. In fact, most hospitals and physicians have stopped allowing vaginal breech births altogether, bringing the 2016 caesarean rate for breech in the US to 93.2% (Dekker, 2018). (We discuss breech birth in Chapter 19.)

In the USA, the 2013 caesarean rate for live twin births was 74.8% (Bateni et al., 2016). For triplets and higher, the CS rate was 93.9% in 2006 (Lappen, Hackney & Bailit, 2016). As with VBAC and breech births, finding a care provider who will support a vaginal birth for twins or higher-order multiples can prove difficult, if not impossible.

When accredited birth centres do not offer planned vaginal breech or twin births, the choice becomes a homebirth or a non-accredited birth centre. The only collation of US-wide regulations, which control access to midwife-supported breech and multiple homebirth, was a document we found which was undated but approximately five years old from the Arizona Department of Health Services (n.d.). Licensed homebirth midwives can freely attend breech and multiple gestations in only a small number of states; most states either prohibit or restrict these options. Table 1.3 shows our findings after we added a few recent changes from states that altered their regulations.

Breech presentation is often discovered in the last few weeks or days of pregnancy, and as many as 1/4 to 1/3 of all breech pregnancies are undiagnosed when labour begins (Walker, 2013). This last-minute upheaval can be devastating for women. Not only are vaginal breech birth providers nearly impossible to find, women are often left racing against the clock to find someone to help before the baby arrives. If they cannot, an unassisted breech birth at home becomes the only 'choice' other than a caesarean section mandated by the hospital.

In Laura's research, one response highlights how these restrictions can disrupt women's maternity care:

> My third pregnancy was a total shock because we found out at 22 weeks that we were having twin girls. We had been planning a homebirth but knew that the midwife would no longer see us since she did not attend twin births. Added to the fact that I was planning a VBAC, I was sure

> things were going to be more complicated. Thankfully, my pregnancy was not complicated at all … I went into labour at 39 weeks, 1 day, on the day the backup OB had wanted to perform an elective repeat caesarean, which I refused. I did not show up for the scheduled caesarean and instead gave birth to two 7 1/2 lb healthy babies in my bedroom in the company of 2 midwives I had never met before in my life. I had planned to birth alone but when the midwives found out that I had been abandoned by my midwife (long story, went through three different midwives who all discharged me from care, the last doing so at 38 weeks) they drove 7 hours from two states away to be with me.
>
> (Anonymous, 39, mother of six, Tanner, unpublished)

Notably, midwifery licensure/regulation in the US presents a double bind. While it permits midwifery practice without the risk of prosecution for practising without a licence, licensure can impose restrictions on women's choices and force midwives to abandon or refuse care for some types of pregnancies. Additionally, because vaginal breech/multiple births are not considered standard practice, fear of the non-medical consequences (e.g. blame, stigma, increased state regulation, medical board review) can have a chilling effect on providers' willingness to support those births, regardless of the law. Midwives are being prosecuted for attending breech/multiple births at home; the most recent example being in Australia, where an unlicenced midwife was prosecuted for manslaughter after attending a twin pregnancy and a breech birth in the home. (The midwife was acquitted of both charges three years later.)

Racial bias and racialised outcomes

Lack of cultural competency and racial discrimination in mainstream maternity care can constitute factors pushing women towards freebirth. As noted earlier, US maternal and infant mortality rates are significantly higher for women of colour, particularly black women, when compared to white women (Maternal Infant Strategy Group, 2019). The US maternal mortality rate for white women is currently 12.4 per 100,000 live births. This rate rises to 17.8 for non-black women of colour, and spikes to 40 for black women (CDC, 2018). Black women also have higher caesarean section and morbidity rates, and have longer hospital stays (Tangel, White, Nachamie, & Pick, 2019). These disparities hold true across income, education, age, insurance and receipt of prenatal care (Harper et al., 2004; Tangel et al., 2019). Research points to two factors that contribute significantly to these poor outcomes: accumulated lifetime stress from being targeted by racism, and racial discrimination and race-based bias in health care (Alhusen, Bower, Epstein, & Sharps, 2016; Novoa & Taylor, 2018).

Some black women respond to these disparities by seeking less-medicalised care in a more culturally competent environment. Roughly 0.5% of black women choose birth outside of hospital, largely opting for midwife-attended homebirths (MacDorman, Mathews, & Declercq, 2014). Unfortunately, they face the same policy and regulation limitations to maternity care discussed above. In addition to the regulatory barriers, black women may face a lack of culturally competent homebirth care providers.[3]

According to statistics collated by Midwives Association of North America, in 2011 only 21% of CPMs are women of colour and just 5.2% of all CPMs serve populations that are predominantly non-white (Cheyney et al., 2015). Some of the black women will choose freebirth as their best option.

There is also evidence that, for black women, poor birth outcomes and racial discrimination are important factors to choosing freebirth. While the overall number of black women filling out Laura's survey was low ($n = 6$), 66% indicated that avoiding racial or cultural discrimination from care providers was either fairly important ($n = 1$) or very important ($n = 3$) to their decision to freebirth (Tanner, 2019). Anecdotes and testimonials online also suggest this to be the case. For example, journalist Imani Bashir reports on her fear of race-discrimination in mainstream maternity care driving her decision to freebirth:

> From almost the moment I found out I was pregnant, I worried. Every mom-to-be worries – Will I have pregnancy complications? Will my child be healthy? Will I poop during labor? – but with my being a black woman in America, the realization quickly set in: Being pregnant meant putting my well-being, even my life, on the line in a way that white moms, statistically, don't have to … The prevailing theory as to why this gross inequity exists? Black women are often ignored and dismissed when it comes to health issues, including ones that can turn fatal … This racial bias weighed heavily on my mind – with stories like [Kira] Johnson's and [Serena] Williams' happening more often than I could stomach, how could I feel safe having a hospital birth?
>
> (Bashir, 2019)

After her search for a midwife proved unfruitful, Bashir planned a freebirth. Having had a complication-free 'perfect birth', Bashir still wished for the option of a supportive midwife to attend to her in birth:

> Looking back, I would have also preferred a pro was on hand to examine us both immediately after birth so that the anxiety of possible unknowns – like infection – wouldn't have been gnawing at the edges of our blissful moment. A midwife with birthing expertise would have been the icing on the cake of my son's entry in the world.
>
> We should live in a world where black women don't have to feel afraid of giving birth in a hospital – every woman should be able to have a safe birth on her terms. Until then, we have to keep advocating for ourselves. We have to keep demanding better.
>
> (Bashir, 2019)

Black women are at increased risk within a system in which all women struggle for self-determination and respect and where refusing care or countermanding doctor's orders during pregnancy and labour can result in police arrests, forced medical intervention and reports to child protection services (Paltrow & Flavin, 2013). Opting out of maternity care may offer protection from both discriminatory medical care and increased state surveillance. It is, however, worth noting the flip side of this coin: black women are more likely to face censure and prosecution if their freebirths result in tragedy. They certainly face suspicion and punitive treatment by medical providers when seeking post-natal care. Thus, for black women, both the push factors for, and the risks of, freebirth may be intensified.

History of negative birth experiences (*push-T*)

Childbirth, as a shared experience and a normal physiological function of the female body, is as mundane as life gets. Equally, it can function as a 'peak experience' of transcendence and transformation (Schwartz, 2014) or leave a woman feeling disempowered and suffering from doubt, sadness, or worse. Giving birth has been called a 'rite of passage' due to its profound social importance (Robbie Davis-Floyd, 1992). It is also an intense embodied experience that can call on all of a woman's physical and psychological reserves. Her experience of birth may affect how she conceives of herself as a woman and mother, and her personal integrity, long-term mental health, parenting, relationships and future reproductive decisions (Simkin, 1991, 1992; Elmir, Schmied, Wilkes, & Jackson, 2010).

The impact of birth – good and bad – can be seen in the words of women who planned freebirths:

> I felt completely empowered as a person and mother. It changed my sense of my own intelligence, intuition, and power.
>
> (Tanner, 2019)

> My hospital birth was the most traumatic stressful thing I have ever been through. I still have nightmares about it and cry every time I talk about it. I wish I could go back and choose differently. My next birth will be at home, I will not transfer.
>
> (Tanner, 2019)

Every woman experiences birth differently. What qualifies as a push factor away from mainstream maternity care varies from a relatively mild sense of frustration or dissatisfaction to an intense feeling of violation. The spectrum of reactions is seen in both Rixa's and Laura's research. In the extracts below, note the way that restrictions imposed on VBAC, breech, twins and midwives are woven into women's stories:

I didn't like having a hospital birth. I didn't like how the caregivers (nurses) changed shifts and no matter where I was in the birth process I had to adjust to completely new people … The doctor was not around very much until the baby was actually coming out. Then everyone was there. It was like a circus. So dramatic.

(Tanner, 2019)

We considered home birth primarily as a result of my wife's very short first labour (< 4 hours) and so our oldest son could be present. As we studied, other reasons (home environment safety, personal responsibility, easier labours) convinced us. The first home birth was not unassisted. We had a very experienced midwife. She was able to just watch while we had our baby. This gave us the confidence to have only friends at the last two home births.

(Freeze, 2008)

I could never imagine giving birth in a hospital. I believe birth is a private and natural bodily function. But my first midwife-attended birth was traumatic and left me with a lot of fear and lack of confidence in myself. But after researching UC [unassisted childbirth], I realized that the difficulties I had in my first birth were caused by lack of preparation on my part, and by interference on the part of the midwife. I realized I could have a safer, more satisfying birth experience by preparing myself and listening to my intuition about whom to have present.

(Freeze, 2008)

[I] had an unmedicated birth that seemed to be fine until pushing when I was utterly abused by nurses AND doctors, culminating in being fisted to 'check for tears' immediately after even when begging for the Dr. to stop. He told me to be quiet and he HAD to, even though I had no tears and he had no reason to be inside me like that.

(Tanner, 2019)

My baby turned footling breech during birth, and I was forced to go to the hospital where I was pushed into accepting another caesarean. I felt like a failure and like I wasn't even a person while they were getting me ready for surgery, just a body to be manhandled. The surgery was so painful – they kept pushing extremely hard on my stomach to get my baby to turn, and while she was perfectly fine before it all, she came out floppy and not breathing, due to all the abuse to make her turn. She's fine now, but it was terribly traumatic to all of us. I do not trust doctors anymore. I barely trust midwives, because I was let down by mine.

(Tanner, 2019)

> My first birth resulted in a traumatic episiotomy without my consent and horrible PTSD from previous sexual assault. My second birth resulted in me being discharged from care by my homebirth midwife for being postdates. I ended up having a completely unnecessary caesarean without any labour, listed in my medical records as an 'elective primary caesarean.' I was/am outraged. That is what led me to freebirth.
>
> (Tanner, 2019)

These stories highlight the variety of abuses birthing women face from their care providers and the institutions in which they labour. Mainstream maternity care in the United States claims to be the best and safest option for birth. Both statistical outcomes and women's stories, however, challenge this assertion. In addition to having some of the worst maternal and infant health outcomes of any high-income country (Martin & Montagne, 2017), the medical system is producing dissatisfied, frustrated and traumatised women at an alarming rate. Of the women in Laura's survey who said a negative previous birth was a very important factor in freebirthing, one in four explicitly described their previous births as 'traumatic'.

Birth trauma and obstetric violence

Public discussions describing maternity care as abusive or cruel initially surfaced in the late 1950s, when nearly all births occurred in hospital and twilight sleep in labour was common (Mathews & Zadak, 1991).[4] In 1957, after a nurse called for an investigation into 'cruelty in maternity wards' in the *Ladies' Home Journal*, hundreds of letters from readers followed detailing cruel, callous, abusive, or uncaring treatment by doctors and nurses (Robbins, 1998), two of which are extracted below.

> I have seen doctors who have charming examination-room manners show traces of sadism in the delivery room. One I know does cutting and suturing without anaesthetic. He has nurses use a mask to stifle the patient's outcry. Some doctors still say, 'Tie them down so they won't give us any trouble.'
>
> (Obstetrical Nurse)

One woman wrote that she was strapped to a delivery table for over 24 hours:

> Far too many doctors and hospitals seem to assume that just because a woman is about to give birth she becomes a nitwit, an incompetent, reduced to the status of a cow. I was strapped to the delivery table on Saturday morning and lay there until I was delivered on Sunday afternoon. When I slipped my hand from the strap to wipe sweat from my face I was severely reprimanded by the nurse.[5]

(See also Chapter 8: in Jordan, birth continues to be managed with a form of twilight sleep and holds a different meaning for women there.)

In her study of birth trauma narratives between 1940 and 1980, historian Paula Michaels notes that women's complaints about treatment in childbirth have remained remarkably consistent over time. Trauma caused by provider in institutional care has proven an intractable problem resistant to efforts to soften, humanise or reform hospital delivery (Michaels, 2018).

Worse, women are shamed about their feelings and concerns when it comes to their births. After experiencing anything from disappointment to trauma, women are wounded a second time when they are told to 'get over it' and be grateful for the arrival of a 'healthy baby'. Feminist philosophers Sara Cohen Shabot and Keshet Korem refer to this as a 'gendered shame' in which:

> [W]omen are primed to experience obstetric violence as a normal part of being … an all-giving mother. Obstetric violence is thus perpetuated, turning laboring women into objects and depriving them of the opportunity to experience labor as an integrated, embodied, fully sensual experience.[6]
>
> (2018, p. 394)

Women want to protect their babies and they are willing to put their own needs second. This is what makes them vulnerable within a medical system that is indifferent to their pain and a society that both valorises their sacrifices and minimises their suffering (Rich, 1976; Hays, 1998; Davis-Floyd, 2004; Owens, 2017; Dusenbery, 2018). Comments like 'Baby comes first' and 'All that matters is a healthy baby' illustrate this.

Birth rape and obstetric violence

In the 1990s, women began framing mistreatment in childbirth in a specifically *sexual* sense.[7] Some used the term *birth rape* to describe the dynamics of abuse in childbirth. This term is used to portray, in a literal sense, the sexual violence associated with hands or objects being inserted into vaginas without consent, cuts to the genital area and being forcibly held down with legs spread. It may also be employed in a figurative sense to describe women's lack of power or autonomy during childbirth.

> A woman who is raped while giving birth does not experience the assault in a way that fits neatly within the typical definitions we hold true in civilised society. A penis is usually nowhere to be found in the story and the perpetrator may not even possess one. But fingers, hands, suction cups, forceps, needles and scissors … these are the tools of birth rape.
>
> UK writer, mother, and reproductive activist Amity Reed
> 'Not a happy birthday', *The F-Word* (March 2008)

Some women choose an elective caesarean to avoid the trauma and violence they associate with another vaginal birth (Reed, 2008). Others leave the hospital system altogether in favour of a birth centre or midwife-attended homebirth. But what of the women who experienced abuse at the hands of their homebirth midwives? Freebirth may be the only safe place left.

> When birth was moved from the home to the public arena of a hospital delivery room, and turned into an industrial process with the aim of assembly-line efficiency, our technocratic culture brutalized it. A woman may be immobilised, tethered to machines and surrounded by strangers whose eyes are all apprehensively fixed on the lower end of her body. In striving to make birth safer, an intimate experience that used to take place with the support and encouragement of women friends has been transformed to an act of violence. Medical control of women's bodies turns into 'iatrogenic rape'.
>
> Sheila Kitzinger, PhD, British anthropologist,
> *Birth Crisis* (2006, p. 56)

Birth rape terminology has proven controversial and, consequently, not found much traction outside alternative birth communities (with notable exceptions like Kitzinger). In the twenty-first century, however, activists and scholars have been successful with raising awareness using the less-threatening terminology of *obstetric violence*. The most commonly used definition of obstetric violence is one taken from a 2007 Venezuelan law intended to give women the right to a life free of violence, including obstetric violence, defined as

> the appropriation of the body and reproductive processes of women by health personnel, which is expressed as dehumanized treatment, an abuse of medication, and to convert the natural processes into pathological ones, bringing with it loss of autonomy and the ability to decide freely about their bodies and sexuality, negatively impacting the quality of life of women.
>
> (Pérez, 2010; Borges, 2018)

While the term *obstetric violence* lacks explicit reference to the sexual nature of the term 'birth rape', it is sufficiently broad to recognise the full spectrum of abusive treatment and, importantly, the inherent harms associated with medicalizing childbirth.

Birth Monopoly, an advocacy group, adapted the 'rape culture pyramid' (11th Principle Consent, 2019) (Figure 1.1) to describe the hierarchy of obstetric violence practices, ranging from abusive or manipulative behaviours

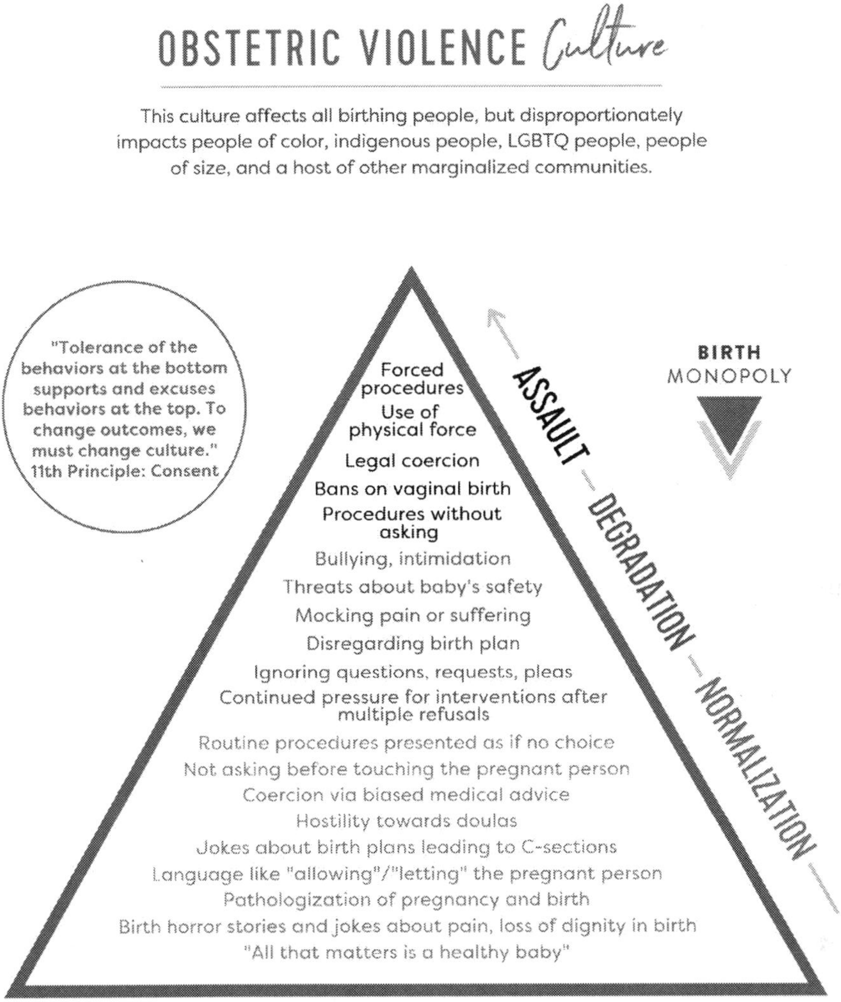

Figure 1.1 Hierarchy of obstetric violence practices
Source: http://birthmonopoly.com/obstetric-violence. Copyright 2019 Birth Monopoly.

(viewed as normal) to the maternity healthcare practices that constitute assault and abuse (Birth Monopoly, 2019a).

PTSD and mental health

Birth trauma has drawn the attention of another discipline: psychologists, who are investigating Post-Traumatic Stress Disorder (PTSD) as a response to traumatic childbirth. (Chapter 12 deals with this issue in greater depth.)

Research has shown that some women suffer mental health morbidities following birth, exhibiting symptoms of PTSD and trauma-induced stress (PTS) and postpartum anxiety, depression or psychosis. In this literature, between 20% and 48% of women describe their births as traumatic (Simpson & Catling, 2016). In one study, 9% of women fulfilled the screening for full PTSD and an additional 18% reported elevated levels of PTS (Beck, Gable, Sakala, & Declercq, 2011; Kendall-Tackett, 2014). An analysis of 68 studies of postpartum PTSD in ten countries calculated a conservative prevalence rate for clinical PTSD of 3.1% in community samples and a rate of 15.7% for women assumed to be at high risk of developing trauma (Grekin & O'Hara, 2014).

Personal risk factors for women include pre-existing mental health disorders and prior traumatic events. Research into birth-related PTSD, however, reports that women's perceptions of trauma often have more to do with the *subjective* experience of birth (Beck, 2004). These subjective experiences are informed by women's perception of their relationship with medical staff, a feeling of loss of control during the birth, fear and pain and medical interventions, especially caesarean section (Grekin & O'Hara, 2014). In one survey of 748 women describing their birth as traumatic, 66.7% named the actions of their care providers as the source of that trauma (Reed, Sharman, & Inglis, 2017).

Freebirth for well-being (*pull*)

Freebirth is not only a rejection of harmful birth practices, it is also a move towards a positive and empowering experience. Freebirth can help heal trauma from previous births and positively affects women's lives in the long term. Women who freebirth view birth as an inherently normal body process and an opportunity for personal growth. In Laura's survey, nearly all women rated the following reasons as 'Very' or 'Fairly' important in their decision to freebirth (Table 1.4).

Table 1.4 Pull factors for choosing freebirth (Tanner, 2019) ($n = 235$, rounded)

Reason	*N/A*	*Not really*	*Slightly*	*Fairly*	*Very*
Believing freebirth is the safest option for me and my baby (*pull*)	8 (3%)	4 (2%)	16 (7%)	47 (20%)	160 (68%)
Wanting to be 100% responsible and in charge of my birth (*pull*)	2 (<1%)	2 (<1%)	9 (4%)	26 (11%)	196 (83%)
Believing that birth is a normal, non-medical process (*pull*)	0	0	5 (2%)	23 (10%)	206 (88%)
Wanting an intimate, private birth (*pull*)	2 (<1%)	6 (3%)	13 6%	36 (15%)	179 (76%)

Another way to think about this is through the lens of Self-Determination Theory (SDT), a term developed by psychologists to identify the innate psychological needs that ground personal growth, integrity and well-being (Ryan, Huta, & Deci, 2008). Psychologists Ryan and Deci argue that humans feel a sense of personal and interpersonal well-being in environments that support and nurture three basic needs of autonomy, competence and relatedness. Environments that actively thwart or frustrate these needs can crush the human spirit (Ryan & Deci, 2000; Bartholomew, Ntoumanis, Ryan, Bosch, & Thøgersen-Ntoumani, 2011). We explain each basic need below and apply examples from Laura's dissertation research to illustrate how freebirth fulfils these needs.[8]

Autonomy

We all need to feel a sense of control over our own lives or, at least, our own behaviour. Autonomy can equate with individual choice, but is more complex than merely selecting from available options and is not necessarily individualistic. When autonomy is satisfied, we experience willingness, volition and responsibility for our own behaviour. When autonomy is frustrated, we have a sense of being controlled by outside forces or of losing the ability to determine our own behaviour or what happens to us (Ryan & Deci, 2000; Chen et al., 2015). Women who freebirth point to feelings of autonomy when they describe themselves as both responsible and able to make decisions and be in charge during their births.

> It was a profoundly liberating experience. Sticking up for myself and my choices, taking FULL RESPONSIBILITY for any outcome was empowering.
>
> (Tanner, 2019)

Competence

Through competence, humans feel effective in what we do and are able to work towards our goals. We have a sense of mastery – we have important knowledge, skills, or abilities – and others recognise our capability. We also have opportunities to demonstrate our competence. Competence frustration leaves us feeling like failures and doubting our abilities and effectiveness (Chen et al., 2015). When women talk about feeling strength and empowerment, they are demonstrating how freebirth nurtures their need for competence:

> I know exactly how strong I am & what I'm capable of, without anyone's help. That's incredibly empowering. I don't really have words for it.
>
> (Tanner, 2019)

Relatedness

Our need for relatedness is satisfied through intimacy, connection and sense of belonging with others, i.e. when we feel embedded in meaningful social relationships. Relatedness is frustrated when we feel excluded, lonely, let down or betrayed, or when our relationships are not as imagined or expected (Chen et al., 2015). Women who freebirth talk of how privacy and intimacy in birth made them feel closer to their loved ones, and strengthened their relationships and sense of connectedness.

> It was amazing! I felt a burning sensation, and in that moment, I felt so connected to other people who had done this before me. I felt so powerful.
>
> (Tanner, 2019)

> I think giving birth to my son at home did change my relationship with my partner. It made me realize how strong I was and how much I loved his son. When his violent tendencies took over during the next year, I had the strength to leave him. I'm not sure if I could've had that strength without experiencing homebirth with my baby and the intensity of that bond.
>
> (Tanner, 2019)

Women's experiences of birth are pivotal moments when their psychological needs are either profoundly nurtured or denied. By maintaining a biomedical or technocratic paradigm of birth, US mainstream maternity care fails to recognise and account for women's subjective experience of birth, consequently denying them their psychological needs. Autonomy, competence and relatedness are not just the needs of a handful of women. They are *the innate requirements of all women*. Women who freebirth are, in part, seeking an environment that will nurture these human capacities.

Finally, some women freebirth even where homebirth midwives or progressive hospitals are available. Others prefer to have a care provider but are effectively locked out of maternity care due to inflexible hospital policies, midwifery regulations, or a medical model of birth.

All women deserve a birth free from violence that nurtures their basic psychological needs, no matter where or with whom they give birth.

The way forward

(1) Provide trauma-informed care to all women by approaching women respectfully and never entering their physical space or performing a procedure without explicit permission and clear, prior consent

(2) Vigorously uphold maternal autonomy. This includes a woman's right to informed consent and right to informed refusal and the right to access maternity care free from coercion

(3) Support liberal rather than restrictive midwifery regulations, which allow midwives and women room for autonomy. Allow midwives to provide care that falls outside guidelines rather than abandon their clients
(4) Provide flexible hospital options for physiologic birth, VBAC, breech and multiple births that are supportive of women's needs
(5) Respect the mother–baby dyad and trust that a mother has her baby's best interests in mind

Notes

1 Birth was just one of Carter's interests: she also ran the first free public library in Titusville. She was recognised by the National Organization of Women and the American Association of University Women for this work. From Betty Sue Cummings' 'Memorial to Pat Carter', submitted by Carter's daughter Mary Winn on 11 May 2002 and available from http://archiver.rootsweb.ancestry.com/th/read/WEAVER/2002–05/1021160999 [accessed 1 September 2008].

2 87.6% among homebirths in England; 87% among homebirths in the USA; 87% in US birth centres.

3 There is a rich history of black women serving their communities as midwives and healers both during and after slavery in the USA. These 'Granny' midwives continued to practise into the twentieth century when midwifery was mostly stamped out through racially targeted anti-midwifery public health campaigns (Hays, 2015).

4 Twilight sleep was a morphine–scopolamine cocktail widely used as an anaesthetic/amnesiac during labour. It caused women to be unable to consciously remember labours in which they became highly agitated and were in tremendous pain yet were unable to actively communicate or participate. Twilight sleep typically necessitated large episiotomies and forceps deliveries followed by resuscitation of morphine-drugged babies. Twilight sleep was promoted as feminist progress, a release from the pains of labour. For about a year in 1914–15, upper-class white women led a campaign for access to twilight sleep. Although it became quickly apparent that it was in fact bad for mothers and babies, it took decades to end the practice.

5 Quotations originally found in Gladys Denny Shultz's article 'Journal Mothers Report on Cruelty in Maternity Wards', *Ladies' Home Journal* (May 1958): 44–45, 153–154 and (December 1958): 58–59, 135, 137–139.

6 Note that Shabot and Korem are here locating the trouble in the social expectations of femininity and motherhood. They argue that the only way to eliminate obstetric violence is to create new models of femininity not centred on intensive motherhood. However, locating the problem of birth trauma in the medical system and non-physiological birthing practices rather than in the social expectations of maternal sacrifice, and rather than rejecting intensive motherhood and mother-identity, women who freebirth are often reclaiming this position as their own and in their own image. Reframing the struggle to birth in positive and empowering terms, these women are often seeking a space where they can be free to embrace the process of birth and intensive mothering practices without interference.

7 Rixa's 2008 dissertation explores the evolution of birth rape as a term and concept. She also conducted an internet survey about birth rape.

8 Although we focus here on the US, Self-Determination Theory has shown that these basic needs are cross-cultural and their importance to human functioning remains across cultures that value things like autonomy or relationships differently. See, for example, Chen et al. (2015).

References

ACNM. (2017). Comparison of Certified Nurse-Midwives, Certified Midwives, Certified Professional Midwives Clarifying the Distinctions Among Professional Midwifery Credentials in the U.S. Retrieved from: www.midwife.org/acnm/files/ccLibraryFiles/FILENAME/000000006807/FINAL-ComparisonChart-Oct2017.pdf [accessed 19 April 2019].

ACOG. (2019). Vaginal birth after cesarean delivery. *ACOG Practice Bulletin No. 205, 133*(2), e110–127.

Alhusen, J. L., Bower, K., Epstein, E., & Sharps, P. (2016). Racial discrimination and adverse birth outcomes: An integrative review. *Journal of Midwifery & Women's Health, 61*(6), 707–720.

Arizona Department of Health Services. (n.d.). Midwifery scope of practice by state: VBAC, multiple births, breech births in non-hospital settings. Retrieved from: https://azdhs.gov/documents/licensing/special/midwives/committees/mspac/additional-resources/state-laws-chart-vbac-br-mg.pdf [accessed 19 April 2019].

Baker, J. P. (1974). *Prenatal yoga & natural birth*. Albion, CA: Freestone.

Baker, J. P. (2001). *Prenatal yoga & natural childbirth*, 3rd edn. Monroe, UT: Freestone.

Baker, J. P. (2002). Hygeia. Retrieved from: http://web.archive.org/web/20150820051255/http://www.freestone.org/hygieia/ [accessed 19 April 2019].

Bartholomew, K., Ntoumanis, N., Ryan, R., Bosch, J., & Thøgersen-Ntoumani, C. (2011). Self-determination theory and diminished functioning: The role of interpersonal control and psychological need thwarting. *Personality & Social Psychology Bulletin, 37*(11), 1459–1473.

Bashir, I. (2019). I chose to have a totally unassisted home birth. *Glamour*. 1 March. Retrieved from: www.glamour.com/story/i-chose-an-unassisted-home-birth [accessed 19 April 2019].

Bateni, Z. H., Clark, S. L., Sangi-Haghpeykar, H., Aagaard, K. M., Blumenfeld, Y. J., Ramin, S. M., ... Shamshirsaz, A. A. (2016). Trends in the delivery route of twin pregnancies in the United States, 2006–2013. *European Journal of Obstetrics and Gynecology, 205*, 120–126.

Beck, C. T. (2004). Birth trauma: In the eye of the beholder. *Nursing Research, 53*(1), 28–35.

Beck, C. T., Gable, R. K., Sakala, C., & Declercq, E. R. (2011). Posttraumatic stress disorder in new mothers: Results from a two-stage U.S. national survey. *Birth (Berkeley, California), 38*(3), 216–227.

Birth Monopoly. (2019a). Obstetric violence. Retrieved from: https://birthmonopoly.com/obstetric-violence/ [accessed 19 April 2019].

Birth Monopoly. (2019b). VBAC bans: vaginal birth bans: interactive map of the US. Birth Monopoly. Retrieved from: https://birthmonopoly.com/vbac-bans/ [accessed 19 April 2019].

Borges, M. T. R. (2018). A violent birth: Reframing coerced procedures during childbirth as obstetric violence. *Duke Law Journal, 67*, 36.

Brown, L. A. (2009). Birth visionaries: An examination of unassisted childbirth (MA thesis). Boston College, Boston, MA.

Buckley, S. J. (2009). *Gentle birth, gentle mothering: A doctor's guide to natural childbirth and gentle early parenting choices*. Berkeley, CA: Celestial Arts.

Cameron, H. J. (2014). Expert on her own body: Contested framings of risk and expertise in discourses on unassisted childbirth (MA thesis). Lakehead University, Ontario. Retrieved from: http://knowledgecommons.lakeheadu.ca/handle/2453/526 [accessed 8 January 2020].

Carter, P. C. (1957). *Come gently, sweet Lucina.* Titusville, FL: Self-published.

CDC. (2018). Pregnancy mortality surveillance system. Centers for Disease Control and Prevention. 7 August. Retrieved from: www.cdc.gov/reproductivehealth/maternalinfanthealth/pregnancy-mortality-surveillance-system.htm [accessed 28 April 2019].

Chen, B., Vansteenkiste, M., Beyers, W., Boone, L., Deci, E. L., Van der Kaap-Deeder, J., … Verstuyf, J. (2015). Basic psychological need satisfaction, need frustration, and need strength across four cultures. *Motivation and Emotion*, *39*(2), 216–236.

Cheyney, M., Olsen, C., Bovbjerg, M., Everson, C., Darragh, I., & Potter, B. (2015). Practitioner and practice characteristics of Certified Professional Midwives in the United States: Results of the 2011 North American Registry of Midwives Survey. *Journal of Midwifery & Women's Health*, *60*(5), 534–545.

Childbirth Connection. (2012). *Vaginal or cesarean birth: What is at stake for women and babies? A best evidence review*. New York, NY: Childbirth Connection. Retrieved from www.nationalpartnership.org/our-work/resources/health-care/maternity/vaginal-or-cesarean-birth-what-is-at-stake.pdf [accessed 11 December 2019].

Cohen Shabot, S., & Korem, K. (2018). Domesticating bodies: The role of shame in obstetric violence. *Hypatia*, *33*(3), 384–401.

Cox, K. J., Bovbjerg, M. L., Cheyney, M., & Leeman, L. M. (2015). Planned home VBAC in the United States, 2004–2009: Outcomes, maternity care practices, and implications for shared decision making. *Birth (Berkeley, California)*, *42*(4), 299–308.

Craven, C. (2010). *Pushing for midwives: Homebirth mothers and the reproductive rights movement*. Philadelphia, PA: Temple University Press.

Curtin, S. C., Gregory, K. D., Korst, L. M., & Uddin, S. F. G. (2015). Maternal morbidity for vaginal and cesarean deliveries, according to previous cesarean history: New data from the birth certificate, 2013. *National Vital Statistics Reports*, *64*(4), 1–13.

Dahlen, H. G., Jackson, M., & Stevens, J. (2011). Homebirth, freebirth and doulas: Casualty and consequences of a broken maternity system. *Women and Birth*, *24*(1), 47–50.

Dannaway, J., & Dietz, H. P. (2014). Unassisted childbirth: Why mothers are leaving the system. *Journal of Medical Ethics*, *40*(12), 817–820.

Davis-Floyd, R. (1992). *Birth as an American rite of passage.* Berkeley, CA: University of California Press.

Davis-Floyd, R. (2004). *Birth as an American rite of passage*, 2nd edn. Berkeley, CA: University of California Press.

Daviss, B. (2002). Reforming birth and (re)making midwifery in North America. In R. de Vries, C. Benoit, E. van Teijingen, & S. Wrede (Eds.), *Birth by design: Pregnancy, maternity care and midwifery in North America and Europe*. New York, NY: Routledge.

Declercq, E. R., Sakala, C., Corry, M. P., & Applebaum, S. (2007). Listening to Mothers II: Report of the second national U.S. survey of women's childbearing experiences. *The Journal of Perinatal Education*, *16*(4), 9–14.

Dekker, R. (2018). The evidence on: Breech version. *Evidence-Based Birth*. 2 February. Retrieved from: https://evidencebasedbirth.com/what-is-the-evidence-for-using-an-external-cephalic-version-to-turn-a-breech-baby/ [accessed 19 April 2019].

Deneux-Tharaux, C., Carmona, E., Bouvier-Colle, M., & Bréart, G. (2006). Postpartum maternal mortality and cesarean delivery. *Obstetrics & Gynecology*, *108*(3), 8.

Diaz-Tello, F. (2016). Invisible wounds: Obstetric violence in the United States. *Reproductive Health Matters*, *24*(47), 56–64.

Dick-Read, G. (1933). *Natural childbirth*. London: W. Heinemann, Ltd.

Dick-Read, G. (1943). *Childbirth without fear: The principles and practice of natural childbirth*. London: W. Heinemann Medical Books.

Dodd, J. M., Crowther, C. A., Huertas, E., Guise, J., & Horey, D. (2013). Planned elective repeat caesarean section versus planned vaginal birth for women with a previous caesarean birth. *Cochrane Database of Systematic Reviews*, *2013*(12), CD004224.

Dusenbery, M. (2018). *Doing harm: The truth about how bad medicine and lazy science leave women dismissed, misdiagnosed, and sick*. New York, NY: HarperOne.

Elmir, R., Schmied, V., Wilkes, L., & Jackson, D. (2010). Women's perceptions and experiences of a traumatic birth: A meta-ethnography. *Journal of Advanced Nursing*, *66*(10), 2142–2153.

Exposing the Silence Project. (2019). American childbirth: Exposing the silence. Retrieved from: www.exposingthesilenceproject.com/ [accessed 19 April 2019].

Feeley, C. L. (2016a). Giving birth and 'going it alone': Choosing to freebirth in the UK. BMC Series Blog. 12 April. Retrieved from: https://blogs.biomedcentral.com/bmcseriesblog/2016/04/12/giving-birth-going-alone-choosing-freebirth-uk/ [accessed 19 April 2019].

Feeley, C. L. (2016b). Rise in 'freebirthing' suggests women feel midwives and doctors are ignoring their needs. *The Conversation*. 22 September. Retrieved from: http://theconversation.com/rise-in-freebirthing-suggests-women-feel-midwives-and-doctors-are-ignoring-their-needs-65813 [accessed 19 April 2019].

Feeley, C. L., & Thomson, G. (2016a). Why do some women choose to freebirth in the UK? An interpretative phenomenological study. *BMC Pregnancy and Childbirth*, 16.

Feeley, C. L., & Thomson, G. (2016b). Tensions and conflicts in 'choice': Women's experiences of freebirthing in the UK. *Midwifery*, *41*, 16–21.

Feeley, C. L., Burns, E., Adams, E., & Thomson, G. (2015). Why do some women choose to freebirth? A meta-thematic synthesis, part one. *Evidence Based Midwifery*, *13*(1), 4–9.

Freeze, R. A. S. (2008). Born free: Unassisted childbirth in North America (PhD thesis). University of Iowa. Retrieved from: https://ir.uiowa.edu/etd/202/.

Gaskin, I. M. (1977). *Spiritual midwifery*. Summertown, TN: Book Pub. Co.

Green, M. (2019). About us: Maryn Green. Indie Birth. Retrieved from: https://indiebirth.org/about/ [accessed 19 April 2019].

Grekin, R. & O'Hara, M. W. (2014). Prevalence and risk factors of postpartum post-traumatic stress disorder: A meta-analysis. *Clinical Psychology Review*, 34(5), 389–401.

Griesemer, L. M. (1998). *Unassisted homebirth: An act of love*. Charleston, SC: Terra.

Guise, J. M., Denman, M. A., Emeis, C., Marshall, N., Walker, M., Fu, R., … McDonagh, M. (2010). Vaginal birth after cesarean: New insights on maternal and neonatal outcomes. *Obstetrics and Gynecology*, *115*(6), 1267–1278.

Hallgrimsdottir, H., Shumka, L., Althaus, C., & Benoit, C. (2017). Fear, risk, and the responsible choice: Risk narratives and lowering the rate of caesarean sections in high-income countries. *AIMS Public Health*, *4*(6), 615–632.

Hamilton, B. E., Martin, J. A., Osterman, M. J., Curtin, S. C., & Matthews, T. J. (2015). Births: Final data for 2014. *National Vital Statistics Reports*, *64*(12), 1–64.

Harper, M. A., Byington, R. P., Espeland, M. A., Naughton, M., Meyer, R., & Lane, K. (2003). Pregnancy-related death and health care services. *Obstetrics & Gynecology*, *102*(2), 273–278.

Harper, M. A., Espeland, M. A., Dugan, E., Meyer, R., Lane, K., & Williams, S. (2004). Racial disparity in pregnancy-related mortality following a live birth outcome. *Annals of Epidemiology*, *14*(4), 274–279.

Hays, R. (2015). Birthing freedom: Black American midwifery and liberation struggles. In J. C. Oparah & A. D. Bonaparte (Eds.), *Birthing justice: Black women, pregnancy, and childbirth* (pp. 166–175). Boulder, CO: Paradigm Publishers.

Hays, S. (1998). *The cultural contradictions of motherhood*, revised edn. New Haven, CT: Yale University Press.

Hickman, A. (2010). Born (not so) free: Legal limits on the practice of unassisted childbirth or freebirthing in the United States. *Minnesota Law Review*, *94*(5), 1651–1681.

Hollander, M., de Miranda, E., van Dillen, J., de Graaf, I., Vandenbussche, F., & Holten, L. (2017). Women's motivations for choosing a high risk birth setting against medical advice in the Netherlands: A qualitative analysis. *BMC Pregnancy and Childbirth*, *17*(423), 1–13.

Hollander, M., Holten, L., Leusink, A., van Dillen, J., & de Miranda, E. (2018). Less or more? Maternal requests that go against medical advice. *Women and Birth*, *31*(6), 505–512.

Holten, L., & de Miranda, E. (2016). Women's motivations for having unassisted childbirth or high-risk homebirth: An exploration of the literature on 'birthing outside the system'. *Midwifery*, *38*, 55–62.

Jackson, M., Dahlen, H., & Schmied, V. (2012). Birthing outside the system: Perceptions of risk amongst Australian women who have freebirths and high risk homebirths. *Midwifery*, *28*(5), 561–567.

Kendall-Tackett, K. (2014). Birth trauma: The causes and consequences of childbirth-related trauma and PTSD. In D. L. Barnes (Ed.), *Women's reproductive mental health across the lifespan* (pp. 177–191). New York, NY: Springer International Publishing.

Klassen, P. E. (2001). *Blessed events: Religion and home birth in America*. Princeton, NJ: Princeton University Press.

Kline, W. (2019). *Coming home: How midwives changed birth*. Oxford: Oxford University Press.

Lappen, J. R., Hackney, D. N., & Bailit, J. L. (2016). Maternal and neonatal outcomes of attempted vaginal compared with planned cesarean delivery in triplet gestations. *American Journal of Obstetrics and Gynecology*, *215*(4), 1–6.

Lieberman, E., Ernst, E. K., Rooks, J. P., Stapleton, S., & Flamm, B. (2004). Results of the national study of vaginal birth after cesarean in birth centres. *Obstetrics and Gynecology*, *104*(5), 933–942.

Lindgren, H. E., Nässén, K., & Lundgren, I. (2017). Taking the matter into one's own hands – Women's experiences of unassisted homebirths in Sweden. *Sexual & Reproductive Healthcare*, *11*, 31–35.

Liu, S., Liston, R. M., Joseph, K. S., Heaman, M., Sauve, R., Kramer, M. S. & Maternal Health Study Group of the Canadian Perinatal Surveillance System. (2007). Maternal mortality and severe morbidity associated with low-risk planned cesarean delivery versus planned vaginal delivery at term. *Canadian Medical Association Journal*, *176*(4), 455–460.

Lundgren, I. (2010). Women's experiences of giving birth and making decisions whether to give birth at home when professional care at home is not an option in public health care. *Sexual & Reproductive Healthcare*, *1*(2), 61–66.

MacDorman, M. F., Mathews, T. J., & Declercq, E. (2014). Trends in out-of-hospital births in the United States, 1990–2012. NCHS data brief No. 144. US Department of Health and Human Services. Retrieved from: www.cdc.gov/nchs/data/databriefs/db144.pdf [accessed 11 December 2019].

MacDorman, M. F., Declercq, E., Cabral, H., & Morton, C. (2016). Is the United States maternal mortality rate increasing? Disentangling trends from measurement issues. *Obstetrics and Gynecology*, *128*(3), 447–455.

Martin, N., & Montagne, R. (2017). U.S. has the worst rate of maternal deaths in the developed world. NPR. 12 May. Retrieved from: www.npr.org/2017/05/12/528098789/u-s-has-the-worst-rate-of-maternal-deaths-in-the-developed-world [accessed 19 April 2019].

Maternal Infant Strategy Group. (2019). Mother infant health and equity improvement plan. Retrieved from: www.michigan.gov/documents/mdhhs/MIHEIP_Final_Draft_Approved_2_25_19_647304_7.pdf [accessed 1 May 2019].

Maternal Safety Foundation. (2019). Caesarean rates. Retrieved from: www.cesareanrates.org/ [accessed 16 April 2019].

Mathews, J. J., & Zadak, K. (1991). The alternative birth movement in the United States: History and current status. *Women & Health*, *17*(1), 39–56.

Metz, T., Berghella, V., & Barss, V. (2019). Choosing the route of delivery after cesarean birth. Up To Date. 4 April. Retrieved from: www.uptodate.com/contents/choosing-the-route-of-delivery-after-cesarean-birth [accessed 20 April 2019].

Michaels, P. A. (2018). Childbirth and trauma, 1940s–1980s. *Journal of the History of Medicine and Allied Sciences*, *73*(1), 52–72.

Miller, A. C. (2009). 'Midwife to myself': Birth narratives among women choosing unassisted homebirth. *Sociological Inquiry*, *79*(1), 51–74.

Miller, A. C., & Shriver, T. E. (2012). Women's childbirth preferences and practices in the United States. *Social Science & Medicine*, *75*(4), 709–716.

Moran, M. A. (1981). *Birth and the dialogue of love*. Leawood, KS: New Nativity Press.

Moran, M. A. (Ed.) (1986). *Happy birth days: Personal accounts of birth at home the intimate, husband/wife way*. Leawood, KS: New Nativity Press.

Moran, M. A. (1997). *Pleasurable husband/wife childbirth: The real consummation of married love*, Leawood, KS: New Nativity Press.

Morgan, K. P. (1998). Contested bodies, contested knowledges: women, health, and the politics of medicalization. In S. Sherwin (Ed.), *The politics of women's health: Exploring agency and autonomy* (pp. 83–121). Philadelphia, PA: Temple University Press.

Morgan, L. A. (2002). *The power of pleasurable childbirth*. Michigan: AuthorHouse.

Novoa, C., & Taylor, J. (2018). Exploring African Americans' high maternal and infant death rates. Center For American Progress (pp. 1–13). Retrieved from: https://cdn.americanprogress.org/content/uploads/2018/01/29114454/012918_MaternalInfantMortalityRacialDisparities-brief.pdf [accessed 26 April 2019].

OBoyle, C. (2016). Deliberately unassisted birth in Ireland: Understanding choice in Irish maternity services. *British Journal of Midwifery*, *24*(3), 181–187.

Oregon Health Authority. (2019). Division 15: Definitions & licensing (proposed rule). 9 January. Retrieved from: www.oregon.gov/oha/PH/HLO/Proposed%20Rules/DEM-Proposed-Rules-09–01–19.pdf [accessed 1 May 2019].

Owens, D. C. (2017. *Medical bondage: Race, gender, and the origins of American gynecology*. Athens, GA: University of Georgia Press.

Paltrow, L. M., & Flavin, J. (2013). Arrests of and forced interventions on pregnant women in the United States, 1973–2005: Implications for women's legal status and public health. *Journal of Health Politics, Policy and Law*, *38*(2), 299–243.

Paul, P. (2009). The trouble with repeat cesareans. *Time*, *173*(8), 36–37.

Pérez, D. R. (2010). Obstetric violence: A new legal term introduced in Venezuela. *International Journal of Gynaecology and Obstetrics*, *111*(3), 201–202.

Plested, M. (2014). Freebirth in pursuit of normal birth: A quest for a salutogenic framework? *Essentially MIDIRS*, *5*(10), 16–19.

Plested, M., & Kirkham, M. (2016). Risk and fear in the lived experience of birth without a midwife. *Midwifery*, *38*, 29–34.

Reed, A. (2008). Not a happy birthday [The F-Word]. 7 March. Retrieved from: https://thefword.org.uk/2008/03/not_a_happy_bir/ [accessed 19 April 2019].

Reed, R., Sharman, R., & Inglis, C. (2017). Women's descriptions of childbirth trauma relating to care provider actions and interactions. *BMC Pregnancy and Childbirth*, *17*(21), 1–10.

Reid, M. (1989). Sisterhood and professionalization: A case study of the American lay midwife. In C. S. McClain (Ed.), *Women as healers: Cross-cultural perspectives* (pp. 219–238). New Brunswick, NJ: Rutgers University Press.

Rich, A. C. (1976). *Of woman born: Motherhood as experience and institution*. New York, NY: Norton.

Rigg, E. C., Schmied, V., Peters, K., & Dahlen, H. G. (2018). A survey of women in Australia who choose the care of unregulated birthworkers for a birth at home. *Women and Birth* (in press, corrected proof).

Robbins, J. (1998). *Reclaiming our health: Exploding the medical myth and embracing the sources of true healing*. Tiburon, CA: H.J. Kramer, Inc.

Rowe, R., Li, Y., Knight, M., Brocklehurst, P., & Hollowell, J. (2016). Maternal and perinatal outcomes in women planning vaginal birth after caesarean (VBAC) at home in England: Secondary analysis of the Birthplace national prospective cohort study. *British Journal of Obstetrics and Gynaecology*, *123*(7), 1123–1132.

Ryan, R. M., & Deci, E. L. (2000). Self-determination theory and the facilitation of intrinsic motivation, social development, and well-being. *The American Psychologist*, *55*(1), 68–78.

Ryan, R. M., Huta, V., & Deci, E. L. (2008). Living well: A self-determination theory perspective on eudaimonia. *Journal of Happiness Studies*, *9*(1), 139–170.

Schwartz, J. A. (2014). Childbirth as a profound experience: Exploring narrative and image of experiences during birth. PhD thesis, California Institute of Integral Studies.

Shanley, L. K. (1994). *Unassisted childbirth*. Westport, CT: Bergin & Garvey.

Shanley, L. K. (2005). 'Freebirth' or 'unassisted'? Mothering.com Forums. 29 April. Retrieved from: www.mothering.com/discussions/showthread.php?t=279140 [accessed 11 December 2019].

Shanley, L. K. (2018). Unassisted childbirth in the 1950s [Unassisted Childbirth]. Retrieved from: www.unassistedchildbirth.com/what-is-uc/unassisted-childbirth-in-the-1950s/ [accessed 19 April 2019].
Silver, R. M., Landon, M. B., Rouse, D. J., Leveno, K. J., Spong, C. Y., Thom, E. A., … Mercer, B. M. (2006). Maternal morbidity associated with multiple repeat caesarean deliveries. *Obstetrics and Gynecology*, *107*(6), 1226–1232.
Simkin, P. (1991). Just another day in a woman's life? Women's long-term perceptions of their first birth experience. Part I. *Birth (Berkeley, California)*, *18*(4), 203–210.
Simkin, P. (1992). Just another day in a woman's life? Part II: Nature and consistency of women's long-term memories of their first birth experiences. *Birth (Berkeley, California)*, *19*(2), 64–81.
Simpson, M., & Catling, C. (2016). Understanding psychological traumatic birth experiences: A literature review. *Women and Birth*, *29*(3), 203–207.
Sousa, M. (1976). *Childbirth at home*. Englewood Cliffs, NJ: Prentice-Hall.
Stewart, D. (1981). *The five standards for safe childbearing: Good nutrition, skillful midwifery, natural childbirth, home birth, breastfeeding*. Marble Hill, MO: NAPSAC International.
Tangel, V., White, R. S., Nachamie, A. S., & Pick, J. S. (2019). Racial and ethnic disparities in maternal outcomes and the disadvantage of peripartum black women: a multistate analysis, 2007–2014. *American Journal of Perinatology*, *36*(8), 835–848.
Tanner, L. (2019). Birthing against the grain: Women's autonomy in birth (PhD thesis in progress). University of California Santa Barbara.
The Big Push for Midwives. (2019). CPMs legal status by state [The Big Push for Midwives]. Retrieved from: http://pushformidwives.nationbuilder.com/cpms_legal_status_ by_state [accessed 19 April 2019].
Torio, P. C. E. (2010). Nature versus suture: Why VBAC should still be in vogue. *Women's Rights Law Reporter*, *31*, 487.
Vedam, S., Stoll, K., MacDorman, M., Declercq, E., Cramer, R., Cheyney, M., … Li, D. (2018). Mapping integration of midwives across the United States: Impact on access, equity, and outcomes. *PLoS ONE*, *13*(2).
Walker, S. (2013). Undiagnosed breech: Towards a woman-centred approach. *British Journal of Midwifery*, *21*(5), 316–322.
Weitz, R., & Sullivan, D. (1985). Licensed lay midwifery and the medical model of childbirth. *Sociology of Health & Illness*, *7*(1), 36–54.
Wendland, C. L. (2007). The vanishing mother: cesarean section and 'evidence-based obstetrics'. *Medical Anthropology Quarterly*, *21*(2), 218–233.
World Bank. (2019). World Bank open data. Retrieved from: https://data.worldbank.org/ [accessed 19 April 2019].

2 Giving birth outside the system in Australia

Freebirth and high-risk homebirth

Melanie Jackson

> I thought home was safer, but for me the real deciding factor was my total and utter fear of going to the hospital again and any of that [abuse] happening to me.
>
> (Woman who had a freebirth)

About the author

In 2008 at the age of 24 and nearing the completion of my training as a student midwife, the clinical educator in the hospital at which I was training said, 'You must get out of here, we will destroy you'. No truer words have been said. They solidified my resolve to stubbornly pursue a career as a private midwife and provide private homebirth services. I have been a private midwife for 10 years, given birth to my two children at home, started a private midwifery group practice and completed my PhD. As my midwifery training drew to a close, I purposefully pursued an experienced private midwife (Robyn Dempsey) to mentor me. For almost a year, and while earning no money at all, I followed her like an awestruck puppy hoping to soak up the magic she sprinkled about with every encounter she had with her clients. She was wise, kind and gentle, and women spoke well of her.

Simultaneously, my aspirations for midwifery sent me down the path of postgraduate study. I met Hannah Dahlen and Virginia Schmied in 2008, and they became my PhD supervisors. After a brief meeting with Hannah, she seemed to almost instantly believe in my ability to complete such a task. So here I was, blessed by the presence of amazing mentors willing to escort me onto my next midwifery adventures. My career path was set, I commenced work as a private midwife while also completing my PhD research in 2014, entitled 'Birthing outside the system: wanting the best and safest'.

Towards the end of my PhD, I gave birth to my first child. I started my pregnancy as a healthy young woman but by the end, I identified as one of the women in my own research. I had repeated bleeds early in pregnancy, was measuring 'small' for gestational age, had declined most of the usual tests and ultimately ended up giving birth to my 36-week-old baby at home, after a lengthy 32-hour labour. He was 2300 g at birth and my midwives advised me that these babies are usually cared for at hospital. I had an intuitive feeling that he was a healthy baby, and I felt confident to care for him at home. I felt strongly that he would thrive under the care I had planned, so I declined their suggestion to move into hospital. I realised, after the fact, that I had used the same rationale as the women in my study as to why I believed home was the best and safest. I confidently went forth and gave him kangaroo care, frequent feeds and kept him skin to skin until he was full-term. I believed that this strategy would be far better for me and my baby, when compared to the experience that would unfold in hospital. This experience gave me a new understanding of the women in my study and, although I wouldn't choose freebirth for myself, I could now intellectualise my way through the decisions that led me to have a high-risk homebirth. To this day, I believe that what I chose was the best and safest for myself and my baby.

Introduction

When I started my PhD (Jackson, 2014), there was very little literature about birth outside the system and only a couple of studies on freebirth (Freeze, 2008; Turton, 2007; Brown, 2009; Miller, 2009). One study that focused on autonomy when choosing high-risk homebirth was exceptional. It changed my thinking about women's autonomy during birth (Symon, Winter, Donnan, & Kirkham, 2010). The 2010 study by Symon et al. included a review of 15 case notes from women's homebirth care where there were significant risk factors that resulted in neonatal deaths or stillbirth. These births were attended by independent midwives in the UK. What was striking about the findings of this study was that midwives reported that the women involved took great responsibility and expressed a willingness to accept a positive or negative outcome provided that they made the decisions. Despite the advice of their midwives, many of the women declined various screening and testing options, and some refused transfer to hospital even when faced with the possibility of a bad outcome. The authors concluded that, 'the women in this review had reportedly accepted the potential consequences of their high-risk situations' and that 'if reality is to match rhetoric about patient autonomy, such decision-making in high-risk situations must be accepted' (Symon et al., 2010). But why would a woman make a decision that could possibly put herself and her baby in danger? This question had not yet been answered by academic literature in Australia. My PhD research aimed to fill this gap.

From home to hospital in Australia

After World War I in Australia, when poverty was common, it was observed that women lacked the basic necessities required to give birth and care for a baby at home, so they were brought to hospital as a way of assisting them with food, clothing and maternity care. The genesis of giving birth in hospital in Australia was not instigated by the desire to make birth safer, but simply as a response to the extreme poverty observed for some birthing women (Barclay,

2008). During this time, wealthy women continued to hire a private midwife and a doctor, and remained at home. In Australia, affluent women continued to have their babies at home with midwives up till approximately 1940, and it wasn't until the 1970s that almost all births in Australia occurred in hospital (Barclay, 2008). This, of course, is limited to the birth history of Australia from the time of colonisation in 1788. One can only imagine the beautiful and rich history of childbirth among Aboriginal and Torres Strait Islander women prior to the colonial invasion.

Currently, the majority of births (97%) in Australia occur in hospitals, while smaller numbers of women give birth in birth centres (1.8%) or at home (0.3%). Around 0.4% of women give birth elsewhere (AIHW, 2017) and these are typically the babies who are born before arrival (BBA) at hospital (Thornton & Dahlen, 2018). There is no formal data collection process currently in Australia to record planned freebirths (Newman, 2008). There appears, however, to be a rise in births outside the system in Australia as the cracks in our medicalised hospital system become more evident.

The Australian maternity care system

Women who plan to give birth in a public hospital are, for the most part, only able to access fragmented maternity care, in which they see a different midwife or doctor at each interaction. There are midwifery group practice (MGP) options slowly developing at some hospitals and each year a small percentage of women (around 8%) (Dawson, McLachlan, Newton, & Forster, 2016) in Australia have access to continuity of midwifery care through MGP models. For the most part, however, women do not have access to their own midwife or a known care provider when accessing maternity care through the public health care system. Although publicly funded homebirth is available in some states and territories in Australia, there are currently just 16 such services across the country (Catling-Paull, Foureur, & Homer, 2012). This circumstance is quite unfortunate as it goes against current evidence on how maternity care should be delivered. That evidence clearly supports improved outcomes for women and babies under continuity of midwifery care. Continuity models are also less costly to operate and lead to greater satisfaction for women, when compared with standard fragmented hospital care (Tracy et al., 2013; Sandall, Soltani, Gates, Shennan, & Devane, 2016). Likewise, homebirth for low-risk women attended by competent midwives who are well networked into the system appears safe for babies and safer for women (Scarf et al., 2018), although this is not the case where significant risk factors exist.

The private Australian healthcare system offers women the option of hiring a private midwife and giving birth at home or in a public hospital, or they can hire a private obstetrician who cares for them throughout their pregnancy and attends their birth in a private hospital (some also birth in public hospitals).

In Australia today, women have very little choice but to birth in hospital, where the process is often managed as a medical event and interventions can be routine. A study undertaken with a group of low-risk group of women found only 15% of first-time mothers in private hospitals and 34% in public hospitals in New South Wales had a normal vaginal birth without intervention (Dahlen et al., 2012). Women with risk factors have little choice but to accept obstetric care as most are unable to access midwifery-led models of care in the majority of hospitals. Overall, there are very few options for women who wish to have a physiological birth and avoid unnecessarily intervention.

Homebirth and private practice midwifery are not well supported in Australia. The politics are complex and becoming more so as the legislative and regulatory parameters that dictate private midwifery practice become more restrictive (Wilkes, Teakle, & Gamble, 2009). Growing regulation around private practice midwifery and homebirth could deter midwives from practising or even registering (Coroner, South Australia, 2012). This is discussed further in Chapters 5 and 11.

Of the women choosing to give birth at home in Australia, some who would be considered 'high-risk' by maternity care providers still choose homebirth, while some reject mainstream maternity care altogether and choose freebirth. It is these two groups of women that will be the focus of this chapter.

Perceptions of hospital-based maternity care options – the hospital cannot provide the best or safest

The women interviewed for my PhD made it clear that they chose to give birth outside the system because they believe it is the best and safest option and they feel hospitals cannot provide them with the best or safest care (Jackson, 2014). Women identified eight specific aspects of giving birth in hospital which subsequently caused them to avoid it. These were: (1) there are not enough resources to cope with demand; (2) the hospital is not like home; (3) it's like a cattle yard; (4) care providers are bound by hospital policies; (5) the hospital intervenes in birth; (6) the hospital fears birth; (7) there is tension when a woman expresses her autonomy; and (8) hospital management of birth is emotionally unsafe (Jackson, 2014). Although the women in this study shunned medical management of birth, they appeared accepting of it when it was obvious to them that it was really needed. In the following sections, 'HB' is used to identify comments from women who birthed at home with risk factors and 'FB' is used to identify women who freebirthed.

Not enough resources to cope with demand

One aspect that contributed to women feeling that hospitals could not cater to their needs is the belief that hospital services have insufficient resources to cope with demand. One woman commented,

> Maybe it's a case of underfunding, short staff, not enough beds ... I don't think that they are an evil corporation trying to deny your life experience, I just think that maybe the system, I feel like the system is really not set up to support the woman.
>
> (HB04)

Another woman made a similar comment,

> It's the volume of women that go through the hospital system, it would be very time-consuming to treat everybody completely individually and holistically with continuity.
>
> (HB05)

By understanding this gap between demand and supply, the women developed a perception that hospitals were incapable of catering to their desire for the best and safest birth. Through their own hospital experiences, the women developed an understanding that hospitals have insufficient resources to cope with demand and they felt that because of the shortfalls, they would suffer. By giving birth outside the system, women thought they could access the resources they desired in order to have a birth that they believed was better than a hospital and the safest option for themselves and their baby.

It's not like home

The birth environment can positively or negatively impact on the course of labour and the outcome of birth (Foureur et al., 2010; Stark, Remynse, & Zwelling, 2016; Howard, 2017). In a relaxing environment, the hormones of labour flow and help to facilitate a physiological labour and birth. Alternatively, where the birth environment is stressful, the ideal hormonal cascade of labour and birth is interrupted and can cause a stalling of labour (Alehagen & Wijma, 2005; Buckley, 2009, 2015). Women chose to give birth out of the hospital to prevent exposure to the negative aspects introduced by the hospital environment (Boucher, Bennett, McFarlin, & Freeze, 2009; Jackson, 2014).

> I remember at the time ... trying to be in my own zone but ... the bright lights and the looking at the clock and then there is the rolling of the eyes and people coming in and out ... so the first thing is, in your average hospital situation its very clinical, it's the least like home you can possibly imagine, there's bright lights there's lots of busy people running around there's machines that go beep ... there is a tension in the environment which is completely opposite to home.
>
> (HB06)

Women who choose to give birth at home feel that a home environment provided the essential elements required to ensure the best possible birth experience and outcome. In contrast, they felt that the hospital could not adequately cater to their needs in labour, birth and postnatally, because the environment was seen as the antithesis of the home context.

> I just didn't feel like I had freedom to move around and I remember just being in labour and not knowing where I wanted to be, if I wanted to be on the toilet or on the bed, it felt like I didn't have an option that felt most comfortable for me and that was a bit frustrating.
>
> (FB07)

A home environment, where a woman is cared for by a known care provider, or none at all, and where she has the power to manage the environment is considered by some women to be a safe and comfortable birth option which likely lends itself to fewer complications in labour and birth. They perceive the hospital as offering the opposite (Jackson, 2014).

It's like a cattle yard

The women who chose to give birth outside the system felt mainstream care was driven by the desire to move women in and out of their institutions in a timely manner (Jackson, 2014). The metaphor most frequently invoked was that of a 'cattle yard', where the hospital's aim is to 'keep them moving through like a cattle yard, keep them moving through like a number' (FB05). One woman reflected on her experience of a hospital birth, noting that if she had her own care provider, her experience would have been enriched:

> … at least I could have skin-to-skin, at least I would have someone there who knew me, knew the baby, would put my best interests first and I wouldn't be just another number in the cattle run.
>
> (HB09)

This metaphor of the cattle yard is also reflected in descriptions offered by a participant in my study who worked as a midwife in a hospital. She contends that in order to maintain productivity, the treatment of women in hospital has become depersonalised,

> There is nothing individual about it, and so staff are, I think, losing the ability to make their own individual choices, they're just going through the process of what they do every day, they just continue to do every day because that's what we've always done and that's what works, that's what gets 300 women in and out every month.
>
> (HB05)

When one woman was asked what could have been done for her at hospital that might have enhanced her experience, she said,

> I'm not sure they really could have done anything better for me just because of the mentality … it's a revolving door and they've got to get this baby out the quickest way possible, whichever way suits us and then get this baby fed, don't care how just get it fed and then get you out the door. I don't know if they could have done anything better.
>
> (HB07)

Having experienced a system, in the past, that treated them as a number rather than a person and having been shuffled through the 'cattle yard', the participants believed that the hospital could not meet their expectations. This led them to pursue birth outside the system.

Care providers are bound by hospital policies

The participants understood that policies and protocols were set up in hospitals to facilitate the smooth running of the system, and, in theory, to get women and babies through as quickly and safely as possible. By affording primacy to productivity, however, the focus shifts away from what is best for the woman and her baby towards what is best for the system and the institution. As one woman explains:

> I sort of feel like when you walk in it's no longer about what you want and what's important to you, it's about what works in the system … you're put into a category and you do things that suit the whole system … it's regimented.
>
> (HB05)

Other women felt that the hospital staff were bound by policy, and thus the service that staff could offer was restricted:

> They are bound by their protocols … I think they have them because they believe that is safety and it is also to guide doctors and midwives in their practice.
>
> (FB06)

In addition to this, the women recognised that their requests fell outside of what was dictated by policy. The women were concerned that their requests would be met with resistance or hostility. Many formed this impression of hospital services as a result of their previous experiences. As one woman recalls:

> [I was met with] quite a strong message there [in hospital], that was, 'we really don't appreciate you making this more difficult, we have a lot of

> women here to get through, just be good, just fit in' … I guess there was a level of threat around anyone that was feeling that the system wasn't going to be good enough … it was just purely a situation of you know, 'this is the way we do things and we really don't have time for you to be trying to ask for any special consideration' … it was met with quite a bit of resistance and defensiveness and I felt that straight away … she [the midwife] just basically was indicating to me that she wasn't interested in any way in looking into that option or giving me that opportunity.
>
> (FB06)

Due to hospital policy boundaries, participants perceived there to be no flexibility in the care offered and that staff were not open to doing something outside of policy within a hospital setting. When one woman was asked what kind of things the hospital was against, she replied:

> I think just generally anything that was going to interfere with standard protocol.
>
> (FB06)

Another woman, when asked why she thought the staff became rude and abrupt when she requested early discharge from hospital, suggested:

> maybe because it didn't fall in line with their policies and procedures.
>
> (FB04)

In one scenario, a woman chose to freebirth rather than birth in hospital after the hospital was unsupportive of her having a midwife-attended homebirth through their programme. She had already had a VBAC at home with their programme in the past. Due to a later policy change, however, they could no longer allow her to do this, despite her lower risk with this third pregnancy. She recounted this story:

> My second baby was a planned homebirth but it's a VBAC homebirth and that went all fine and my third baby, I wanted to have a planned homebirth and the policy changed … therefore I was placed in a high-risk category and they wouldn't allow me to plan a homebirth … it's a strange situation because previously I actually had a homebirth, and this is the ironic part, it was with the same midwife that I had my planned VBAC homebirth and they were under the department of community health and they did a restructure … and the actual midwifery group practice was reshuffled alongside of acute care instead of being under community health … then things like VBACs and those other complications couldn't be dealt with in a homebirth situation, the policies wouldn't allow for it.
>
> (FB03)

Overall, participants felt that the policies and protocols imposed on them by hospitals were restrictive to their requests and preferences. In comparison, birthing outside the system became the clear, better option.

They intervene

Women who give birth at home commonly believe that hospital birth exposes them to a greater number of interventions (Birthplace in England Collaborative Group, 2011). Interference in the birth process is considered by many women to be a hallmark of care offered within a hospital system. The participants in my research expressed an understanding that when you enter the hospital to give birth, 'you are on a timeframe' (HB02): 'Like well, you need to be this many centimetres by this time' (HB03).

Another woman described her experience:

> the clock was there and there was so much talk about hours and minutes and so many vaginal exams and you're this many centimetres and blah blah blah.
>
> (FB01)

Some women explained that they avoided entering the system through fear that they could not satisfy the hospital time limits on labour. Women feared that failure to adhere to hospital time limits would result in interventions designed to expedite the processes of labour:

> [having had 2 previous caesareans], the overall vibe I got [from the hospital] was that I would probably get about eight hours to labour in the hospital and after that they'd get a bit worried. So I just thought well, if I go in there, with the clock ticking, it's just not going to happen, I just don't think I'd be able to do that.
>
> (HB04)

Another woman described interventions as inevitable if she entered a hospital:

> I just can't imagine having a whole hospital staff caring for me and not intervening in some way.
>
> (FB08)

Due to her understanding of how the hospital would manage the birth of her twins, another woman decided to birth at home in order to avoid intervention:

> In hospital, at best if I was 'allowed' to birth vaginally I would have been pressured to have an induction at 38 weeks, with constant monitoring removing the ability to use my body to its best advantage of an active

> birth. I would also have been pressured to consent to an epidural and a forceps removal of the second twin.
>
> (HB13)

The participants believed that intervening in the birth process increased the risk of something going wrong. Because hospitals represented a higher risk of intervention, the women saw giving birth outside the system as the safer option.

They (the maternity system) fear birth

The women who chose to give birth outside the system perceived childbirth to be a normal, natural part of life. Because of this, they did not use the language of fear when describing birth. The participants believed that the hospital system fears birth and thus encapsulates it within a hospital setting where it can be managed. One woman felt that:

> they're [the hospital staff] looking at the worst-case scenario all the time and coming from fear.
>
> (FB02)

One participant was asked why she thought the hospital intervened in the birth process and she responded:

> because they fear that it's a disease process.
>
> (FB05)

The participants also felt that the level of their practitioner's fear of birth was directly proportionate to their tendency to intervene. One woman explained why she believed the hospital staff wanted to use intervention during the birth of her twins:

> because of fear from medical practitioners who have no faith in birth being normal and women's bodies having the innate ability to birth.
>
> (HB13)

The participants' conceptualisation of birth as a natural and normal process, that is best left uninterrupted, makes the women reluctant to enter a system that fears birth and dictates its management with intervention.

Tension about the woman's autonomy

Women who gave birth outside the system expressed a desire to be respected as the authority at their birth and made an assumption that the hospital would not accommodate this. One woman explained her early antenatal experience in the hospital and how it motivated her to disengage from their care:

> there was a real level of tension in my first visit around how much autonomy I would be allowed.
>
> (FB06)

The participants were reluctant to give birth in hospital because they felt there would be tension around how much choice they would be afforded, one woman explained:

> I don't think that choice is there in hospital. Women might choose to birth in hospital but once they are in the hospital I don't think they are getting choice.
>
> (FB05)

For many participants, their previous birthing experiences had taught them that hospital staff would assume control over their body, ultimately challenging and subverting their autonomy:

> Once we were in the room it was just sort of like, okay now we are in charge and this is what you've got to do ... It was just like, okay we are the experts you just do what we tell you to do ... It was sort of disempowering I guess you could call it.
>
> (HB06)

The women's impression that the system 'doesn't trust women at all' (HB04) is embedded in the perception that there is a tension around how much autonomy they are afforded in hospital.

Another woman connected the reasons the hospital gave for why they believed her body would not be able to birth vaginally with the hospitals mistrust in women:

> They kept saying, 'but you are small, your husband's big', cause my husband is like 6 foot something and I'm like 5 foot 1 and they are going, oh – and because I was diabetic, shoulder dystocia, you are going to have a big baby, you're only small, your husband's big, they were just putting it out there, they were just so negative.
>
> (HB03)

Through their experiences within the system, the participants learnt that the system does not trust women to make 'sensible' decisions, and it does not trust their bodies to work effectively. This directly challenges the woman's desire to be respected as the authority at the birth, and conflicts with her belief that her body is naturally capable of birthing. Being respected as the authority was considered by the participants to be something that would offer them a safe birth. The women felt the hospital would not support their autonomy and thus, was not a safe place to give birth.

Emotionally unsafe

Women who give birth outside the system have a broad and rich concept of safety that goes further than mere physical safety in childbirth (Jackson, 2014). In light of their expectations of safety, the care provided to the participants in the hospital system did not appear to meet their emotional needs, with women reporting high levels of dissatisfaction with the emotional experience of being in hospital:

> The hospital doesn't enter into that, they are flat out looking into the physical side let alone the mental and emotional, I don't even think they look at the emotional side.
>
> (FB05)

The women described sustaining trauma (both physical and mental) as a result of the care they received in hospital. The perceived lack of attention to women's emotional needs alienated them and motivated them to pursue something better. Throughout this research, some of the most emotionally difficult moments for me were when the women described the violations they endured at the hands of their maternity care providers. One woman explains:

> My experience with hospital-based care has been incredibly disappointing, and life-changing, but not for the better. The day my first son was born it should have been the best day of my life, instead it has left me scarred, mentally and physically. Part of my treatment in the local hospital included being assaulted by a midwife as she forcibly held me down while I was in pain so that the doctor could poke around in my vagina without my protest.
>
> (FB13)

For another woman, an emotionally traumatic hospital experience was what motivated her to subsequently choose birth outside the system, she explained,

> I decided that should I find myself unable to access a midwife, I would birth at home – alone. Nothing that can happen to me or my baby at home could be much worse than what my second baby and I experienced in hospital. I will never subject myself, my baby or my family to such an ugly, traumatic and dehumanising experience again.
>
> (FB1)

Her choice to give birth at home was motivated by her need to avoid a recurrence of the trauma incurred at her first birth – an experience that she describes as 'birth rape'. She explains:

> I thought home was safer, but for me the real deciding factor was my total and utter fear of going to the hospital again and any of that [abuse] happening to me.
>
> (FB01)

From these recollections, we can see that if a woman is exposed to a traumatising event during a hospital birthing experience, this will predispose her to avoiding the hospital system in the future and force her to consider birthing options that fall outside the system.

A place for giving birth in hospital

Although the participants saw no need to birth in hospital under their regular circumstances, they made it clear that should complications arise, they would not shun the medical system completely. One woman explained,

> [t]here is a need for doctors, [be]cause there are times when things go wrong and they are needed.
>
> (FB02)

The participants acknowledged that the time for medical intervention was when things go wrong. Another woman explained,

> obviously I agree, women do need doctors, I'm not saying that women don't need them, we do need them because there are circumstances where they are needed, you know, they do save some babies.
>
> (HB03)

The participants felt that the hospital and medical interventions should only be used if really needed, rather than as routine in the context of normal birth:

> I think the medical system is really fantastic … it's awesome that it's there if we really need it.
>
> (FB04)

For one woman, birthing at home was only appropriate if it would not compromise her or her babies' safety and she explained that the time to move into the system would be:

> if there is a problem, if there is a risk, there is something possible that is going to affect the mother or the baby and that's their only way of getting

> out a healthy baby, then yeah, that's the advantage of living in today's society.
>
> (HB04)

The resounding message from the women who choose birth outside the system was that if they perceived a problem during their birth, then the best and safest thing to do for themselves and their babies would be to transfer to hospital.

> if I feel like something is wrong, you will not be able to keep me at home … I'll be out the door.
>
> (FB08)

Another participant described how a complication arose following her birth and that remaining at home was no longer the best and safest because it became obvious that they needed more than her midwife and the home environment could provide:

> Even through all its [the hospital's] gripes, there is still some, I mean we had to go to the hospital with the baby, like there was a point where the care we had wasn't enough … so I'm grateful that the hospital was there.
>
> (HB04)

Unlike the participants in Symon et al.'s 2010 study, for the women in my study, homebirth at all cost did not appear to be a thing.

We found that the shortfalls in the Australian maternity care system were a major contributing factor to women's choice to birth outside the system. It can be said that the choice to birth outside the system is an iatrogenic consequence of a maternity care system that does not adequately cater to the needs of some women (Dahlen, Jackson, & Stevens, 2011). These women consider birth in hospitals to be dangerous to them and their babies' well-being. They believe they are taking less of a risk birthing outside the system than within it.

Making Australian maternity care options more acceptable

It is clear that some Australian women feel that hospital-based maternity care options are not fulfilling their need for safe and high-quality care. They want something better. Fortunately, there is a treasure trove of research that has already identified effective safe and satisfying ways to deliver maternity care that is highly acceptable to women, so we need not look far for solutions to the substandard maternity care system that currently prevails in Australia. Government and political approaches that seek to limit women's access to a range of care options will only push many women further out of the system.

If the aim is to encourage women to be more accepting of existing maternity services, then maternity services need to deliver a more satisfactory and acceptable service (Gofen, 2012). Humanising maternity care and expanding birth options are evidence-based strategies to ensure safe and satisfying care is provided to Australian women.

Humanise maternity care

Past experience of traumatising and disrespectful care was one of the major motivators for women choosing to birth outside the system for subsequent births. Therefore, humanising maternity care is what is needed; a move towards humane care is a move away from biomedical models of care (Rattner, Hamouche Abrea, de Olivereira Araújo, & França Santos, 2009). Components of humanised care include non-invasive practices, respect for women's autonomy, providing evidence-based care, valuing family-friendly environments, a focus on relationships between the woman and her care providers, respecting the woman's privacy and ensuring that each woman have adequate birth support (Rattner et al., 2009).

Humanising birth can be achieved in a number of ways, including by implementing midwifery continuity of care models for all women, regardless of risk, providing one-to-one midwifery care during labour and birth, practising woman-centred care and reducing the use of routine interventions.

Midwifery continuity of care models

Midwifery-led continuity of care has better outcomes for mother and baby compared to standard fragmented care in hospitals (Sandall, 2016). Under midwifery-led continuity of care, women experience fewer interventions, greater satisfaction, positive birth outcomes and a heightened sense of confidence and achievement (Fahy, Foureur, & Hastie, 2008; Homer, Brodie, & Leap, 2008; Leap, Sandall, Buckland, & Huber, 2010; Sandall et al., 2016). Continuity of midwifery care is also cost-effective (Tracy et al., 2014) and it has been successfully expanded in other countries so could be effectively implemented in Australia also.

One-to-one midwifery care during labour and birth

Continuous care by a known provider has been shown to improve rates of spontaneous vaginal birth, reduce the use of pharmacological analgesia and improve infant outcomes. It also increases the likelihood of women reporting a satisfying birth experience (Hodnett, Gates, Hofmeyr, & Sakala, 2013). The 2017 UK NICE guidelines for intrapartum care recommend that women in established labour be provided with one-to-one care and not be left on their own except for short periods with the woman's consent (NICE, 2017).

Woman-centred care

Supporting women's autonomy in their birth choices and to have the birth that they believe is best and safest may help protect the safety of women who birth outside the system. One way to promote autonomy for birthing women is for practitioners to provide woman-centred care, a practice model which prioritises treating each woman as an individual and respecting her wishes (Brass, 2012). Woman-centred care in childbirth is a process in which the woman is actively involved, makes choices and has control over her care (Maputle & Donavon, 2013). If a woman who has chosen to birth outside the system knows she will receive woman-centred care while attending her GP or local hospital, she may choose to access timely and necessary medical care when needed. Providing this type of care means that maternity care providers cater to the woman's needs and requests by respecting and facilitating her choices. This may also require providers to exercise flexibility and latitude in relation to hospital policy and procedures. Key aspects of woman-centred care include providing education to promote informed consent (Maputle & Donavon, 2013), while also allowing space for refusal as an acceptable option.

Reduction in routine interventions

A major source of dissatisfaction identified by the women was the number of interventions used in hospitals. The women were opposed to the use of unnecessary interventions and many chose to birth outside the system in order to avoid them. Davis-Floyd and colleagues (2009) argue that the overuse of intervention is a hallmark of birth models that do not work (Davis-Floyd et al., 2009). Bringing hospital-based maternity services into line with current evidence may make hospital birth more acceptable and reduce the number of interventions women and their babies experience during labour and birth (Davis-Floyd et al., 2009). Providing greater access to homebirth with a midwife and the option of midwife-led units is also an effective way of reducing unnecessary interventions (Birthplace in England Collaborative Group, 2011).

Expand birth options

Not all women who gave birth outside the system wanted this from the outset. Some said that if they had access to midwifery-led birth centres, publicly funded homebirth, a private midwife or continuity of care with a midwife, they might have chosen one of these options instead. In order for women to access the model of care and location that they believe is best for them and their baby, service providers need to offer a wide variety of options within the system so women are not forced to birth outside the system. There are a number of birthing options that are safe and evidence-based, and do not require women to birth in hospitals (Birthplace in England Collaborative Group, 2011; Hodnett, Downe, & Walsh, 2012).

Publicly funded homebirth

In Australia, the mainstream belief is that homebirth is more dangerous than hospital birth; this is not supported by research. For example, the 2017 NICE guidelines provide that it is safe for low-risk multiparous women to give birth in a midwifery-led unit (freestanding or alongside) or choose homebirth, because these options offer fewer interventions and very little difference in perinatal mortality and morbidity (NICE, 2017; Scarf et al., 2018).

Birth in standalone or alongside midwifery units

Most birth centres in Australia are annexed to or inside a hospital, with very few standalone birthing units run by midwives. Walsh (2009) suggests that the small-scale approach to birth provided by birth centres and smaller midwifery units provides women with a reprieve from the production-line mentality of larger birthing units. Furthermore, such units allow midwives to provide care that facilitates the involvement of family (Walsh, 2009). Similarly, the NICE guidelines recommend that women plan to give birth in midwifery-led units (standalone or alongside a hospital) because they will experience fewer interventions, and because outcomes are no different than if they birth in obstetric units (NICE, 2017). Hodnett et al. (2012) also concluded that birth centres are associated with lower rates of intervention and higher levels of satisfaction, with no increased risk to either mothers or babies (Hodnett et al., 2012), making them an attractive alternative to obstetric hospital care.

Midwifery care for high-risk women

A major problem in Australia is that women with risk factors have little choice but to birth in a high-acuity setting under obstetric care, or else birth at home with the assistance of a midwife who risks being reported to the regulatory body in the event of a transfer or if an adverse event occurs (Hunter, 2018) (see also Chapter 14). Providing other options – such as continuity of midwifery care – for women with risk factors will broaden the possibilities and lessen the sense that women are faced with an either/or quandary.

An Australian study published in 2013 reinforced the benefits of a midwifery continuity of care model for women of all-risk levels (Tracy et al., 2013). The authors concluded that for women of any risk, caseload midwifery is safe and cost-effective. The authors encourage other maternity care providers to consider adopting this collaborative model, as it would allow higher-risk women to have access to midwife-led care (Beasley, Ford, Tracy, & Welsh, 2012).

Enhanced support for private practice midwifery and private homebirth

The majority of women who chose to freebirth explained that they felt backed into a corner and forced into this situation by the fact that there were no other acceptable options. One way to cater to these women would be to ensure that women have greater access to privately practising midwives (Newman, 2008). Australia needs to make practising as a private midwife less daunting, encouraging more midwives to pursue this professional path. Currently, there is a great deal of cultural and medical hostility towards, and political unrest around, private midwifery practice. As a result, midwives are giving up practising private midwifery and homebirth. Therefore, women who want a midwife at their birth are experiencing difficulty locating an appropriate care provider. Furthermore, vexatious reporting of private midwives to legislative authorities is making midwives afraid when referring complex cases, potentially rendering the practice of private midwifery less safe for women. Policymakers, regulators and government should be making private practice a more welcoming option for midwives by creating a supportive environment, facilitating access to hospitals, providing adequate professional indemnity insurance and offering adequate Medicare funding. This is dealt further with in later chapters.

Conclusion

Women who choose birth outside the system are doing so as a response to a hospital system that is not able to meet their needs on many levels. If the aim is to encourage women to accept maternity care services within the system, then the system must offer care options that work for women, as opposed to what works for the logistical running of the system. Adopting an evidence-based approach to service provision and prioritising midwifery models of care in a variety of settings will go a long way to providing women with what they want and need from their maternity care providers.

The way forward

- We need to humanise maternity care by routinely providing:
  - Midwifery continuity of care for all women
  - One-to-one midwifery care during labour and birth
  - Clinically indicated interventions, rather than routine
- Expand birth options by providing:
  - Publicly funded homebirth
  - Birth units that stand alone or alongside hospitals (not in)
  - Enhanced support for private practice midwifery and private homebirth options

References

Alehagen, S. I. W., Wijma, B., Lundberg, U. L. F., & Wijma, K. (2005) Fear, pain and stress hormones during childbirth. *Journal of Psychosomatic Obstetrics & Gynecology*, *26*, 153–165.

Australian Institute of Health and Welfare (AIHW) (2017) Australia's mothers and babies 2015 – in brief. *Perinatal Statistics Series* no. 33. Cat no. PER 91. Canberra: AIHW.

Barclay, L. (2008) A feminist history of Australian midwifery from colonisation until the 1980s. *Women and Birth*, *21*(1), 3–8.

Beasley, S., Ford, N., Tracy, S. K., & Welsh, A. W. (2012). Collaboration in maternity care is achievable and practical. *Australian and New Zealand Journal of Obstetrics and Gynaecology*, *52*, 576–581.

Birthplace in England Collaborative Group. (2011) Perinatal and maternal outcomes by planned place of birth for healthy women with low risk pregnancies: The Birthplace in England national prospective cohort study. *BMJ*, *343*, doi:10.1136/bmj.d7400.

Boucher, D., Bennett, C., McFarlin, B., & Freeze, R. (2009) Staying home to give birth: Why women in the United States choose home birth. *Journal of Midwifery & Women's Health*, *54*, 119–126.

Brass, R. (2012) Caring for the woman who goes against conventional medical advice. *British Journal of Midwifery*, *20*, 898–901.

Brown, L. A. (2009). Birth visionaries: An examination of unassisted childbirth. Doctoral dissertation, Boston College.

Buckley, S. (2009). *Gentle birth, gentle mothering: A doctor's guide to natural childbirth and gentle early parenting choices*. Berkeley, CA: Celestial Arts.

Buckley, S. J. (2015). Hormonal physiology of childbearing: Evidence and implications for women, babies, and maternity care. Retrieved from: http://childbirthconnection.org/pdfs/CC.NPWF. HPoC.Report.2015.pdf.

Catling-Paull, C., Foureur, M. J., & Homer, C. S. (2012) Publicly-funded homebirth models in Australia. *Women and Birth*, *25*, 152–158.

Coroner, South Australian. (2012). *Finding of Inquest into the deaths of Tate Spencer-Koch, Jahli Jean Hobbs and Tully Oliver Kavanagh*. South Australia: Coroner's Office of South Australia.

Dahlen, H. G., Jackson, M., & Stevens, J. (2011) Homebirth, freebirth and doulas: Casualty and consequences of a broken maternity system. *Women and Birth*, *24*, 47–50.

Dahlen, H. G., Tracy, S., Tracy, M., Bisits, A., Brown, C., & Thornton, C. (2012) Rates of obstetric intervention among low-risk women giving birth in private and public hospitals in NSW: A population-based descriptive study. *BMJ Open*, *2*(5), e001723.

Davis-Floyd, R. E., Barclay, L., Tritten, J., & Daviss, B. A. (2009) *Birth models that work*. Berkeley, CA: University of California Press.

Dawson, K., McLachlan, H., Newton, M., & Forster, D. (2016) Implementing caseload midwifery: Exploring the views of maternity managers in Australia – A national cross-sectional survey. *Women and Birth*, *29*, 214–222.

Fahy, K., Foureur, M., & Hastie, C. (2008) *Birth territory and midwifery guardianship: Theory for practice, education and research*. Edinburgh: Elsevier Health Sciences.

Foureur, M., Davis, D., Fenwick, J., Leap, N., Iedema, R., Forbes, I., & Homer, C. S. (2010) The relationship between birth unit design and safe, satisfying birth: Developing a hypothetical model. *Midwifery*, *26*, 520–525.

Freeze, R. A. S. (2008) Born free: Unassisted childbirth in North America. Doctoral dissertation, Graduate College of the University of Iowa.

Gofen, A. (2012) Entrepreneurial exit response to dissatisfaction with public services. *Public Administration*, *90*, 1088–1106.

Hodnett, E. D., Downe, S., & Walsh, D. (2012) Alternative versus conventional institutional settings for birth. *Cochrane Database of Systematic Reviews*, *2012*(8).

Hodnett, E. D., Gates, S., Hofmeyr, G. J. & Sakala, C. (2013) Continuous support for women during childbirth. *Cochrane Database of Systematic Reviews*, *2013*(7).

Homer, C., Brodie, P., & Leap, N. (2008) *Midwifery continuity of care: A practical guide*. Chatswood: Churchill Livingstone.

Howard, E. D. (2017) Optimizing the birth environment with evidence-based design. *The Journal of Perinatal & Neonatal Nursing*, *31*, 290–293.

Hunter, J. (2018) The experiences of privately practising midwives in Australia who have been reported to the Australian Health Practitioner Regulation Agency: A qualitative study. Honours thesis, Western Sydney University.

Jackson, M. (2014) Birthing outside the system: wanting the best and safest: A grounded theory study about what motivates women to choose a high-risk homebirth or freebirth. Doctoral dissertation, Western Sydney University.

Leap, N., Sandall, J., Buckland, S., & Huber, U. (2010) Journey to confidence: Women's experiences of pain in labour and relational continuity of care. *The Journal of Midwifery & Women's Health*, *55*, 234–242.

Maputle, M. S., & Donavon, H. (2013) Woman-centred care in childbirth: A concept analysis (Part 1). *Curationis*, *36*(1), 1–8.

Miller, A. C. (2009) 'Midwife to myself': Birth narratives among women choosing unassisted homebirth. *Sociological Inquiry*, *79*, 51–74.

Newman, L. A. (2008) Why planned attended homebirth should be more widely supported in Australia. *Australian and New Zealand Journal of Obstetrics and Gynaecology*, *48*, 450–453.

NICE. (2017) Intrapartum care for healthy women and babies. *National Institute for Health and Care Excellence*, clinical guideline. WHO recommendations: intrapartum care for a positive childbirth experience. Geneva: World Health Organization.

Rattner, D., Hamouche Abrea, I., de Olivereira Araújo, M., & França Santos, A. (2009) Humanizing childbirth to reduce maternal and neonatal mortality. In R. Davis-Floyd, L. Barclay, B.-A. Daviss, & J. Tritten (Eds.), *Birth Models that Work* (pp. 385–414). Berkeley, CA: University of California Press.

Sandall, J., Soltani, H., Gates, S., Shennan, A., & Devane, D. (2016) Midwife-led continuity models versus other models of care for childbearing women. *Cochrane Database of Systematic Reviews*, *2016*(4).

Scarf, V. L., Rossiter, C., Vedam, S., Dahlen, H. G., Ellwood, D., Forster, D., … Thornton, C. (2018) Maternal and perinatal outcomes by planned place of birth among women with low-risk pregnancies in high-income countries: A systematic review and meta-analysis. *Midwifery*, *62*, 240–255.

Stark, M. A., Remynse, M., & Zwelling, E. (2016) Importance of the birth environment to support physiologic birth. *Journal of Obstetric, Gynecologic & Neonatal Nursing*, *45*, 285–294.

Symon, A., Winter, C., Donnan, P. T., & Kirkham, M. (2010) Examining autonomy's boundaries: A follow-up review of perinatal mortality cases in UK independent midwifery. *Birth*, *37*, 280–287.

Thornton, C. E. & Dahlen, H. G. (2018) Born before arrival in NSW, Australia (2000–2011): A linked population data study of incidence, location, associated factors and maternal and neonatal outcomes. *BMJ Open*, *8*(3), e019328.

Tracy, S. K., Hartz, D. L., Tracy, M. B., Allen, J., Forti, A., Hall, B., ... Bisits, A. (2013) Caseload midwifery care versus standard maternity care for women of any risk: M@ NGO, a randomised controlled trial. *The Lancet*, *382*(9906), 1723–1732.

Tracy, S. K., Welsh, A., Hall, B., Hartz, D., Lainchbury, A., Bisits, A., ... Tracy, M. B. (2014) Caseload midwifery compared to standard or private obstetric care for first time mothers in a public teaching hospital in Australia: A cross sectional study of cost and birth outcomes. *BMC Pregnancy and Childbirth*, *14*, 46.

Turton, H. (2007). An investigation into unattended birth in the UK and the USA and the clinical, ethical and legal issues surrounding it. Unpublished Master's thesis, University College London, London.

Walsh, D. (2009) Small really is beautiful: Tales from a freestanding Birth Centre in England. In R. Davis-Floyd, L. Barclay, B.-A. Daviss, & J. Tritten (Eds.), *Birth Models That Work*. Berkeley, CA: University of California Press.

Wilkes, E., Teakle, B., & Gamble, J. (2009) Medicare rebates for midwives: An analysis of the 2009/2010 Federal Budget. *Women and Birth*, *22*, 79–81.

3 Understanding women's motivations to, and experiences of, freebirthing in the UK

Claire Feeley and Gill Thomson

> I accepted that like any other mammal, I can give birth so the implicit trust I have in my biology played a fundamental role in this acceptance of birthing alone.
>
> (Cat: Feeley & Thomson, 2016b, p. 8)

About the authors

My (Claire Feeley) interest in the phenomenon of freebirth was sparked when I was a disillusioned second-year midwifery student, where I felt that maternity services often do more harm than good. I had read a lot of online freebirth stories and was struck by the profound sense of joy, wonder and awe of birth that often seemed missing from the births I had facilitated as a student midwife. While freebirthing was not something I had personally considered, I felt a deep sense of understanding as to why some women opted out of the system on offer. My interest led me to carrying out a meta-synthesis for my undergraduate dissertation, which paved the way for carrying out the primary research during my Master's degree. Gill Thomson as my MSc supervisor found resonance with her work on birth trauma. Therefore, our research interests aligned, which provided a valuable contribution to the development of this work.

Introduction

Freebirthing, the intentional decision to birth without midwives or doctor's in attendance, is usually associated with high-income country contexts where women have access to maternity care but choose not to access this care during the birth (Holton et al., 2016). Therefore, freebirthing should not be conflated with other birthing situations such as concealed pregnancies, babies unintentionally born before arrival (BBA) or a lack of access to maternity care services. In the UK, freebirthing also differs from situations where usually available homebirth services or access to birth centres have been temporarily withdrawn, often suddenly and due to staffing issues (Prochaska, 2012). These other situations arise from different circumstances and contexts that generally limit women's choices and decision-making.

Freebirthing is not without risk, with concerns raised regarding maternal/foetal morbidity and mortality. The World Health Organization (WHO) strongly advocates that all women and babies get access to skilled care in pregnancy, childbirth and immediately after (WHO, 2010). The WHO (2010) estimate that 10–15% of pregnancies and/or birth will have obstetric complications that need clinical intervention for optimal outcomes. The risks associated with freebirthing are often perceived as similar to those associated with BBA (where a woman *unintentionally* births before she can access maternity professionals) (Loughney, Collis, & Dastgir, 2006). BBAs are associated with increased morbidity for the mother (e.g. excessive blood loss) or baby (e.g. failure to retain body temperature), although overall outcomes are normally good (Loughney et al., 2006). These risks, however, may not apply for women opting to freebirth as the decision is *intentional*, thereby indicating that women had prepared to give birth without professional support (Jackson, Dahlen, & Schmied, 2012). As such, Jackson et al. (2012) suggest, the risks associated with freebirthing cannot yet be quantified.

Freebirthing is subject to controversy – in recent years there have been heated debates on the topic across international media outlets and social media sites (Twitter, Facebook, etc.). Proponents advocate freebirthing as a legitimate birthing choice while critics argue it is an unnecessarily dangerous decision. From a human rights perspective, we situate freebirthing as an expression of women's autonomy and bodily integrity, both of which should ultimately be respected. However, this perspective does not prevent us from asking important questions about the motivations of women who opt for such a radical birth choice.

Our previous research, a systematic review and metasynthesis (Feeley, Burns, Adams, & Thomson, 2015), identified only four studies that explored women's decision to, or experience of, freebirthing. Most were undertaken in the USA (n = 3), one in Australia and none in the UK. Similar issues were reported across those studies about how women rejected professional intervention, had faith in their bodies to give birth unaided, and how freebirthing offered the means for women to enact choice, control and autonomy over their bodies (Feeley et al., 2015). Given the different maternity model of care and service provision in the UK when compared with the US and Australia, we felt it important to carry out a primary study within a UK context.

Birth and maternity care in the UK

The UK has a National Health Service (NHS) which provides free maternity care for all pregnant women, provided they meet the criteria of residing in the UK for >1 year, otherwise known as 'ordinarily resident' (Maternity Action, 2011). Unlike some high-income countries, in the UK midwifery-led care is the default framework and midwives are the lead professional care provider for healthy women across the childbirth continuum: antenatal, intrapartum, postnatal (DH, 2010a). Midwives are deemed responsible, accountable practitioners who practise autonomously, are skilled at facilitating normal physiological processes of childbirth, as well as the identification, management, or escalation of complications, should they arise (NMC, 2018). They are able to practise in any setting including home, birth centres and hospitals (NMC, 2018). For women who have complicated pregnancies that require obstetric or paediatric input, midwives work alongside other health professionals with a 'coordinator role' to ensure women's needs are met (DH, 2010a). Therefore, regardless of health status, all women are entitled to receive midwifery care and support. Birth in the UK is considered safe (King's Fund, 2008), with low rates of maternal and perinatal mortality, i.e. 9.8 per 100,000 maternal (MBRRACE-UK, 2018b) and 5.65 per 1000 perinatal (MBRRACE-UK, 2018a).

Birth choices: rhetoric versus reality

Since the 1990s, key UK governmental policies have advocated the importance of women making their own choices regarding their maternity care including autonomy over where, and how, to give birth (DH, 1993, 2007, 2010a, 2010b). The concept of choice saw a move away from the passive patient under 'expert' decision makers to a partnership model in which women's needs and preferences are central to decision-making (DH, 2010a). It also included the right to decline care, such as a decision to freebirth, and the right to decline medical intervention in life threatening situations (Birthrights, 2017b, 2017c). In the UK, the concept of 'choice' has been formalised through: legislating women's rights to autonomy (Birthrights, 2017a); governmental policy (DH, 1993, 2007, 2010b) and evidence-based healthcare guidelines (RCOG, 2015; NICE, 2017).

However, critics argue that 'choice' is socially constructed, politically constrained and often inequitable (Kitzinger, 2005; McAra-Couper, Jones, & Smythe, 2012; Budgeon, 2015). It is argued that the combination of dominant medical and risk-averse discourses, within a technocratic culture of maternity care, super-values certain choices over others and creates hegemonic birth practices (Kitzinger, 2005; Walsh, 2009). For example, concerns have been raised regarding the rates of unnecessary interventions, rising caesarean section rates and falling physiological birth rates in the UK (Downe & Finlayson, 2016) and the impact of such on biopsychosocial morbidity rates (Renfrew et al., 2014; *The Lancet*, 2018). While medical interventions can be life-saving, data suggest that overuse can lead to iatrogenic harm (Renfrew et al., 2014). A comparison of birth statistics over a ten-year period in England (NHS Digital, 2018) showed that in 2017–2018, when compared to 2007–2008, the rates of spontaneous onset of labour and birth had declined (52% versus 68%), and that induction rates (32% versus 20%) and caesarean section (28% versus 25%) had increased.

A key issue relating to both declining physiological birth rates and limitations of women's choice is the place of birth. Alternative birth settings, such as birth centres and homebirth, are supported in UK policies and guidelines (DH, 1993, 2007, 2010a; NHS England, 2016) and there is growing evidence of the efficacy, safety, acceptability and cost-effectiveness of non-obstetric birth settings (Brocklehurst et al., 2011; Hodnett, Downe, & Walsh, 2012). For healthy women at the onset of labour, birth outside obstetric units is associated with positive outcomes such as greater levels of physiological births, lower intervention rates (Brocklehurst et al., 2011; Hodnett et al., 2012; Burns, Boulton, Cluett, Cornelius, & Smith, 2012) and women's satisfaction with their birth experience (McCourt, Rayment, Rance, & Sandall, 2016; Olza et al., 2018). However, data from 2017 showed that, while the birth rate for England and Wales was 679,106 (Office for National Statistics, 2018), only 2.1% of births were at home (Office for National Statistics, 2018), approximately 14% were in birth centres (Walsh et al., 2018) and 84% in obstetric units (Office for National Statistics, 2018). While we acknowledge that a hospital (and medicalised) birth is desirable and preferred among some women (Lavender, Hofmeyr, Neilson, Kingdon, & Gyte, 2006; McAra-Couper et al., 2012), these data suggest inequitable access to alternative birth settings. A survey carried out by NCT (2009) found that only 4% of women had access to all four choices of birth place: home, free-standing birth centre, alongside birth centre and obstetric unit. Further research reports multiple factors that limit women's access to a homebirth or birth centre, including local funding sources, staffing levels, organisational structures that prioritise hospital staffing over community, on-call demands, lack of confidence by midwives, lack of support by their wider team (i.e. management) and, in some cases, negative attitudes by the obstetric team (McCourt, Rance, Rayment, & Sandall, 2011; RCM, 2011; NHS England, 2016; Walsh et al., 2018). Therefore, structural, organisational and cultural issues limit women's choices to access non-obstetric settings, which in turn is a limiting factor to achieving a physiological birth.

Despite the UK having strong legislation to supports women's autonomy and bodily integrity (Birthrights, 2017b), barriers exist. Recent research reports that women can face lack of choice or control over decision-making, non-consenting procedures carried out by health professionals and, sometimes, coercion towards particular birthing decisions (Care Quality Commission, 2013; Birthrights, 2013; Care Quality Commission, 2015; Plested& Kirkham, 2016). Coercion can involve steering women towards decisions that comply with maternity professionals' local guidelines and policies, particularly in situations where women are declining recommended care or seeking birth 'outside the guidelines' (Brass, 2012; Shallow, 2013; Scamell, 2014). Coercive practices include repetitive discussions regarding the risks of the woman's decision (Kruske, Young, Jenkinson, & Catchlove, 2013; Birthrights, 2013, 2017a; Plested & Kirkham, 2016), attempting to influence family members (Feeley & Thomson, 2016a), threats of referrals to social services (Plested

& Kirkham, 2016) and the 'dead baby' card (Reed, Sharman, & Inglis, 2017) – an unsubstantiated claim that the baby might die if the woman does not comply with recommendations (Plested & Kirkham, 2016). At the same time, maternity professionals report feeling pressured to conform to local guidelines and policies due to fears of facing disciplinary actions from their employers (Griffiths, 2009; Kotaska, 2011; Robertson & Thomson, 2016). The fear of being accountable for adverse outcomes is associated with maternity professionals practising 'defensively' (Robertson & Thomson, 2016), which in turn can reinforce coercive practices (Griffith & Tengnah, 2010). Therefore, women face conflicts between the rhetoric of choice and the reality of enacting their choices.

Understanding women's motivations

We report on three key themes to highlight what and how different factors influence women's motivation to freebirth. The first theme was framed around 'personal herstories' – where women's decisions to freebirth were based on their own individual, unique psychosocial backgrounds and histories. For some, the decision to freebirth and avoid maternity care during labour and birth related to a history of abuse, a learning/behaviour-related diagnosis, i.e. Asperger's Syndrome, or a difficult upbringing. In all these situations, the participants alluded to an inherent need for control over their bodies and a commensurate lack of faith that their specific needs would be met by maternity care providers. Holly, who had experienced abuse as a child, reported:

> I absolutely hate to feel helpless, lied to or pushed around by people who think they are smarter/better than me, because of this.
>
> (Feeley & Thomson, 2016b, p. 5).

Some women related their freebirth decision to their family history of homebirth. These women wished to replicate the shared familial stories of giving birth within a safe, home environment. For others, their decision related to their previous experiences of childbirth – all bar one had given birth at least once prior to their experience of freebirth. While women's overall reflections of their former birth(s) varied widely, all women recounted 'some' negative experiences of maternity care. Several women described previous traumatic hospital-based births that were characterised by a lack of communication and relationships with care providers and unconsented procedures. Such events, as reflected by Jane (below), led to women feeling a sense of isolation, violation and humiliation:

> I felt violated and humiliated. It ended up with the doctor telling me my baby was stuck and she would try to pull my baby out, in theatre, with an epidural, surrounded by strangers, in case it didn't work in which case

> they would perform an emergency c-section. It was the most awful experience of my life.
>
> (Feeley & Thomson, 2016b, p. 5)

The women blamed themselves for not preventing events from occurring and/or experienced a sense of shame due to how they had behaved:

> I felt ashamed, the only other thing I have ever felt ashamed of uh through the whole process, I was ashamed that I sounded like a pig that's being slaughtered.
>
> (Cat: Feeley & Thomson, p. 6)

Several women experienced positive, out-of-hospital births, i.e. at a birth centre or at home with midwives. In their accounts women referred to how the midwives had helped create a calm, safe and peaceful environment, where women felt free and able to achieve a physiological birth. Despite this positive aspect, the women considered what they deemed as 'unnecessary', clinical checks, monitoring and/or the midwife's interactions as detracting from their birth experience. Nicky reported:

> Well the fascinating thing is that because the midwife was talking to me regularly during contractions, I was very irritated by her presence (laughs).
>
> (Feeley & Thomson, 2016b, p. 7)

Diverging paths of decision-making

The second theme explores how women's backgrounds and/or previous experiences of childbirth influenced their decision to freebirth. Only one participant had been expecting her first baby. She made an instinctive decision to freebirth early in her pregnancy. Claire related this decision to her behavioural diagnosis where she believed that the presence of maternity professionals, at the time of birth, would induce stress and increase the likelihood of 'things more likely to go wrong'. Freebirthing therefore offered the best solution for her needs.

Some of the women who'd had a previous traumatic birth initially booked for a homebirth to avoid a recurrence of their former ordeal. Negative interactions with community midwives during antenatal appointments, however, led them to change their decision to freebirth. These women complained about midwives 'manipulating' or 'bullying' them about their homebirth decision, leading to high levels of stress and a lack of faith that their needs and preferences for birth would be met. Holly reported:

> I felt no faith whatsoever in my local maternity service in 2006. No trust. No support. Nothing but revulsion for their attitudes and revolving

> door policies, and for the lies and pressure they put me under without understanding I am a smart and educated girl.
>
> (Feeley & Thomson, 2016b, p. 6)

As there was no guarantee as to who the woman's attending midwives would be, the concern of having unsupportive caregivers who could interfere and potentially jeopardise their birth experience meant that freebirthing was the only viable option. Cat reported:

> The obstructive behaviour by the community midwives, the lottery of who would turn up at the birth. If their behaviour was indicative of many of the midwives in the Trust then I could not trust that they were supportive of home births. I actually became fearful that they would turn up in time for the birth as they seemed more scared of attending a home birth than I felt about having a home birth.
>
> (Feeley & Thomson, 2016b, p. 6)

Conversely, some women with a history of traumatic birth had at least one successful homebirth prior to freebirthing. These women recounted that while freebirthing had always appealed, their traumatic ordeal had eroded their faith in their capacity to give birth. A homebirth thereby provided them with the middle ground of being cared for by midwives in an environment more aligned with normality and to 'prove' they could give birth physiologically:

> I think in hindsight I probably needed to prove to myself I was capable of doing it before contemplating doing it alone.
>
> (June: Feeley & Thomson, 2016b, p. 7)

Whereas for the women who had only had previous positive experiences of childbirth (either at home or in a birth centre), a freebirthing decision was based on their embodied knowledge that they could 'do it'. As reflected by Jenny, these women trusted their instincts and their bodies:

> I already knew from the first birth that when I have space to internalise, to tune into that super strong survival instinct a birthing mother has, that I know whether all is well, or not.
>
> (Feeley & Thomson, 2016b, p. 7)

The converging path of decision-making

The third theme relates to how women validated their decision to freebirth. All the women stressed that their freebirth decision was carefully considered and based on their inner convictions and intellectual reasoning. Alex stated:

> I do not believe that freebirth is a choice for everyone and it is something that I worked towards, rather than made hard, fast decisions about but I think it is crucial to stress that my choices were born out of positivity, a deep understanding of myself and intelligent reasoning.
>
> (Feeley & Thomson, 2016b, p. 7)

All the women discussed how they had undertaken extensive research into their legal rights regarding freebirthing, and birth physiology. A deeper understanding of mammalian biology helped to reinforce the women's belief that they could give birth without intervention or midwives in attendance:

> I accepted that like any other mammal, I can give birth so the implicit trust I have in my biology played a fundamental role in this acceptance of birthing alone.
>
> (Cat: Feeley & Thomson, 2016b, p. 8)

This greater understanding of birth also highlighted their knowledge of how non-evidenced-based practices can create iatrogenic harm – thus serving to strengthen their freebirth decisions. Jenny stated:

> But the more I thought about it, the more, um, the more I started reading into the iatrogenic injuries that happen because you know there's this practice if baby need resuscitation, the guidelines that you cut and clamp immediately. And I really began to be quite concerned about that, everything I could get my hands on in terms of papers, on this, the evidence was saying you need to resuscitate with the cord intact.
>
> (Feeley & Thomson, 2016b, p. 9)

Contrary to the critique that freebirthing women are irresponsible risk-takers, most of the women had accessed 'some' antenatal care to ensure, and provide ongoing reassurance of, their low-risk status. Women who had experienced more than one freebirth tended to access less professional antenatal care. They did, however, report undertaking their own physiological assessments such as blood pressure and urinalysis in order to check for and mitigate against risks. All the women (and many partners) educated themselves about complications such as haemorrhage, cord prolapse and post-birth resuscitation, and felt confident they could manage these situations while waiting for expert help:

> Yes, it is seen that if you freebirth, you would stay at home regardless and that you know you don't have anything else in place. I gave my husband a few things to read so in an emergency he would know what to do while we waited for help.
>
> (Jane: Feeley & Thomson, 2016b, p. 9)

The women used this knowledge to inform a personal assessment of what they considered to be unacceptable or acceptable risks:

> In the end, it was a risk assessment. We weighed up the likelihood of all the risks that mattered to us, and made a decision based on our level of comfort with each of those risks.
>
> (Jenny: Feeley & Thomson, 2016b, p. 9)

For most women, the decision to freebirth was made with their partners. The women's intention was not to give birth alone, but with partners who were supportive and able to provide what women needed – a safe space to give birth, unheeded by distractions and for any emergency to be actioned as needed. June reported:

> Having gone through the wonderful homebirth together I knew that I could give birth normally and that I could trust my husband to protect and support us through the labour. He was also comfortable with things, now knowing what he needed to do and what would happen. I opted with this pregnancy to use maternity care at a minimum.
>
> (Feeley & Thomson, 2016b, p. 8)

Tensions and conflicts in choice

The women in our study encountered a number of challenges with professionals either during pregnancy or during the postnatal period (Feeley & Thomson, 2016a). The challenges included misinformation from midwives, conflict with their midwives and reprisals and recriminations. These experiences continued to occur, despite the women's awareness of their legal rights concerning freebirth and the fact that their engagement with maternity services was voluntary.

Several women felt that their rights were violated when their decision to freebirth was met with suspicion and prejudice, and that their midwives lacked knowledge regarding the legalities of freebirthing (Feeley & Thomson, 2016a). Midwives' perceived lack of knowledge could result in a mistaken conflation of a decision to freebirth with child protection concerns – that is, that the women were supposedly putting their unborn at risk. This was highlighted by Claire:

> Not being willing to engage with health services at every point they want you to is not necessarily a precursor to putting your child at risk, and they need to learn to make that distinction better.
>
> (Feeley & Thomson, 2016a, p. 18)

Despite women being aware of their rights, they recognised that opting out of the norms of maternity care placed them in a precarious situation. The majority of women interviewed had heard of situations (via online forums or personal networks) where freebirthing women were reported to organisations with enforcement powers, such as child protection services or the police. The women reported using strategies to pursue the birth they wanted while circumventing conflicts and reprisals with maternity caregivers. For some, this included a conscious decision to not share their freebirthing plans with maternity professionals. However, as June reports below, not being able to have open conversations with their midwives could be experienced as stressful:

> You know, you keep talking about reducing stress and that, but if you can't have an open conversation with your midwife because you are afraid of what she is going to say or what she is going to do, you know bringing in social services. That is a stressful situation and it is not a positive thing for a mother or a baby.
>
> (Feeley & Thomson, 2016a, p. 19)

Some women planned a BBA, in that they had booked a homebirth but planned to contact the midwives after the birth. These women had a pre-prepared explanation such as the 'birth progressed too fast' to avoid arousing suspicion. When interacting with midwives postnatally, the women adopted an apologetic stance to mitigate against potential recriminations from the professionals. Jenny illustrates:

> In fact, maybe I was a little bit aware, and my tactic with the midwives that we called three or so days later was to be very agreeable, be very kind of apologetic, kind of argh yea. Just helpful and agreeable, that we're not being contrary or irresponsible, it just kind of happened like this and it was all ok and you know, saved the placenta for you to check and do all the checks to show we've nothing to hide.
>
> (Feeley & Thomson, 2016a, p. 19)

The women's strategies to avoid potential reprisals were not always successful. Four women were reported to child protection services for allegedly putting their unborn child at risk. While all reports were subsequently resolved, two women described their engagement with child protection services (including a police presence) as a highly stressful, terrifying and threatening experience. They felt coerced into accepting welfare checks for fear of having their baby removed, as described by Alex:

> Then that evening about seven o'clock social worker came again with two police officers, you know looking out of the window with two police officers on your door step, I've got a 7-day-old baby and a 3-year-old daughter, and I just had no idea why these people were in our lives. I was absolutely terrified, and um, my husband answered the door and they said they wanted to a welfare check.
>
> (Feeley & Thomson, 2016a, p. 19)

Experiences of freebirthing

We report below the women's experiences of freebirthing that highlights the reported feelings of positivity and empowerment (Feeley, 2015).

Most of the women reported using water, music, visualisation and/or movement to help them relax during labour:

> I choose the birthing day session on the CD and it took me into deep relaxation straight away. The water was wonderful in supporting me as I moved around for each pressure wave, alternating positions.
>
> (Julie: Feeley, 2015)

Many described how their birth partners helped them to facilitate a 'safe and secure' birth space so they were able to succumb to their physiological forces: 'I felt able to totally let go in labour and to be myself'. On one occasion, Jenny described how her husband 'intuitively' recognised when she needed a supportive presence and when she needed to be left unattended:

> I love how it panned out, the fact that they were both there [husband and son] with me, but that at the moment of her being born it was just me and her, just like I'd fantasised. It was incredibly empowering and I love the fact that X [partner] intuitively gave me that perfect first moment with her.
>
> (Jenny: Feeley, 2015)

Holly had a prior arrangement with an independent midwife, where she would request support only if needed:

> I enjoyed an easy labor, listening to music, dipping in and out of the bath and called her when things got intense. She arrived 30 mins after I delivered a healthy daughter in the bath, into my own hands.
>
> (Holly: Feeley, 2015)

Women frequently said the uninterrupted and relaxed birth space (i.e. 'nobody bothering me. I just did my thing') enabled them to embrace and 'walk with' their contractions, which, in turn, helped to alleviate or eradicate their labour pains. Cat stated:

> I tried to imagine these calm waves and you know the shores. These waves just crashing in front of me, that is what my labour was like, these crashing waves. But for me, I only figured it out, that this pain, like it was next to me and I had to embrace it and walk with it, walk with it. I just walked with it until the contractions subsided. Then at one point I went, I was over my ball and that was the last pain I'd had, it was painless from that point.
>
> (Cat: Feeley, 2015)

A number of the women were physically alone at the time of birth through choice. In some cases, however, this was due to either the doula's late arrival or the husband being on a telephone call with the midwife. One woman's recent ex-partner arrived 'five minutes after he was born', leaving her to give birth with only her older children present. This mother reflected that while this situation had not been intended, it had been an ideal scenario as it was a 'really bonding' and 'really stabilising' experience for her children, in the midst of their emotional, family upheavement.

Women's freebirthing stories frequently depicted an embodied mother–baby union such that they 'knew' what was happening with their babies *in utero*: 'I knew that my baby was moving down through my cervix and would be here soon' (Julie). They also knew what was needed to progress their labour:

> She was out in three contractions and that was just optimal fetal positioning and being in water and being on my knees and I didn't even push. […] My body did it, and it was completely painless.
>
> (Cat: Feeley, 2015)

The physical and emotional mother–baby unification was also experienced during the birth. Julie used a visceral description: 'it felt like my cervix was a golden circle that the baby swam through'; others described it as a 'perfect', 'wonderful', 'beautiful' and 'intimate' moment in which they welcomed new life:

> I think you know that moment when they haven't taken the first breath, and you are holding them waiting for them to breathe, it is just (…) the moment that nobody can take away, or ought to take away. You know, you hold your baby and you watch them cross over.
>
> (Cat: Feeley, 2015)

Many women expressed a sense of pride in what they had achieved during their freebirth; 'I'd done it … all by myself'. Others, such as Claire, referred to feeling more 'competent' and 'capable' due to the sense of control she had over 'my body and choices'. Jane also reflected on how her freebirth had helped to heal her previous trauma:

> It was perfect, and kind of healing in a way, I perhaps felt after my 2nd that I couldn't give birth and um, you know to actually do it by myself I realised that I could.
>
> (Feeley, 2015)

While all women in the study reported positive experiences of freebirthing, June reported that the midwife's presence after the birth had been disruptive, because she provided unwelcome advice which culminated in June having to transfer to the hospital for postnatal care:

> The midwife who turned up turned our home and peaceful birth upside down because a trained professional hadn't been there and she said there was too much blood and I was bleeding out. I wasn't [...] we ended up with a transfer.
>
> (Feeley, 2015)

In a different situation, Alex who had been reported to social services (highlighted earlier) found comfort from her birth experience which gave her strength to manage the distressing situation:

> And I feel so grateful for the birth experience that I had, because again it was that kept me grounded, in the same way X's [daughter] birth had. And again I'd had this incredibly powerful experience where, the level of consciousness was great this time um, it just kept me focussed on that. Nobody, no matter what happens to you according to people's structures of beliefs, nothing can take away your own kind of experiences.
>
> (Feeley, 2015)

Discussion/implications

Our study found that women's freebirthing decision-making can be broadly categorised in two ways: (1) women with a philosophical view that undisturbed birth is a safer birth option; and (2) women who are dissatisfied with the maternity system. While for some women this dissatisfaction was due to a traumatic birth with negative and long-lasting implications on maternal well-being, for others, it represented a misalignment between the views/attitudes of the woman and maternity professionals. In the latter cases, maternity professionals were perceived to be interfering with what the women wanted to achieve. Previous negative experiences of care were compounded, either in subsequent pregnancies where poor care was experienced, or where midwives demonstrated inaccurate knowledge or understanding regarding the legalities of freebirth. The negative impact of previous birth experience(s), and poor-quality care, on women's subsequent birth decisions is equally reflected in women choosing either elective caesareans for a subsequent birth (Lavender et al., 2006) and a homebirth following a traumatic caesarean birth (Keedle, Schmied, Burns, & Dahlen, 2015). Our findings echo those in previous metasynthesis (Feeley et al., 2015; Holton & de Miranda, 2016) where women's former experiences of birth led them to reject any form of maternity care that they perceived would interfere with normal birth processes. Additionally, where women reported greater knowledge of their rights than their midwives, there was a further erosion of trust leading women to either not share their freebirthing plans or 'play the game' to ensure they achieved the birth they wanted. Planning a 'BBA' was a strategy deployed to reduce unnecessary conflicts or reprisals with maternity staff, and to guard against statutory referrals to social services. Unfortunately, some women were unable to circumvent the conflict, which led to deeply distressing reprisals and recriminations. Poor communication, enacting reprisals and recrimination and using enforcement process when women are seeking to enact their autonomy is a far cry from the woman-centred rhetoric asserted in relation to UK maternity services.

While some women's postnatal freebirthing experiences were experienced as challenging due to unwanted 'interference' by professionals, their experience of having a freebirth was positive. Descriptions were characterised by a safe, relaxed atmosphere, which was supported by responsive and intuitive birth partners that enabled an embodied mother–baby union. This was where women felt inherently connected to their babies and their physiological responses. Freebirthing was often depicted as an empowering experience that enhanced women's confidence and self-esteem. For women who had a previous traumatic birth, freebirth represented a 'redemptive' birth (Thomson & Downe, 2010): an experience that allowed them to heal them from their previous distressing ordeal. Contrary to the claim that freebirthing women are irresponsible risk-takers, we found that freebirthing was in fact a careful and consciously mediated decision, often made in conjunction with partners. Women actively developed a knowledge and understanding of birth physiology and considered/prepared their own risk assessments. It was not the case that women rejected medical care; rather, the decision to engage medical care was based on their judgement as to when and what types of help would be sought. The balancing of, on the one hand, being low-risk, knowledgeable about birth physiology, confident in abilities to give birth unaided and being prepared for risk with, on the other hand, the potential to be cared for by professionals who may interfere, not support what women want to achieve and create iatrogenic risks meant that, for these women, freebirthing was the safer option.

These insights into women's motivations and experiences of freebirthing points again to the benefits of a continuity relational model of midwifery care (Sandall, Soltani, Gates, Shennan, & Devane, 2016). These models of care provide women and midwives the opportunity to forge mutually trusting relationships, where women's needs are prioritised and clinical outcomes are optimised (Sandall et al., 2016). Even women who choose freebirth can derive some benefit from developing a trusting relationship with a known midwife. This would help mitigate against postnatal reprisals. Our study highlights that fragmented care, lack of support for women's homebirth plans and a perceived lack of professional skill in facilitating homebirth influenced some women's decisions to freebirth. These insights echo the wider literature that we reported earlier. Conceivably, a meaningful relationship with midwives who are skilled and supportive of physiological births could offer a positive alternative to freebirth. For example, midwives report that where they have met the needs of women through proactive support, co-created care plans (see Chapter 15) and positive communication, they retain women's engagement with their services (Feeley, 2019; Feeley, Thomson, & Downe, 2019). Meeting the needs of women, even in complex situations such as a twin homebirth, is perceived as preferable to women birthing alone (Symon, Winter, Donnan, & Kirkham, 2010; Feeley, 2019). From the midwives' perspectives, safe care was personalised care characterised by mutual trust (Symon et al., 2010; Cobell, 2015; Feeley, 2019). Women who nevertheless pursue plans to freebirth would still benefit from having a trust-based mother–midwife relationship for support as needed. For example, midwives could work with women to negotiate reduced antenatal care and to create an optimum birth plan which informs women about key risk factors and actions to take in case of an emergency. Where communication is positive and non-judgemental, in our view, full disengagement with services are unlikely.

Conclusion

Our study highlights that women's decision to freebirth is influenced by personal and individual factors including beliefs that an undisturbed birth is a safer birth. However, women's decision-making is also informed by their experiences with UK maternity services, which did not provide individualised woman-centred care. Negative experiences either occurred during previous births that were experienced as traumatic or through unsupportive interactions with professionals during a subsequent pregnancy. Such negative experiences influenced the women's decision-making to freebirth and/or compounded negative views about their local maternity services. The rejection of midwifery care also related to the women's concerns that clinical care would interrupt and disturb the normal processes of birth. As such, the women reported to feel safer birthing without professional attendance, preferring instead to rely upon their embodied knowledge to determine if and when help was required. We suggest that providing women access to continuous relational midwifery models of care will help mitigate against negative experiences and increase women's trust in their care providers. Even where women continue their plans to freebirth, the benefits of a positive relationship with a midwife can bolster women's assurance in maternity services and encourage access, should the women want or need clinical care. Retaining positive open and non-judgemental communication is paramount to retaining women's confidence in their local care providers. Maternity services and health professionals have a collective responsibility to ensure that the care they offer is respectful, dignified and in accordance with legislation, regardless of women's choices.

The way forward

- All women should have access to a known midwife, where relational trust-based care can be actualised, regardless of women's intended birth decisions
- Maternity services should offer meaningful choices, including access to skilled midwives to support homebirth services
- All maternity professionals require training and awareness on women's ethical, legal and moral frameworks related to respectful maternity care
- If a woman discloses her intention to freebirth, maternity professionals must provide factual evidence-based information, including the legal requirements following the birth such as birth notifications/registrations to support her
- Communication with women should be positive, non-judgemental and supportive to facilitate trust and provide access to maternity services if it is wanted/needed

References

Birthrights. (2013). *Dignity in childbirth: The Dignity Survey 2013 Women's and midwives' experiences of dignity in UK maternity care*. Birthrights.

Birthrights. (2017a) *Consenting to treatment* [Homepage of Birthrights] [Online]. Retrieved from: www.birthrights.org.uk/library/factsheets/Consenting-to-Treatment.pdf [accessed 9 May 2017].

Birthrights. (2017b) April – last update, *Human rights in maternity care* [Homepage of Birthrights] [Online]. Retrieved from: www.birthrights.org.uk/library/factsheets/Human-Rights-in-Maternity-Care.pdf [accessed 13 March 2016].

Birthrights. (2017c) *Unassisted birth: The legal position* [Homepage of Birthrights] [Online]. Retrieved from: www.birthrights.org.uk/library/factsheets/Unassisted-Birth.pdf [accessed 23 November 2016].

Brass, R. (2012) Caring for the woman who goes against conventional medical advice. *British Journal of Midwifery*, *20*, 898–901.

Brocklehurst, P., Hardy, P., Hollowell, J., Linsell, L., Macfarlane, A., McCourt, C., … Stewart, M. (2011) Perinatal and maternal outcomes by planned place of birth for healthy women with low risk pregnancies: The Birthplace in England national prospective cohort study. *British Medical Journal*, *343*.

Budgeon, S. (2015) Individualized femininity and feminist politics of choice. *European Journal of Women's Studies*, *22*, 303–318.

Burns, E., Boulton, M., Cluett, E., Cornelius, V., & Smith, L. (2012) Characteristics, interventions, and outcomes of women who used a birthing pool: A prospective observational study. *Birth*, *39*, 192–202.

Care Quality Commission. (2013) *National findings from the 2013 survey of women's experiences of maternity care* [Online]. Retrieved from: www.cqc.org.uk/sites/default/files/documents/maternity_report_for_publication.pdf [accessed 26 January 2016].

Care Quality Commission. (2015) *2015 survey of women's experiences of maternity care.* Care Quality Commission [Online]. Retrieved from: www.cqc.org.uk/sites/default/files/20151215b_mat15_statistical_release.pdf [accessed 25 January 2018].

Cobell, A. (2015) What are midwives' experiences of looking after women in labour outside of Trust guidelines? Unpublished Master's thesis, King's College London.

DH. (1993) *Changing childbirth.* London: Department of Health.

DH. (2007) *Maternity matters. Choice, access and continuity of care in a safe service.* London: DH Publications.

DH. (2010a) *Midwifery 2020: Delivering expectations.* Cambridge: Jill Rogers Associates.

DH. (2010b) *White Paper; Equity and excellence: Liberating the NHS.* London: Department of Health.

Downe, S. & Finlayson, K. (2016) *Interventions in normal labour and birth.* London: Royal College of Midwives.

Feeley, C. (2015) Making sense of women's childbirth choices; Exploring the decision to freebirth in the UK. Unpublished Master's thesis, University of Central Lancashire.

Feeley, C. (2019) Practising outside of the box, whilst within the system': A feminist narrative inquiry of NHS midwives supporting and facilitating women's alternative physiological birthing choices. University of Central Lancashire.

Feeley, C., Burns, E., Adams, E., & Thomson, G. (2015) Why do some women choose to freebirth? A meta-thematic synthesis, part one. *Evidence Based Midwifery, 13*, 4–9.

Feeley, C. & Thomson, G. (2016a) Tensions and conflicts in 'choice'. Women's experiences of freebirthing in the UK. *Midwifery, 41*, 16–21.

Feeley, C. & Thomson, G. (2016b) Why do some women choose to freebirth in the UK? An interpretative phenomenological study. *BMC Pregnancy and Childbirth, 16*, 59.

Feeley, C., Thomson, G., & Downe, S. (2019) Caring for women making unconventional birth choices: A meta-ethnography exploring the views, attitudes, and experiences of midwives. *Midwifery, 72*, 50–59.

Griffiths, R. (2009) Maternity care pathways and the law. *British Journal of Midwifery, 17*, 324–325.

Griffith, R. & Tengnah, C. (2010) *Law and professional issues in midwifery (Transforming Midwifery Practice Series).* Exeter: Learning Matters Ltd.

Hodnett, E., Downe, S., & Walsh, D. (2012) Alternative versus conventional institutional settings for birth. *Cochrane Database of Systematic Reviews, 2012*(8), CD000012.

Holton, L. & de Miranda, E. (2016) Women's motivations for having unassisted childbirth or high-risk homebirth: An exploration of the literature on 'birthing outside the system'. *Midwifery, 38*, 55–62.

Jackson, M., Dahlen, H., & Schmeid, V. (2012) Birthing outside of the system; Perceptions of risk amongst Australian women who have freebirths and high risk homebirths. *Midwifery, 28*, 561–567.

Keedle, H., Schmeid, V., Burns, E., & Dahlen, H. (2015) Women's reasons for, and experiences of, choosing a homebirth following a caesarean. *BMC Pregnancy and Childbirth, 15*, 206.

King's Fund. (2008) *Safe births: Everybody's business.* London: King's Fund.

Kitzinger, S. (2005) *The politics of birth*. London: Elsevier.

Kotaska, A. (2011) *Guideline-centered care: A two-edged sword*. Malden, MA: Blackwell Science Inc.

Kruske, S., Young, K., Jenkinson, B., & Catchlove, A. (2013) Maternity care providers' perceptions of women's autonomy and the law. *BMC Pregnancy and Childbirth*, *13*, 84.

Lavender, T., Hofmeyr, G., Neilson, J., Kingdon, C., & Gyte, G. (2006) Caeserean section for non-medical reasons at term. *Cochrane Database of Systematic Reviews*, *2006*(3).

Loughney, A., Collis, R., & Dastgir, S. (2006) Birth before arrival at delivery suite: Associations and consequences. *British Journal of Nutrition*, *14*, 204–208.

Maternity Action. (2011) Entitlement of free NHS maternity care for women from abroad. Retrieved from: www.maternityaction.org.uk/sitebuildercontent/sitebuilderfiles/entitlementtonhscareinfo.pdf [accessed 8 March 2017].

MBRRACE-UK. (2018a) *MBRRACE-UK Perinatal Mortality Surveillance report for births in 2016*. Oxford: NPEU.

MBRRACE-UK. (2018b) *MBRRACE-UK: Saving lives, improving mothers' care. Lessons learned to inform maternity care from the UK and Ireland Confidential Enquiries into Maternal Deaths and Morbidity 2014–16*. Oxford: NPEU.

McAra-Couper, J., Jones, M., & Smythe, L. (2012) Caesarean-section, my body, my choice: The construction of 'informed choice' in relation to intervention in childbirth. *Feminism and Psychology*, *22*, 81–97.

McCourt, C., Rance, S., Rayment, J., & Sandall, J. (2011) *Birthplace qualitative organisations case studies: How maternity care systems may affect the provision of care in different birth settings. Birthplace in England research programme*. London: NIHR Service Delivery and Organisation Programme.

McCourt, C., Rayment, J., Rance, S., & Sandall, J. (2016) Place of birth and concepts of wellbeing. *Anthropology in Action*, *23*(3), 17–29.

NCT. (2009) *An investigation into choice of place of birth*. London: NCT.

NHS Digital. (2018) *NHS Maternity Statistics, England 2017–18*. Retrieved from: https://digital.nhs.uk/data-and-information/publications/statistical/nhs-maternity-statistics/2017–18 [accessed 1 November 2018].

NHS England. (2016) *National Maternity Review. Better births; Improving outcomes of maternity services in England*. London: NHS England.

NICE. (2017) Intrapartum care for healthy women and babies [Homepage of NICE] [Online]. Retrieved from: www.nice.org.uk/guidance/cg190/chapter/recommendations#pain-relief-in-labour-nonregional [accessed 9 March 2017].

NMC. (2018) *Standards for competence for registered midwives*. London: Nursing & Midwifery Council.

Office for National Statistics. (2018) Births in England and Wales: 2017. Retrieved from: www.ons.gov.uk/peoplepopulationandcommunity/birthsdeathsandmarriages/livebirths/bulletins/birthsummarytablesenglandandwales/2017 [accessed 10 January 2019].

Olza, I., Leahy-Warren, P., Benyamini, Y., Kazmierczak, M., Karlsdottir, S., Spyridou, A., … Nieuwenhuijze, M. (2018) Women's psychological experiences of physiological childbirth: A meta-synthesis. *BMJ Open*, *8*(10), e020347.

Plested, M. & Kirkham, M. (2016) Risk and fear in the lived experience of birth without a midwife. *Midwifery*, *38*, 29–34.

Prochaska, E. (2012) Enforcing birth choices. *AIMS Journal*, *24*(2), 6–7.

RCM. (2011) *Survey of current midwives thinking of homebirth*. London: RCM.

RCOG. (2015) *Obtaining valid consent*. Norwich: Royal College of Obstetricians and Gynaecologists.

Reed, R., Sharman, R., & Inglis, C. (2017) Women's descriptions of childbirth trauma relating to care provider actions and interactions. *BMC Pregnancy and Childbirth*, *17*(21), 1–10.

Renfrew, M., Homer, C., Downe, S., Muir, N., Prentice, T., ten Hoope-Bender, P., & McFadden, A. (2014) Midwifery, an executive summary for the *Lancet*'s series. *Lancet* [Online]. Retrieved from: www.thelancet.com/pb/assets/raw/Lancet/stories/series/midwifery/midwifery_exec_summ.pdf [accessed 1 October 2018].

Robertson, J. H. & Thomson, A. M. (2016) An exploration of the effects of clinical negligence litigation on the practice of midwives in England: A phenomenological study. *Midwifery*, *33*, 55–63.

Sandall, J., Soltani, H., Gates, S., Shennan, A., & Devane, D. (2016) Midwife-led continuity models versus other models of care for childbearing women. *Cochrane Database of Systematic Reviews*, *2016*(4).

Scamell, M. (2014) 'She can't come here!' Ethics and the case of birth centre admission policy in the UK. *Journal of Medical Ethics*, *40*, 813–816.

Shallow, H. (2013) Deviant mothers and midwives: Supporting VBAC with women as real partners in decision making. *Essentially MIDIRS*, *4*(1), 17–21.

Symon, A., Winter, C., Donnan, P., & Kirkham, M. (2010) Examining autonomy's boundaries: A follow-up review of perinatal mortality cases in UK independent midwifery. *Birth: Issues in Perinatal Care*, *37*, 280–287.

The Lancet. (2018) Stemming the global caesarean section epidemic. *Lancet*, *392*(10155), 1279.

Thomson, G. & Downe, S. (2010) Changing the future to change the past: Women's experiences of a positive birth following a traumatic birth experience. *Journal of Reproductive and Infant Psychology*, *28*, 102–112.

Walsh, D. (2009) Childbirth embodiment: Problematic aspects of current understandings. *Sociology of Health*, *32*, 486–501.

Walsh, D., Spiby, H., Grigg, C., Dodwell, M., McCourt, C., Culley, L., … Byers, S. (2018) Mapping midwifery and obstetric units in England. *Midwifery*, *56*, 9–16.

WHO. (2010) Skilled birth attendants. Retrieved from: www.who.int/maternal_child_adolescent/topics/maternal/skilled_birth/en/ [accessed 1 February 2019].

4 Birthing 'outside the system' in the Netherlands

Martine Hollander

When we, as professionals, refuse to make any concessions, the result is not that women will fall in line, but rather that they turn their backs on us and end up taking more risks than they initially set out to. It seems a change in paradigm is in order.

(Martine Hollander)

About the author: an obstetrician with the heart of a midwife

As far back as I can remember I have wanted to be a doctor and deliver babies. The first memory I have of this wish was around the time I was 8 years old. At 18, I went to medical school with the sole aim of becoming an obstetrician. In 1999, I graduated from medical school at the age of 24. Like most young doctors, I was full of ambition and zeal to provide the very best care for my patients, and 'help people'.

I managed to secure a job as a house officer (junior doctor) in obstetrics and gynaecology in a regional teaching hospital and set to work learning how to deliver babies. I loved my job on the labour ward and in the outpatient clinic, seeing pregnant women. However, I also saw some general gynaecology, which did not inspire quite the same enthusiasm. I understood that if I wanted to specialise in obstetrics, I would also have to train in gynaecology. In addition, I quickly realised, from working with the residents who had already secured a training post, the road to achieving such a coveted position was long and hard, with no guarantee of success. The only thing that significantly increased one's odds of being successful in attaining such a post was finishing a PhD. This was a difficult process which I really didn't want to do.

One evening, while on call and waiting at the nurses' station for some action, I began discussing my misgivings with a local community midwife who was there to deliver one of her clients and was taking a coffee break. She thought about this for a minute and then suggested, 'Why don't you retrain as a midwife? Then you only have to do obstetrics, there is no PhD required and you can be your own boss'. At that time, there was a shortage of community midwives, so a job would have been easy to come by.

I thought about this for a few days and then made a call to the nearest school of midwifery. To my surprise and happiness, I was told that, due to previous training and work experience, they would be happy to have me and I could start in the final year. After a quick meeting with my bank manager, I quit my job and went back to school full-time. I graduated at the end of the year with the rest of my class and found a job in a lovely rural part of the country, in a group midwifery practice with four colleagues.

In retrospect, these were the happiest years of my life. Our clientele was friendly and down to earth, and almost everybody desired a homebirth. The obstetricians in the hospital were good colleagues and cooperation was fine. However, after a few years on the job and about 300 homebirths, I realised that I had learned all I could learn in a home-based midwifery setting. I began to feel the urge to do more for my clients than hand them over to the hospital staff when trouble arose. I wanted to be an obstetrician again. I secured a job as house officer at the local hospital, and started working on my CV in order to secure a training post. This was, as expected, no mean feat. It took a diversion to Belgium for me to finally be able to call myself a gynaecologist.

As my primary interest was still obstetrics, I secured a fellowship in perinatal medicine and afterwards a staff position in obstetrics at a university hospital. Until then, I had no special ideas about what kind of care I wanted to provide (other than 'good', or 'excellent'). That changed when I first heard the story of a woman in our area who, against medical advice, had her second baby at home after her first was born by c-section. A previous c-section means a scar on the uterus, which is at risk of rupturing during a subsequent labour. If this happens, the foetus is in acute danger and needs to be delivered immediately. Therefore, as in other countries, in the Netherlands a previous c-section means a hospital birth is recommended. This woman had apparently decided to ignore that advice and chosen a homebirth. I was intrigued. Does this really happen in the Netherlands? With homebirth and community midwives being an integral part of our maternity system, is there really a need or desire to go against medical advice? Together with some colleagues, I decided to study the phenomenon of women who decline medical advice in their birth choices, and a PhD project was born. During the following four years, I not only got the answers to my questions, but I also learned to view the care we deliver as health professionals in a whole new light.

Setting the scene of birth in the Netherlands

Each time I interact with midwives, birth activists or clients from other countries, I am told that the Netherlands is the Valhalla, for pregnant women and midwives alike, because we have an integrated homebirth system with primary care midwives as gatekeepers to secondary (hospital) care. However, whenever I speak to obstetric colleagues from other countries on social media, or at medical conferences all over the world, I receive ridicule for this exact same system. Statements are made to the effect that we (i.e. the Netherlands) are stuck in the Middle Ages, and that the Netherlands is the only high-income country where the natural course of pregnancy and childbirth can still be seen to unfold. While Dutch midwives are generally proud to be from the Netherlands and revel in the praise for their system, many Dutch obstetricians blush and mumble when confronted with the opinions of their colleagues from abroad, as they not infrequently feel the same way.

This duality is illustrative of the fact that midwives and obstetricians worldwide can have diametrically opposite views about which maternity care system is optimal or desirable. Both sides make several assumptions about maternity care in the Netherlands and most of these assumptions are actually incorrect. For instance, midwives elsewhere assume that most healthy women who carry normal term vertex babies have homebirths in the Netherlands. Obstetricians, on the other hand, seem to believe that, due to complications during homebirths, our maternal and perinatal outcomes are inferior to similar countries which have (almost) exclusively hospital-based maternity services.

In order to understand what is currently going on in Dutch maternity care (more on that later), we have to look at the history. For centuries, midwives were present at most births, which usually took place at home. In most developed countries, this changed gradually in the first half of the last century, with midwives losing their primacy, even in physiological births. With the increase in medical knowledge and treatment options for the prevention of adverse maternal and perinatal outcomes, maternity care moved into the domain of hospitals, where doctors and nurses took control over what is, in essence, a natural process. Midwives were still involved, but no longer in the capacity of lead caregiver. In the Netherlands, however, this move towards hospital care did not occur, at least not at the time and to the extent that it did elsewhere. Midwives retained their primacy as gatekeepers to second-tier maternity care. This development can perhaps be explained by the nature of Dutch people, seen as sober and down to earth. Another driving force has been the influence of insurance companies, who were (and are) loath to fund hospital care that could be delivered as well, and much more cost-effectively, at home. To this day, low-risk women who opt for a hospital birth have to pay a certain amount out of pocket for 'using more (expensive) care than they need'. Over the past six decades, midwives' insistence on their role as gatekeepers has caused an unabated string of clashes between their professional organisation and that of obstetricians.

To determine who is entitled to secondary (hospital, obstetrician-led) care, insurance companies in the 1950s, together with professionals, devised a list comprised of 39 reasons for secondary maternity care. Naturally, this list has evolved and expanded over the years, with the most recent version (from 2003) containing 143 reasons for referral. More indications result in more referrals, such that the 8.5% of women meeting criteria for hospital care in 1958 have evolved to 71.2% in 2017 (Ministry of Health, 2017). In addition to more women being referred by midwives for medical reasons, many of these referrals are also patient-driven, such as a substantial increase in requests for pharmacological pain relief (only available in secondary care in the Netherlands) and more women being unwilling to accept slow progress in labour.

Other developments in Dutch maternity care relate to the composition of midwifery and obstetric practices. In 1980, in the Netherlands, more than two-thirds of community midwives worked as solo practitioners and only 8.8% of midwives worked in a group of three or more. By the year 2015, there was a complete turnaround, with only 5% of midwives working solo and 80% in a group of three or more (Netherlands Institute for Health Services Research, 2016). In addition, group practices are growing in size, with groups of six to eight midwives becoming common in recent years. The same phenomenon occurs in hospitals, where, due to several factors such as feminisation of the profession, an increase in part-time roles and mergers between different hospitals, women are now likely to see groups of obstetricians of not just three to five, but frequently between ten and 20. In 1980, there were 7.5 maternity care providers per 1000 pregnant Dutch women. By the year 2015, the number of care providers had grown to 24.3. Therefore, the number of representatives of both professions that women encounter has more than tripled in the past four decades.

All of the above is illustrative of the fact that the idealised image of Dutch women having a cosy homebirth with their known midwife, in this day and age, is the exception rather than the rule. In spite of this, the Netherlands is still the world leader in homebirths in the developed world, with 12.7% of all births occurring at home in 2017 (Ministry of Health, 2017). Another 15.1% occur in midwife-led birthing centres or hospital units, at the woman's own request.

Another myth that needs dispelling is the claim that homebirths in the Netherlands are responsible for more adverse outcomes when compared to other European countries. In fact, in a large study comparing maternal and perinatal outcomes in 743,070 low-risk women, no difference was found for any outcomes, except for a *lower* incidence of Apgar scores below 7 and NICU admissions for homebirths in parous women (de Jonge et al., 2015). It appears, therefore, that the position of the Netherlands in the middle range of European perinatal mortality statistics (Euro Peristat Project, 2018) is not due to the availability of homebirth for low-risk women, but rather to a number of other factors.

In summary, the picture exalted by midwives around the world, of the Netherlands as a haven of physiological (home) birth is not strictly accurate (any more), but neither is the notion of obstetricians elsewhere that in the Netherlands babies are at increased risk of dying because we insist on birthing them at home.

The road to enlightenment: you can never go back

As stated at the start of this chapter, I embarked on a PhD looking at why some women in the Netherlands, with 'everything on offer', choose to birth outside the system. During our research into why women choose to go against medical advice in their birth choices, I discovered a whole new world. We talked to 28 women who had all made choices against medical advice (Hollander et al., 2017a). In order to not 'muddy the waters' with 'light cases', we focused on women who had made choices that would really upset most maternity care professionals. This was when I first heard about the phenomenon of 'unassisted childbirth' (UC), or 'freebirth'. After speaking with seven women who had decided not to call anyone when labour started, I began to question several instances of 'born before arrival' (BBA) which I had encountered in my own practice as a midwife. The thought that my tardy appearance might have been purposefully planned by my client had never entered my mind at the time.

The other 21 women we spoke with for the study had all had homebirths in high-risk pregnancies, with the majority attempting a vaginal birth after caesarean (VBAC), a twin or a breech birth at home. Their stories made me question everything I had always taken for granted about the way we deliver care. Many of these women had had a previous traumatic childbirth experience, and had lost their trust in the maternity care system and in their providers. Themes we found during those interviews centred around a pathway of a traumatic experience, followed by self-education through access to medical literature, books, blogs and social media (Holten, Hollander, & De Miranda, 2018). The women used the information gathered to weigh the evidence underpinning medical advice, such as it was, sometimes coming to a different conclusion. The next step was to prepare a birth plan that did not quite fit within medical protocol. Discussion of this plan with their providers would meet with a paternalistic style of decision-making and a 'my way or the highway' approach. The women then chose the highway, opting for either a homebirth or a freebirth. In most cases, they would have been willing to give birth in hospital if only (some of) their wishes had been met. The final result was women assuming a higher medical risk than they originally set out to do because they encountered no flexibility from their provider to negotiate the birth plan and no willingness to make concessions. One of the women I talked to was Jeske, whose story I will reproduce here, in her own words.

Jeske is expecting her first child. She has had a difficult childhood, and not many friends or family. The pregnancy is complicated by severe pelvic pain and she has difficulty walking. Around the due date, labour starts suddenly and one contraction quickly follows another. She calls her midwifery practice, and a locum midwife, whom she has never seen before, comes to her house. After several hours and only 2 cm of dilation, she asks her midwife for pain relief and she is transported to the hospital for an epidural. Jeske feels that the anesthetist is in a hurry. 'I was forced to sit cross-legged and couldn't move. Meanwhile it was one contraction after another.' Pain relief is suboptimal and Jeske is surrounded by unknown people. She remembers being told to lie on her back without much explanation, and an electrode is placed on the baby's head. When she reaches complete dilation, she is told to start pushing, even though she feels no urge. She is left pushing with a nurse for 45 minutes, after which an obstetrician enters. All she remembers of this is him saying: 'I am here to help you.' The next thing she remembers is that he 'pushes the ventouse in', without much in the way of explanation. She has no idea what to do, but tries to push. It is in vain. She is taken to the operating theatre for an emergency caesarean section.

At the follow-up appointment six weeks later, Jeske has recovered well physically, but nobody asks her how she feels about the birth. She has recurring nightmares, and has been experiencing vaginismus ever since, which was never an issue for her before.

A year later, Jeske is pregnant again. This time she is resolved to do things differently. She reads books about natural childbirth and joins several social media groups. She wants to have a homebirth and discusses this with her midwifery practice. They advise against it because of her previous caesarean section, but arrange for Jeske to speak to an obstetrician, in a different hospital this time. The conversation goes well. Jeske is open to discussing a hospital birth, but does not want foetal monitoring. She wants to deliver with her own midwife, and have a water birth. Most of all, she wants to stay in control and be left alone during labour. Even though the obstetrician is willing to meet her halfway, and will allow for all of her wishes, except no foetal monitoring, Jeske decides to pursue a homebirth. She feels that the risk of unnecessary interventions due to false positive foetal monitoring readings, during which she will again lose her autonomy, far outweighs the risk of complications due to uterine rupture. This means that, in the third trimester of her pregnancy, she has to find another midwife to assist her. After several weeks of frantic phone calls, she finds a midwife about an hour away, who agrees to be by her side.

Jeske has 'a glorious water birth at home, with confidence and trust'. She feels that, as opposed to her first labour, she did this one by herself. Even the fact that she has to go to the hospital in the end for a manual removal of the placenta does not bother her in the least.

Jeske's story is reflective of the stories many women told us about what had happened to make them decide to go a different way.

What do partners say about birthing outside the system?

We also talked to the partners of the women we interviewed. The most noteworthy finding from these conversations was the fact that, in almost all cases, the idea to go against medical advice originated with the women. They had done the research and convinced their partners of the merit of their plans. Once convinced, the partners became fierce advocates for the women and the birth choices they made together, both when interacting with their respective families and with maternity care providers. Some partners even went as far as confronting medical staff during a hospital appointment, which they attended instead of their spouse, as this quote illustrates:

> The last week before the due date the doctor wanted another meeting. [Wife] felt like: 'I don't want to talk unless he has something [new] to

> offer.' [...] She didn't want to go, so I said: I will go and talk to him. [...] It was a pretty stressful meeting. I was glad [wife] wasn't there. She had gone through enough.

All partners were in support of the final plan, although one regretted this in hindsight.

What do the midwives who support high-risk women to birth at home say?

All women who had a homebirth and had a high-risk pregnancy were attended by a midwife. As discussed before, high-risk pregnancies are outside the scope of community midwifery practice, so these midwives were operating well outside their mandate. Most community midwives are very cautious about attending such births, fearing a bad outcome and disciplinary action from the medical review board. However, there is a small group of Dutch midwives, mostly working in case-load practice, who are willing to attend these births. We interviewed 24 of them, which make up the majority of this group nationwide (Hollander, de Miranda, Vandenbussche, van Dillen, & Holten, 2019). When asked why and how they practise, they told us that they consider themselves the last safety net between these women and an unassisted high-risk homebirth. They attend the birth because, once these women have decided that the hospital is no longer an option, there isn't anybody else that will support them. These midwives forge a close bond of mutual trust with their clients, in circumstances where continuity and the client–provider relationship are central. Their clients have to trust them enough to be willing to be referred if things go awry. They spend a great deal of time talking with their clients in order to ascertain that the woman understands all the risks her choice entails, and that she can 'carry herself', even if things do not work out the way they hope, as the following quotes illustrate:

> And so in some way I was the final destination, because after me there was nobody else who could say: oh well, go to the next midwife, she will do it, she will help you. [...] Yes, someone had to be with that woman, somebody had to do it, you know.
>
> If a client approaches me the first thing I ask myself [about her] is: can you carry yourself? Are you [...] prepared to deal with your process and reflect on it? And are we capable of establishing a meaningful relationship?

What do midwives and obstetricians say about women who birth outside the system?

We also interviewed many mainstream midwives and obstetricians who had been involved in one or more high-risk cases in order to understand their take on what happens when a woman choses to birth outside the system. Many expressed great surprise at the choices their clients make and are mystified as to where it had all gone wrong. Several obstetricians expressed profound disbelief that women were willing to endanger themselves and their baby in order to have the kind of birth they 'desired', although others said they understood how the system did not meet the needs of some. The obstetricians also discussed ways health professionals could do more to retain the trust and confidence of their clients, as the following quote illustrates:

> What I am realising more and more, is that we are slowly moving from 'informed-consent' to 'shared decision' to 'informed choice'. In which the patient makes an informed choice, and that you … that I find myself respecting that more and more.
>
> I also feel that we are learning a lot from this. I think that […] patients are having trouble recognising themselves in hospital care as it is sometimes offered. Too impersonal, not involved enough. That they really miss that [the personal involvement] and opt for a caseload midwife to monitor their pregnancy and … I actually feel that you can make tremendous use of that model and still have a good basic outcome for these women.

Looking at the impact of birth trauma on the choice to birth outside the system

Because a traumatic experience, either during a previous birth or during the current pregnancy, was a common theme in our interviews with women and their partners, we decided to conduct a second study in order to elucidate the origins of this trauma (Hollander et al., 2017b).

We designed an online questionnaire and asked more than 2000 women with a self-reported traumatic experience about: (a) the nature of their trauma; and (b) what professionals might have done differently to prevent this. The results were surprising. As we expected, women mentioned interventions and adverse events during childbirth as causes of their trauma. However, when asked how we, as professionals, might have prevented the traumatic experience, the women said that we should have communicated better, supported the women more by staying with them during birth, and explained what was happening and why.

As it turns out, it wasn't so much the occurrence of complications as the lack of communication surrounding these events which made it a traumatic experience. In addition, women told us how unprepared they were for the realities of childbirth and how they were not aware of the odds that the complications would actually happen to them in hospital. There were lessons to be learned here. For the past 15 years, I had always been convinced that we, as care providers, were doing a good job in taking care of our clients. Here were thousands of women who had ended up being traumatised and dozens who felt so unsafe in our hospitals they would rather have a high-risk homebirth with a midwife. All this made me thoroughly rethink everything

I thought I knew about my job. It made me realise that, when doctors and patients disagree, the patient is the one who has the final say. When we, as professionals, refuse to make any concessions, the result is not that women will fall in line, but rather that they turn their backs on us and end up taking more risks than they initially set out to do. It seems a change in paradigm is in order.

The trials and tribulations of a dedicated clinic

The realisation that trying to force women into a protocol only results in driving them further away from the care that we as providers feel is optimal was a turning point in my professional life. I had heard of a clinic in Amsterdam which used a special approach to support women with birth plans that were (far) outside recommendations, and, together with a colleague, we decided to start a similar clinic in our own hospital in Nijmegen.

Women are referred to our clinic by primary care midwives from the community, in-house by colleagues, or by hospital staff elsewhere. Women are seen at the clinic a minimum of three times. The community midwife providing care for the woman in each case is encouraged to attend all clinic visits with the woman. Visits are structured according to a predetermined plan, but are flexible because no two 'cases' are identical. The first visit lasts approximately one hour and is reserved exclusively for listening to the woman's plans and ideas for the upcoming birth, and determining what motivates certain refusals or requests. Because previous trauma has been shown to be an important part of women's reasons for wanting to deviate from advice, much time is spent exploring a woman's past obstetric history, with emphasis on how women feel about these births in hindsight, and how those feelings influence her current plans and ideas. We also seek to determine the extent of the woman's understanding of relevant risks and chances, without immediately countering these cognitions with our own interpretation of the evidence.

During the second visit, if we are convinced that enough trust has been earned for the woman to feel that she wants to hear our advice, the relevant guidelines are discussed. In this conversation, the evidence (and also sometimes lack of evidence) behind these recommendations is presented in a non-threatening way. The aim is to inform, not to frighten her into consenting to protocols. Risks and chances are presented with actual numbers and percentages, not odds ratios, and both numbers needed to treat and numbers needed to harm are used in discussions. In addition, levels of evidence are discussed, with more emphasis placed on high-level evidence than on recommendations through professional consensus.

Finally, in the last visit, solutions are explored. If the woman still wishes to deviate from recommendations, alternative solutions are discussed. These can consist of a medical birth with fewer interventions than recommended, a hospital birth with a community midwife, or a homebirth with a community midwife. The purpose, throughout the entire process, is to find a solution that is acceptable to the woman, with minimum risk for her and her child.

If an agreement is reached which is deemed a challenge for the maternity department team, a 'moral case deliberation' is called. This meeting is chaired by a member of the hospital ethics staff, and all maternity care team members, including the community midwife, are invited. The woman and her partner are invited to present their wishes to the team and answer a few questions. Then the team continues the meeting behind closed doors, where all team members can discuss their feelings about the plan. In these discussions, the autonomous preferences of the woman (and partner) are weighed against the professional responsibilities of the maternity team. However, the team is legally obliged to respect the woman's refusal, except when an alternative hospital can be found that is more comfortable with the birth plan. In very rare cases, when several team members are very uncomfortable with the plan, my colleague at the clinic and I may offer to be on call for a particular birth. All information given to the woman and her partner, as well as the content of their objections and the final plan are documented extensively in the chart. All passages are copied in an email and sent to the woman. There is no need for signatures, as making her/them sign anything is not considered conducive to the mutual trust required for the birth.

This clinic, unfortunately, meets with a lot of resistance from colleagues around the country. They feel that guidelines and protocols are there for a reason: they provide the best odds for a 'good' outcome for both mother and child. They believe we should not deviate from our protocols, and if a woman will not accept this, she is free to go elsewhere. This, of course, is the same attitude that was encountered by most of the women we interviewed. Professionals are afraid of a bad outcome. They feel that, if they accept what they view as second-best care and there is an unfavourable outcome, they can be held responsible by both the disciplinary board and a civil or even criminal court. This way of thinking is also quite prevalent among community midwives, many of whom are hesitant to accept a client for homebirth when the woman has a high-risk pregnancy.

Legally, both groups of care providers are incorrect. Dutch law and jurisprudence from the disciplinary board clearly state that assisting a woman in labour on her own terms can be deemed as 'emergency assistance' and must always be provided, as long as it is clear from the case notes that the provider recommended against this course of action on several different occasions and the woman is well aware of the risks involved with her birth plan. In addition, if a woman decides to have a homebirth when experiencing a high-risk pregnancy because she has found no possibility of compromise in her hospital and there are complications leading to a bad outcome, it is possible that disciplinary action can be initiated against the hospital for being unwilling to accommodate her wishes. This scenario has yet to happen.

The challenges of working the way we do continue. In the meantime, our clinic has seen around 40 women in the past four years who had birth plans that did not align with medical advice. Many, if not most, of these women wanted a homebirth when they had a high-risk pregnancy or were prepared to have one if they encountered a resistant or more rigid approach. There were a few cases in which women desired a homebirth for its own sake to such an extent that nothing we could offer would change their minds. However, in the greater majority of cases, we were able to reach a compromise and arrive at a birth plan, in hospital, which was acceptable to all parties. In two cases, the final birth plans were so far outside protocol that my colleague and I were on call for those births. All outcomes so far have been good, with no perinatal or maternal deaths or serious morbidity. As an example of the difference this clinic can make for women, I will share with you the story of Karen.

Karen was pregnant for the third time, and this time it was twins. She had experienced her second birth as a traumatic event. She had had a very quick labour in her local hospital, with contractions coming hard and fast. The only position in which she could manage her contractions was on her hands and knees. Every time a midwife tried to get her to lie on her back for a vaginal exam, the next wave of contractions rushed through her. At one point she had been forced on her back and examined, just when she started to feel the urge to push.

It had taken Karen a long time to process this traumatic experience. When she found herself pregnant again and discovered it was twins, she felt dread, because she knew that this would mean another hospital birth, but also more pressure to birth on her back, as it would be easier to keep a close eye on the condition of the twins that way. She was convinced she could not give birth on her back.

Karen really wanted a homebirth, but realised that a twin pregnancy was indeed high-risk, and therefore considered going to a hospital.

When her local hospital had turned down her entire birth plan, she came to our clinic because she had heard that perhaps we might be willing to accommodate some of her wishes. She explained she wanted no vaginal exams, no foetal monitoring, no IVs or active management of the third stage, and to give birth to both babies on her hands and knees. We followed the steps of our clinic, and explained to her why we as providers felt that all of those interventions were indicated for a twin birth, while at the same time reassuring her that she had the right to refuse any and all of them, if she was convinced she didn't want them. In addition, we went over all possible scenarios with Karen, from placental abruption and foetal malposition in the inter-twin interval, to management of postpartum haemorrhage, right up to a hysterectomy for intractable bleeding, so that if something untoward started happening during the birth, she would know what all the steps would be, and there would be no precious time lost in discussions.

After several consultations it was clear that Karen's mind was made up. She wanted to stick to her plan, and if we were not willing to honour her refusal she would stay at home. This plan caused great discomfort among our colleagues, who believed it increased the possibility of a bad outcome for both Karen and her twins to the extent that they felt unable to deliver care in her case. Therefore, I attended Karen's birth on my day off.

It was a quick labour. At several points I again offered foetal monitoring and vaginal exams, and made notes in her chart when she declined. This had also been discussed in the clinic beforehand, and she knew I would be doing so. Karen gave birth to both of her babies in quick succession, on her hands and knees, just like she wanted. A baby boy and baby girl were born in good health. When the placenta also arrived in short order and with minimal blood loss, I was relieved and very happy for Karen. However, while I was writing up my case notes 45 minutes later, I was called back by the nurse because Karen had started to bleed. In no time at all, she lost a lot of blood. I told her: 'This is what we discussed in the clinic. It is happening now. We need to take the necessary steps', and she said 'Fine. Do whatever you think is necessary.' We had to take her to theatre, and managed to stop the bleeding with a tamponnade. When it was over she had lost 2600 millilitres. Luckily she remained stable throughout and was able to leave the hospital with her twins after 2 days.

Karen's story illustrates several points. First, if we hadn't discussed all possible steps of the postpartum haemorrhage protocol beforehand, she might not have agreed to everything as quickly as she did and would likely have lost even more blood. Second and most importantly, if we had not treated her and her birth plan respectfully, we would not have gained her trust to the extent that she was willing to come to the hospital when her labour started. If she would have stayed at home, she would very likely have lost much more blood and the situation could have turned life-threatening very quickly. Third, and in my opinion, Karen's case illustrates the importance of being willing to honour birth plans that are against medical advice, not because that will make care more dangerous but because it actually makes care safer.

Where do we go from here?

Because there is no reporting of high-risk birth at home, it is currently unknown how many women decide to have a homebirth with a high-risk pregnancy each year in the Netherlands. There are also no data on the annual number of unassisted births; however, estimates in the freebirth community range around 200 (from a total of 170,000 births annually nationwide). The general impression among maternity care providers is that these numbers are increasing, due to growing dissatisfaction with the system, women's greater access to medical information and social media and a change in perception towards medical authority. In addition, it is safe to assume that for every woman who takes the big step to go against medical advice in this way, there are many others with similar misgivings who hold their tongues and just hope for the best.

As stated above, maternity care in the Netherlands, too, has gradually been shifting to more hospital and medicalised births. This puts a strain on the system of community midwives as gatekeepers to secondary (hospital) care. If most community midwives only attend a very small number of homebirths per year, are they still safe? Can homebirths still be called 'the norm' if only a small minority of women actually end up having one? How should we, as professionals, address the lack of continuity associated with antepartum or peripartum transfers of care, a known risk factor for traumatic birth experiences? What is clear to me is that the current Dutch system of hosting two parallel but vastly different echelons of care, each of which maintain a strict wall of separation and impose black-and-white selection criteria for the allocation of care, has become unsustainable. When the majority of primiparous women who start labour with a community midwife are transferred to a different location and an all-new team during birth triggering a known risk of trauma, it is time to break down that wall and aim for integrated care.

In the past eight or nine years, this realisation has also dawned on governing bodies and organisations regulating maternity care in this country. Pathways and structures for integrated maternity care are being implemented. This is a very slow process for several reasons. First, there are different concepts of what integrated care looks like, ranging from midwife-led care for all women (the UK model), to midwives employed by hospitals who work under the supervision of an obstetrician (obstetrician-led care, the US model). Second, there is of course the issue of money. About half of all Dutch obstetricians are salaried, while the other half are self-employed in group practices. Community midwives are usually self-employed and earn several times the amount their hospital-based, salaried colleagues earn. Many plans for integrated care pathways have become stranded around the issue of money. If both midwives and obstetricians care for the same woman, who gets to bill the insurance company? They are certainly not willing to pay two claimants who both delivered half the care, as both parties can only bill for the full amount. And are community midwives prepared to become salaried in an integrated birth facility, if that means losing approximately half their income? Last but not least, there is the issue of medical responsibility. Who is legally responsible for which care, if we all work as a team and there is no longer a strict division between-low risk and high-risk? These are the issues occupying Dutch maternity care professionals at this point in time.

I am not claiming I have all the answers. What I do know is that we can't go on the way we have been, where a lack of flexibility, continuity, time and respect for women's wishes and so many decisions based on fear are traumatising so many women.

The relationship between provider and client will have to be a truly equal partnership, in which we as professionals are not the ones who decide but rather guide the client in reaching the decision that is most in line with her views and values. This means that the protocol or guideline is the starting point of the conversation, instead of the bottom line. We will have to practice actual shared decision-making, as shared decision-making is an art often avowed but rarely practised, and not, as is so often the reality, 'I share my decision with you'. We need to counsel with absolute risks, numbers needed to treat and numbers needed to harm instead of using odds ratios, and we need to learn to communicate risk without appearing to be 'shroud waving' (threatening women with the prospect of a dead baby). We need to start realising the importance of the language we use when talking to or about our clients, and learn to refer to them not as 'the c-section in room 1', but 'the woman who delivered by c-section in room 1'. When discussing birth plans, we will have to learn to start with the question: 'What matters to you?', and refrain from using phrases such as 'you can't' (yes, she can) and 'you have to' (no, she doesn't). Finally, if a woman has decided to have a homebirth in a high-risk pregnancy with a holistic midwife, we will have to accept that this midwife is the only assistance the woman wants. Our professional organisations (and healthcare insurance companies) will have to work harder to achieve consensus on the importance and definition of continuity of care, in order to better establish a relationship of trust between ourselves and our clients, because that is an important contributing factor to our joint ability to reach a compromise. Finally, we are going to have to try to teach all the above to our residents and midwifery students, who, despite being in this era of 'putting the client first', are being trained to follow protocol more than ever before. Indeed, if we are successful in teaching flexibility and the relative value of protocol-based care, this may benefit not only women who decline recommended care, but all women in maternity care.

The view of a Dutch midwife

Ank de Jonge, Professor of Midwifery Science, AVAG/Midwifery Science, Amsterdam Public Health, Amsterdam University Medical Center and practising primary care midwife at Midwifery Practice 'Vondelpark' in Amsterdam

It is great to read how an obstetrician is as passionate about the need to provide continuity of care to women as I am. This is crucial for reducing birth trauma and enhancing women's birth experience. Low-risk women in the Netherlands benefit from having continuity of care from their primary care midwife and have choices in place of birth which includes homebirth; however, many women are transferred to hospital care and most of them are looked after by clinical midwives and obstetric nurses in hospital who often look after more than one woman.

Midwives, obstetricians, other maternity care professionals, insurance companies and policy-makers have to work out a way to implement continuity of care by one midwife or a small team of midwives for all women. The challenge is to focus on *continuity of carer*, which is not the same as all professionals working in one system. Experiences in many countries show that cost-effective continuity of care projects that lead to good outcomes are discontinued if obstetric units need the staff and resources. Separate resources may therefore need to be allocated to continuity of care given by midwives to ensure its viability.

The current caseload of primary care midwives in the Netherlands is more than double the caseload of midwives in other countries who provide continuity of care. The fee for intrapartum care is based on attending to women in labour for an average length of time and referring a considerable number of them. Some midwives take on a higher caseload than is the norm for a full-time midwife. However, others try to continue looking after women after transfer of care, although they are not paid to do so, and several are paid based on a part-time caseload. Important questions for the Netherlands are: are all midwives prepared to provide continuity of care in the community and in hospital? How do we optimise collaboration between professionals so that all women can receive continuity of care? Are we prepared to allocate adequate resources to the provision of continuity of care? If we want to reduce the numbers of women traumatised by their births and re-engage women to birth within our system of maternity care we need to get our models of care right and relationship-based care is the best way to do this.

The way forward

- In the case of birth plans that go against medical advice, being willing to compromise as providers actually makes birth safer
- A change in paradigm is needed: providers in the Netherlands need to restructure maternity care with an emphasis on continuity of caregiver and counselling without fear
- The attitude of 'my way or the highway' must stop as it is driving women to choose the highway and take additional unnecessary risks
- Guidelines and protocols are important, but must never usurp women's right to make a choice, even if it is outside current recommendations
- Having a designated multidisciplinary clinic to advise women who have significant risk factors and make high-risk choices can help avert poor outcomes and trauma

References

De Jonge, A., Geerts, C. C., Van Der Goes, B. Y., Mol, B.W., Buitendijk, S. E., & Nijhuis, J. G. (2015) Perinatal mortality and morbidity up to 28 days after birth among 743 070 low-risk planned home and hospital births: A cohort study based on three merged national perinatal databases. *British Journal of Obstetrics and Gynaecology*, *122*, 720–728.

Euro Peristat Project. (2018) European Perinatal Health Report: Core indicators of the health and care of pregnant women and babies in Europe in 2015. Retrieved from: www.europeristat.com/images/EPHR2015_web_hyperlinked_Euro-Peristat.pdf.

Hollander, M., De Miranda, E., Van Dillen, J., De Graaf, I., Vandenbussche, F., & Holten, L. (2017a) Women's motivations for choosing a high risk birth setting against medical advice in the Netherlands: A qualitative analysis. *BMC Pregnancy and Childbirth*, *17*, 423.

Hollander, M., Van Hastenberg, E., Van Dillen, J., Van Pampus, M., De Miranda, E., & Stramrood, C. (2017b) Preventing traumatic childbirth experiences: 2192 women's perceptions and views. *Archive of Women's Mental Health*, *20*, 515–523.

Hollander, M., de Miranda, E., Vandenbussche, F., van Dillen, J., & Holten, L. (2019). Addressing a need. Holistic midwifery in the Netherlands: A qualitative analysis. *PLoS ONE*. https://doi.org/10.1371/journal.pone.0220489

Holten, L., Hollander, M., & De Miranda, E. (2018) When the hospital is no longer an option: A multiple case study of defining moments for women choosing home birth in high-risk pregnancies in the Netherlands. *Qualitative Health Research*, *28*, 1883–1896.

Ministry of Health. (2017) Ministry of Health statistics on location of all Dutch births in 2017. Retrieved from: www.staatvenz.nl/kerncijfers/bevallingen.

Netherlands Institute For Health Services Research (2016). Netherlands Institute for Health Services Research: Self-reported midwife registration of working situation in 2016. Retrieved from:www.nivel.nl/sites/default/files/cijfers-uit-de-registratie-van-verloskundigen-peiling-jan-2016.pdf.

5 The rise of the unregulated birth worker in Australia

The canary flees the coal mine

Elizabeth Rigg

> A birth worker's behaviour is more aligned to the midwifery philosophy of 'woman centred care' than a registered midwife. They don't have hospital policy or supervisors to deal with and so they can actually be 'with women'.
>
> (Woman who chose an unregulated birth worker, Rigg et al., 2018b, p. 7)

About the author

In 1992, I (Elizabeth Rigg) immigrated to Australia. I trained as a midwife in the UK and worked my way up the ranks to my dream job as midwife in the community. In this role, I experienced tremendous respect from colleagues and the medical profession who seemed to really value midwives, ethical practice and the provision of quality maternity services that not only met women's needs but also reflected what women wanted. I wanted to continue my role as a woman's advocate and midwife in Australia. However, I quickly realised that Australian midwives do not enjoy the same level of respect or autonomy in practice as their European counterparts. The Australian system seemed like a very hostile place, with limited respect for women or acknowledgement of midwives' capabilities. The reasons for this were not clear to me, but there seemed to be a focus on maintaining ownership of the commodity (*the pregnant woman*) and ensuring sustainability of health providers' financial security in a medically dominated system.

The stimulus for my research occurred in 2010, when I was caring for a woman who was admitted following a homebirth with an unregulated birth worker (UBW). The woman presented in a critical condition. She had given birth several hours earlier on a rural property and transferred to hospital in the UBW's car. The UBW reported to the hospital staff that the woman had an uneventful birth but lost approximately 500 millilitres of blood post-birth. The UBW departed the hospital and was not seen again. The woman required life-saving care and was transferred to the operating theatre for a manual removal of her placenta. Her condition remained serious for approximately 48 hours and she required a transfusion of several units of blood. The woman was unwilling to identify or share information about the UBW. I had not come across UBWs previously, so I asked the hospital midwives about them. They acknowledged, to my surprise, the existence of UBWs practising in the area. This experience made me question why a woman might choose a UBW over a registered midwife to facilitate birth at home and prompted me to understand a woman's motives for not identifying the UBW, given the severity of the complications she experienced.

In 2012, I commenced my PhD under the supervision of Professors Hannah Dahlen and Virginia Schmied, seeking to investigate the role of UBWs in Australia from the perspectives of women and birth workers. My study used a mixed-methods, sequential exploratory design, and is the first of its kind in Australia to explore UBWs as a distinct group.

The rise of UBWs

As the option for midwife-supported homebirth becomes increasingly restricted in countries like Australia and the USA, there appears to be a rise in UBWs attending birth at home. A UBW can be anyone who provides support services to women during pregnancy and childbirth. They have no regulatory requirements for formal or supervised training that would enable them to have recognition as a registered midwife or doctor; however, they may have knowledge and experience of childbirth. UBWs normally work as independent birth workers with no formal or informal organisational structure. This means UBW practice is not regulated. UBWs can include doulas, lay-midwives, childbirth educators, hypnotherapists, nutritionists, naturopaths and ex-registered midwives or overseas-trained midwives who are not eligible or who chose not to register with the Australian regulatory authority, the Australian Health Practitioner Regulatory Authority (AHPRA) (Schapel, 2012; Rigg, Schmied, Peters, & Dahlen, 2015). While most UBWs do not call themselves a midwife, many practise skills and provide services that resemble midwifery. UBWs practise and provide services similar to a midwife across all states in Australia and their numbers appear to be rising. The largest numbers of UBWs seem to reside in Queensland, New South Wales and Victoria, which are also the most populated states (Rigg, Schmied, Peters, & Dahlen, 2018a).

The rise of UBWs in Australia represents a significant and concerning phenomenon. The underlying reasons for this increase appear to be a lack of support for homebirth and a limited or small number of midwives who provide homebirth services (Dahlen, 2012; Rigg, Schmied, Peters, & Dahlen, 2017). We previously argued that the regulation of midwives in Australia is excessive, which prevents them from practising to their full scope of practice (Rigg, Schmied, Peters, & Dahlen, 2018b). While midwifery models of care are becoming more available in Australia, access to these models, including publicly funded homebirth,[1] is restricted to women who are low-risk. Women in Australia must demonstrate they satisfy strict medical eligibility selection criteria to access a publicly funded homebirth choice and they must remain low-risk throughout their childbirth journey to continue to enjoy the service (Royal Australian and New Zealand College of Obstetricians and Gynaecologists (RANCOG), 2017). Not all states in Australia provide a publicly funded homebirth service, and the numbers of privately practising midwives who can provide this service have dwindled significantly, mainly due to issues related to the lack of an insurance product to cover intrapartum care since 2002. The maternity service reforms in Australia in 2010 promised women greater access to midwives and midwifery models of care by enabling midwives access to Medicare[2] and the Pharmaceuticals Benefits Scheme,[3] but these came with significant problems. Privately practising midwives experienced significant difficulties meeting the new regulatory requirements for indemnity insurance and collaborative working agreements with medical service providers as there has been reluctance to work with privately practising midwives or to give them access to hospital services (Nursing and Midwifery Board of Australia, 2016). Essentially, these issues have limited women's access to midwives even more, with many privately practising midwives either ceasing practice altogether or surrendering their registration in order to work as UBWs (Schapel, 2012).

The drivers in the Australian maternity system

The dominant model of maternity care provided to women in Australia is a medical model, which is characterised by high rates of intervention and limited options. The current caesarean section rate for Australia is high (33%), which is one of the highest in the world (Organisation for Economic Cooperation and Development, 2018). Intervention in birth can place a woman at greater risk of experiencing a complication as a result of that intervention. It also means women carry a label of being high-risk in future pregnancies (Rigg et al., 2017, 2018a). From a woman's perspective, this can feel like the system and professionals are manipulating them to secure a future need for medical care. From a midwife's perspective, the consequences of not practising in accordance with professional regulations can mean the threat of disciplinary action, which can include the loss of registration and livelihood. In turn, this can lead to defensive practice rather than woman-centred practice. When women feel their wishes are not being met or feel disrespected by caregivers, this can lead to feeling they have no other option but to avoid the mainstream system and medical model of care. By choosing a UBW, women may feel they can avoid a repeat negative experience and it may present their only chance at having a homebirth (Rigg et al., 2017).

Exposing the issue of UBWs through coronial enquiries

A high-profile coroner's case involving an ex-registered midwife in South Australia (SA) has generated significant media attention over the past seven years (Mamamia News, 2012; Schapel, 2012). This ex-registered midwife had migrated to Australia from the UK in 2003. She worked as a midwife in charge of a labour ward in a SA private hospital for two years before setting up her private practice in 2005 as an independent midwife providing homebirth services to women in Adelaide (Barrett, 2013). The midwife became well-known as a homebirth advocate through her practice and a blog she developed (Barrett, 2013). However, she increasingly provided homebirth services to women with high-risk pregnancies, at a time when midwives were either restricted from caring for those women or were not available. In early 2011, six months after the Australian National Law[4] was introduced in South Australia, this midwife relinquished her registration as a midwife. She asserted that the new legislative regulations prevented midwives from supporting women. Between 2007 and 2009, three infants died following a homebirth attended by this UBW, and all three mothers had risk factors (Schapel, 2012). According to the description given by the deputy coroner examining the infant deaths, the UBW had commenced practice as a birth advocate working privately within the 'homebirth industry' (Schapel, 2012). Two separate planned homebirths in 2011, with mothers who were high-risk and attended by this UBW, resulted in the deaths of a further two infants. Deputy Coroner Schapel's (2012) inquest investigated the deaths of three of the babies delivered by this UBW, as one of the infant deaths occurred outside SA's jurisdiction. The coroner found the infants would have survived if the mothers had birthed in hospital. While there have been other cases in Australia that have not resulted in coronial inquiries, the coroner in this case found the UBW practised midwifery skills despite her claims that her role was to support the mothers' homebirth choice and provide labour support (Schapel, 2012, p. 94).

Literature has highlighted how the existence of underground midwifery practices occurring in Australia only becomes evident when charges are laid against practitioners (Barclay, Brodie, Lane, Reiger, & Tracy, 2003). Coroner Schapel highlighted deficiencies in the Health Practitioners Regulation National Act 2009, which made it possible for UBWs to circumvent requirements of the National Law (2009) regarding insurance for intrapartum care and compliance with codes and midwifery standards of practice (Schapel, 2012). He made recommendations for the urgent introduction and adoption, at the National level, of legislation that would 'render it an offence for a person to engage in the practice of midwifery, including its practice in respect of management of the three stages of labour, without being a midwife or a medical practitioner registered pursuant to the National Law' (Schapel, 2012, p. 3; Government of South Australia, 2013). While this proposal was presented as a public safety initiative to protect women and their infants' health and well-being, it also worked to further deny Australian women their right to choose how and with whom they give birth (World Health Organisation, 2018). This is at odds with Australia's international obligations to protect women's human rights to equality, dignity and the highest attainable level of health (United Nations, 2015). It can also serve to drive homebirth underground.

A proposal to protect midwifery practice in SA

In January 2013, the SA government published a *Proposal to Protect Midwifery Practice in SA Consultation Paper* and sought public consultation over a three-month period (Government of SA, 2013). The Consultation Paper expressed concerns about the increasing numbers of UBWs providing support to women birthing at home and the need to protect the public from harm (Government of SA, 2013). The proposed legislation was intended to restrict the practice of midwifery to registered midwives who fulfil all regulatory requirements and further restrict women's access to homebirth services from UBWs.

Despite the high-profile media coverage of the events that inspired this proposed legislation, the SA Health Department only received 33 submissions (Rigg et al., 2015). Of these, 30 submissions were publicly available, which we analysed. Twenty-five (78%) of these submissions supported the legislation, five (16%) opposed it and two (6%) were neither for nor against the legislation. Respondents included: professional midwifery, nursing and medical organisations, individual midwives (13), consumer organisations (three), a General Practitioner, a hospital-based registered nurse and an individual consumer. One overarching theme we entitled 'not addressing the root cause' was identified in the submissions, comprising seven themes and five subthemes. This overarching theme suggested the legislation being proposed did not address the underlying reasons why women choose UBWs to attend their birth at home (Figure 5.1). The rest of the themes and subthemes related to the barriers and effects of a broken system including legislative, regulatory and health system barriers which women experienced as traumatising, as well as the unintended consequences, unclear boundaries and a need for a better way forward.

Following the public consultation process, further legislation was introduced in SA to amend existing legislation in 2013 entitled 'Health Practitioner Regulation National Law (SA) (Restricted Birthing Practices) Amendment Act 2013', and an additional amendment to the 'Health Community Services Complaints Act 2004'. The Restricted Birthing Practices Amendment Act 2013 defined a restricted birthing practice as:

> An act that involves undertaking the care of a woman by managing the 3 stages (or any part of these stages) of labour or child birth and, for the purposes of this definition, the Minister may from time to time, on the joint advice of the Medical Board of Australia and the Nursing and Midwifery Board of Australia, by notice in the Gazette, specify activities that will be conclusively taken to constitute the management of any part of 1 or more of these stages of labour or child birth.
>
> (South Australian Government, 2013, p. 3)

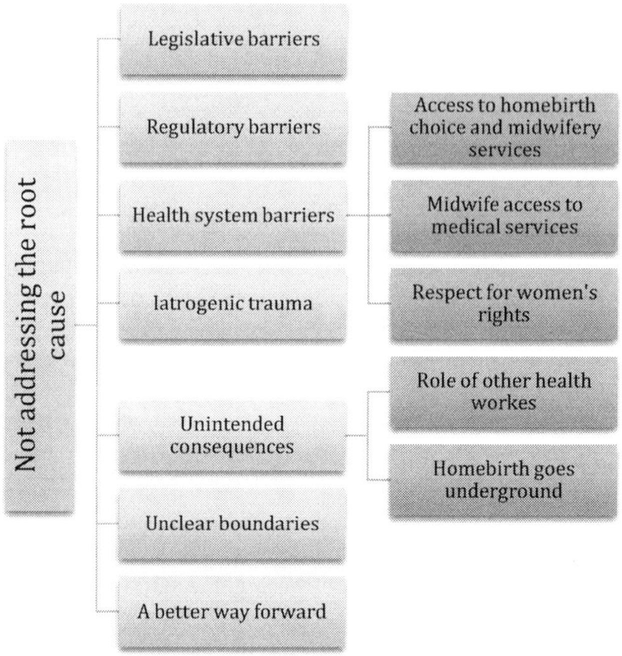

Figure 5.1 Relationship of themes
Source: Rigg et al. (2015, p. 3).

The legislation prohibits a person from carrying out a restricted birthing practice (as defined) unless they are:

- A medical practitioner, midwife or student undertaking their clinical training and acting under the supervision of a medical practitioner or midwife and in accordance with standards, codes or guidelines issued by the National Registration Board for the relevant profession, or
- Acting under a form of delegation authorised or conferred by a registered midwife and still working in accordance with relevant standards, codes and guideline, or
- Rendering assistance to women who are in labour or giving birth or who have given birth to a child where the assistance is provided in an emergency

The maximum penalty for breaching this legislation is $30,000 or imprisonment for 12 months (South Australian Government, 2013).

A new Code of Conduct for Unregistered Health Care Practitioners (Health Care Complaints Commission (HCCC), 2012) was introduced through amendments to the Health Community Services Complaints Act 2004. In October 2012, the HCCC issued a public health warning on the UBW involved in the SA coroner's case to 'cease giving advice about clinical or medical matters, cease performing clinical or medical tasks and cease participating in planned medically unassisted homebirth, being a homebirth that is not attended by a medical practitioner or registered midwife' (Tully, 2013). Shortly after the issue of the public health warning, another infant death occurred under the care of the UBW in December 2012. This resulted in a Prohibition Order being issued against the UBW, banning her from providing any services to pregnant women (Tully, 2013). Further, any mothers knowingly engaging her services contrary to the order were also committing a criminal offence (Tully, 2013; Hunt, 2014). The UBW was placed under covert surveillance as part of an extended investigation conducted by SA Police and the Office of the Director of Public Prosecutions. In August 2017, the UBW was arrested and charged with two counts of manslaughter. In June 2019, she was acquitted of both charges. The Court stated, in relation to the charges: 'Although I find the accused's conduct was less than competent, I am not satisfied that her conduct merits criminal sanction' (Vanstone, 2019, p. 35).

The case exemplified the problems that can arise when an ex-registered midwife practises as a UBW and is no longer accountable to regulatory and professional standards. While the UBWs' intentions may be well-meaning and it could be argued they are the product of a system that does not support women's choice, women can be misled into a false sense of security and trust (Tully, 2013). Professional midwifery standards and codes for safe practice can be sidelined with resulting detriment to woman and baby. It can make the battle to secure a legitimate, professionally supported homebirth choice for women even more difficult, as it casts a negative shadow on the midwifery profession as a whole.

Why do women choose UBWs?

In our next study, we interviewed nine women in Australia: five women who had previously experienced a UBW-supported homebirth and four UBWs who provided homebirth services (Rigg et al., 2017). All but one woman had intentionally chosen a UBW-supported homebirth without a midwife present. All participants had previously accessed pregnancy care and birth through mainstream care options and reported experiences as limited, inflexible, disempowering, impersonal and unsupportive of their choice to have a normal birth. This resulted in women feeling abandoned, disrespected and ultimately traumatised. Based on their prior experiences of care and the narratives shared with other women on social media networks, they concluded that mainstream care options provided suboptimal treatment of women, consistently disrespected women's wishes and made women feel traumatised. These experiences motivated women to seek an alternative care option with a UBW in order to avoid a repeat negative birth experience within mainstream care.

Women reported that UBW care provided them greater flexibility, autonomy and a more personalised birth experience that resulted in them feeling more satisfied and empowered by their UBW-supported homebirth experience.

> She really empowered me and gave me lots of autonomy but in the crucial moment of birth, I didn't want autonomy ... like in that moment, she did mother me, you know. Yeah, I am very lucky.
>
> (Woman, Rigg et al., 2017, p. 9)

> It was amazing; she would do whatever so I could stay at home.
>
> (Woman, Rigg et al., 2017, p. 9)

> Birth workers who work as doulas ... have a lot more trust in the birthing process. They are a lot more willing to allow the woman to make her own decisions rather than taking control.
>
> (UBW, Rigg et al., 2017, p. 9)

UBWs' attendance at homebirths exist partly as a result of the over-regulation of midwifery and governments' allocation of control over childbirth to the medical profession who view birth as a highly risky, life-threatening event for the woman and baby. Decision-making about what is best for women irrespective of women's wishes or what the research evidence demonstrates is dominated by medical professionals' views, beliefs and traditions.

What do UBWs do?

We undertook two national surveys in Australia to elicit the practices of UBWs and the experiences of women who used their services. In the survey of UBWs (n = 39), we sought to establish the role, practices and training of UBWs in Australia and find out what they would do if legislation prevented them from practising.

> I generally work with 'low-risk' women but I also simply work with anyone that I felt comfortable with who wanted me by their side. This included so many 'high-risk' situations that I cannot even begin to list them all. Please note that my stats are very telling in the magnitude of positive outcomes for all, despite risk status.
>
> (UBW, Rigg et al., 2018a, p. 5)

> She [birth worker] was more woman-centred, care felt focused on me and my needs rather than general policies and procedures. I felt [the] birth worker was better at knowing when to step in or step back and truly trusted the birth experience. Birth worker was there to empower me to birth my own baby.
>
> (Woman, Rigg et al., 2018b, p. 7)

We found that UBWs provide a range of maternity services to women with both high- and low-risk pregnancies. This included:

- Women wanting a vaginal birth after a caesarean (VBAC)
- Women whose pregnancies have reached more than 42 weeks
- Women who have diabetes
- Women whose babies are in a breech position
- Grandmultipara (women who have had more than five pregnancies)
- Women with twin pregnancies

Other potential medical risks factors included:

- A history of shoulder dystocia
- Obesity/high BMI
- Sexual abuse
- Obstetric cholestasis or depression

Specifically, UBWs provide homebirth services when the women are either denied this choice or offered unacceptable alternatives in mainstream service provision options (Rigg et al., 2018a). Women were more likely to choose a UBW for care at home if they had a previous unassisted homebirth and/or witnessed abusive or coercive care provided by medical and/or midwifery staff.

Individuals are motivated to become UBWs for a number of reasons, for example, a strong belief that mainstream maternity care unnecessarily interferes with birth and provides limited choice and access or support for women who seek a natural undisturbed birth experience supported by midwives. There are a number of terms that UBWs can use interchangeably to describe themselves and what they do, for example, 'body or birth worker' and 'childbirth educator'; however, the dominant term is doula' – a Greek work used to describe a female woman servant.

> As a birth worker I support women who ask me to be with them, during their birth, through their pregnancy and birth, but that can be in many different forms, it's usually however much they want me to do. I have worked like in a doula kind of arrangement before with women who are having hospital births; and I have also helped women have their babies at home as well for homebirths when they haven't had a registered midwife attending.
>
> (UBW)

> Even though I remind them that I am working as a doula. They believe that I am their midwife, simply because I am with them. Which after all is what the word midwife means.
>
> (UBW, Rigg et al., 2018a, p. 5)

Characteristics of the work of UBWs

In Australia, UBWs provide birthing services to women at home without a midwife present. They can also provide doula support during a hospital birth, although some UBWs will only ever work in the home environment. Experience levels can be extensive, with many having practised between 10 and 20 years, attending between five and 36 births per year. This number may exceed the number of women a hospital or privately practising midwife might attend in a year. UBWs charge women a private fee for their services. There are no formal agreements in place to determine what these fees should be; therefore, these UBW fees can range from as little as $200 to $3000 Australian dollars. These rates can be flexible and negotiated, dependent upon a woman's means and needs, with some UBWs providing services for barter.

Categories of services

The care or service that UBWs provide can be categorised into three broad areas: complementary therapies, emotional support and what would be deemed the clinical skills and practices midwives or obstetricians are trained to provide. Complementary therapies or 'bodywork' predominately involves some form of physical manipulation of the woman's body. This can be techniques such as massage or Robozo to release pelvic tension, make space for the baby and create optimal foetal positioning. Some UBWs use therapies for which they either have previous experience or received training. Acupressure and acupuncture are an example of this. Herbalism is a common therapy that UBWs use. In our study, however, only two UBWs had completed training to support use of this therapy (Rigg et al., 2018a).

Emotional support includes general 'doula support, advocacy in health care, counseling, coaching and grief work, meditation, breath work and self-development workshops' (Rigg et al., 2018a, p. 6). UBWs also provide general doula support to women. This involves the provision of information to assist women's decision-making and provide moral support for the woman's wishes. UBWs described this as 'guarding the woman's space'. Advocacy in health care is another feature of emotional support that UBWs provided when working with women having a hospital birth. This involves advocating for women's wishes with hospital staff. Counselling and coaching was also seen as an essential element of UBW care. This helped support women to overcome trauma previously experienced within the mainstream system of care and was achieved when the UBWs debriefed with the woman about previous birth experiences. Through discussion, meditation and self-development workshops, they aim to realign the woman's inner strength and confidence in her ability to have a positive birth experience.

Finally, the skills and practices of UBWs were very similar to the skills and practices that a registered midwife would normally practice; for example, conducting assessments on the mother and baby antenatally (listening to the foetal heart, measuring the growing uterus), during labour (vaginal examinations) and in the early postnatal period (temperature, weighing) and using hand-on skills to support the mother.

> I am usually watching as the baby is coming, making sure there is no tearing, making sure the baby is coming out gently, in a good position, not getting stuck, that she is in a good position as well ... checking there is no bleeding, no problems, so then the baby is coming through. Once the baby is born, checking he's responsive enough. If the mother doesn't catch the baby herself or the father doesn't, then I would be there to catch the baby, just bring the baby up on the mother's chest and keep them together.
>
> (UBW)

Hands-on skills can include performing an abdominal palpation, listening to the foetal heart and one UBW mentioned how she was skilled at performing an external cephalic version, a skill that not even an experienced obstetric doctor with several years of training and experience would attempt without the support of ultrasound and access to operating theatre services. Other skills identified included nutritional education specific for pregnancy, breastfeeding support, lotus birth and placental encapsulation.

Education of UBWs

UBWs in this study were well-educated, with many holding a university degree. They had a variety of experiences, commonly having previously undertaken nursing and/or midwifery training. This included lay midwifery training in Australia or overseas via online courses in America. Most undertook up to four additional training courses, such as doula training, complementary therapy, adult and child CPR and first aid training to support their role.

What UBWs believe

The role and practice of UBWs can vary considerably and is dependent upon the UBWs personal views of practice. A UBW's practice is driven by a strong belief and trust in women's ability to birth naturally and feminist approaches to support women's choice in achieving this. While UBWs do not generally call themselves a midwife, women interviewed and surveyed for this study viewed and referred to them as their midwife. This is most likely because they practise like a midwife, carrying out similar tasks within a holistic paradigm of care. UBWs provide childbirth education and information services regarding care options as well as strong emotional support that is respectful of women's individual choices regarding pregnancy and childbirth.

> The services that I offer are a good rounded service that they feel comfortable to come to me about pretty much any problem and if I can't help them I can help them get to whoever they need to help them … They are very comfortable with me.
>
> (UBW)

UBWs view the regulation of midwifery practice as limiting women's access and experience of care. Regulation of practice is seen as an enabler for medical and midwifery professionals to claim exclusivity over care which subsequently removes a woman's ability to have autonomy over her own body. Currently, UBWs operate in covert ways to protect their practice and avoid scrutiny. If further legislation were to be introduced in Australia to restrict or prevent their practice, the homebirth services they provide could potentially go even further underground. It is highly likely that UBWs would seek ways to circumvent this type of legislation and continue to provide homebirth services to woman regardless.

> If that legislation came in to my state, I don't know that it would necessarily stop me from doing what I do.
>
> (UBW)

UBWs can view the practices of midwives as tasks that anyone can perform and therefore see no need for formal training or permission to practice. Working outside regulation enables UBWs greater freedom to practice in ways they and their clients feel are necessary and required. Anecdotally, evidence to support the practices of UBWs seems to weigh more heavily on views, opinions and discussion derived from certain websites, social medial groups and blogs in preference to scientific evidence.

Services UBWs provide

UBW services are accessed through informal self-referral systems such as word of mouth, social media and/or doulas and midwives. UBWs normally commence seeing woman in the second trimester of pregnancy. Not many women access UBW services in the first and third trimesters. Both antenatal and postnatal visiting schedules can be similar to visiting schedules in the mainstream system; however, more often, UBWs' visiting schedules offer women a high level of flexibility to accommodate women's wishes, visiting them in their own homes as often, and for as long as, the woman wishes.

Most UBWs believe that accessing medical support and having an emergency back-up plan is an important safety consideration for a homebirth; however, not all UBWs will develop an emergency back-up plan with women. In our study, UBWs reported that most births they attended proceeded normally; however, when asked about how frequently they transferred women to hospital following a birth at home, a significant number reported high transfer rates following a UBW-supported birth at home (46%). The most common reasons for transferring women to hospital was a postpartum haemorrhage (34%) and an unresponsive baby at birth (34%). UBWs can have their own system of support if unfamiliar situations present. This involves consulting with other more experienced UBWs, midwives and occasionally doctors if they feel safe to do so. One UBW mentioned she would discontinue care if she felt uncomfortable, pushed beyond her boundaries of practice or if the women failed to follow her guidance. This seemed contradictory to proclamations of being supportive of women's choice irrespective of risks. While some UBWs will call for medical support within 30 minutes (42%) or an hour (24%) of a medical concern arising, significant numbers report having no protocol in relation to timeframes for seeking professional medical support (34%). Despite this, significant numbers of UBWs said they had needed to call an ambulance and transfer women to hospital (42%) in the past. While most UBWs are willing to stay with women once transferred (42%), some can be unwilling to accompany or stay with the women if transferred to hospital (11%). The reason for this can be an inability to accept, acknowledge or engage with the medical paradigm of birth and a fear of drawing attention to their practice with potentially negative consequences. For this reason, if a UBW remains with the woman when transferred, they are more likely to present as a support person (66%) or a doula (55%), as this role identification camouflages the true nature of their role. In addition, UBWs have reported that they use code language to communicate their services to women, for example:

> I will support you in whatever choice you make, that's like the underground code for I'll assist you to have an unassisted homebirth.
>
> (UBW)

Paradigm of care

UBWs work within a holistic paradigm of care providing non-medical, community-based, flexible childbirth services that support the natural physiological processes of birth. Key features of their interpretation of holistic approaches include spending extensive time with a woman and getting to know her and her holistic needs, in particular her social, emotional, spiritual and community needs, not simply her physical needs. UBWs seemed genuine in their approach, exercising kindness, supportive listening and simple uninvasive remedial therapies that relaxed the woman and kept her calm. All approaches supported the development of a strong relationship based on absolute trust and respect. The woman was seen as central to everything; she held the power and made all the decisions. The UBW acted like the woman's servant, performing tasks as requested and often without question. By avoiding and redefining clinical and medical language, the UBW demedicalised the language of childbirth and helped to humanise and reposition birth as a normal physiological process. Explaining medical and midwifery terms used by the health professions helped women to better understand their bodies and empowered them to be more confident and autonomous. UBWs believe that labelling birth with clinical language and treating it as a medical event disempowers women and enables the medical profession to control woman and birth.

Equipment and consumables

Most UBWs carry a range of equipment similar to what a registered midwife might carry in preparation for a homebirth. This can include: birthing pools, stools, Pinnard, stethoscope and/or electronic Doppler/foetal heart monitor, sphygmomanometer and stethoscope to record blood pressure, suturing equipment, sterile bowls, a measuring jug and consumables such as sterile disposable gloves, antiseptic solution or lubricant. Some UBWs carry resuscitation equipment such as suction, oxygen and a thermal blanket. Others carry very simple comfort measures such as drinking straws; face flannels and massages oils. UBWs do not normally carry or have access to supplies of oxytocic drugs; however, anecdotally women may obtain a prescription for this drug from a local general practitioner.

What motivates women to choose a UBW-supported homebirth

We surveyed 82 women who had experienced a UBW supported homebirth to explore their experiences and views of UBW care. We used social media and word of mouth to distribute the survey. Most women were born in Australia or New Zealand, well-educated (i.e. holding a tertiary qualification), were in a relationship and had middle to low levels of personal income. At the time of undertaking the survey, three women were pregnant and planning to have another UBW birth at home. The majority of respondents came from Queensland, New South Wales and Victoria, which are the most populated Australian states.

The main motivator for women to choose a UBW-supported homebirth include:

- A previous negative experience with mainstream services in either a hospital, birth centre, and/or with a private midwife at home
- A belief that mainstream service providers unnecessarily interfered in birth
- Inflexible maternity services
- Concern about being coerced or bullied into unwanted treatments or interventions by hospital and homebirth midwives
- Not being able to afford or access a privately practising midwife
- The risk of having care terminated at the last minute by privately practising midwives if complications developed
- No access to a publicly funded homebirth

Features of disrespectful hospital care and care provided by private midwives included women being pressured or coerced into unwanted medical procedures and interventions or care that women have not consented to and choices not being supported. When this happens, women can feel that care is disrespectful, abusive, traumatising and not supportive of normal birth. This leads to mistrust of the system and a perceived need to avoid the medical model and system of care for future births.

Women's views of UBW care

In our research, we found that most women viewed UBWs very positively, describing them as trustworthy, convenient and flexible care providers who are both knowledgeable and supportive of normal birth and homebirth. They provide very flexible services to women in their private practice (Rigg et al., 2018b). Women view UBWs as natural birth advocates who are always available, able to establish a more personal relationship with women and provide a more attentive level of care than the women experienced with registered midwives. Women responded in the survey that they saw UBWs as non-registered workers, who are not inhibited by regulatory or employer responsibilities to restrict their practice. Women viewed UBW care as having less red tape, paperwork and interference in the woman's birth than registered midwives.

> UBWs aren't bound by regulation, bookkeeping and that accountability to a higher power … that affects our scope of what we can do.
>
> (Woman, Rigg et al., 2017, p. 9)

Women also viewed the UBWs not being limited by registration requirements and/or the need to answer to institutional rules or guidelines as a positive element. They felt this enabled UBWs to be more flexible with care provision and thus to better meet the care choices and needs of women:

> A birth worker does what I want them to do. A registered midwife does what they have to do to maintain registration and cover themselves.
>
> (Woman)

> A birth worker is there to support and respect the choices a birthing mother makes in the best interests for her and her family … A registered midwife should do the same but is tethered by certain restrictions, which are not always based on the best or most current available evidence. Registered midwives are forced to work within a system that does not support the wide range of normal that exists in birth.
>
> (Woman)

When a woman engages a UBW, the contractual arrangement is between her and the UBW. As the woman is the principal (i.e. recipient of contractual services), she sets the contractual parameters and terms for her care with the UBW. This means she dictates what and how care will happen and for how long. This enables the women to have full control over their birth experience. Women believe UBWs can better support their informed choices and provide a different, more positive birth experience than mainstream service providers. This they saw as occurring in an authentic continuity of care service model.

> A birth worker's behaviour is more aligned to the midwifery philosophy of 'woman centred care' than a registered midwife is. They don't have hospital policy or supervisors to deal with and so they can actually be 'with women'.
>
> (R33)

> Having a registered midwife was like having a medical professional at your birth. No matter how friendly they are, there is always a power difference. A midwife steers the ship. Having a birth worker at your birth is like having a caring aunt hold the space as you do your thing. Nothing was ever done without my requesting it first. A birth worker adjusts the sails.
>
> (R31, Rigg et al., 2018b, p. 7)

Features of care that made women view their experience positively included a care provider who could support:

- A natural, non-medical, non-intervention homebirth experience
- Woman's choice and control over the birth experience itself without conditions
- Flexibility with birth positions and with who was present
- Women to feel in control of their birth and only carry out tasks requested by the woman and
- A relaxed birth environment that supported an uninterrupted labour and birth

One significant finding from our study was that 70% of the women who participated identified as having moderate to high-risk medical or obstetric factors, which would exclude them from most publicly funded homebirth options in Australia. While over 50% (n = 48) of the women did not experience any medical issues throughout their UBW homebirth experience, 41% (n = 34) needed to seek medical treatment for either themselves or their baby (n = 34) and three women said their baby died. Hospital transfer rates for a UBW-supported homebirth were high.

When things go wrong it is devastating

When everything goes well with the woman's UBW-supported homebirth experience, there is a tendency for women to idealise their birth choice and to be triumphant in their achievement against the odds (Rigg et al., 2018b). In research by Keedle, Schmied, Burns and Dahlen (2013), 12 women who had a VBAC at home reported how they felt victorious and 'like superwoman' (Keedle et al., 2013). However, when things go seriously wrong in maternity care, there can be devastation. The three women who reported they lost babies articulated significant regrets for choosing a UBW-supported homebirth and strongly advised women who may be contemplating this choice against it. They criticised their UBW for presenting as skillful and suggested their trust had been misguided; they blamed both themselves and their UBW for the death of their baby, highlighting the dangers of this scenario:

> My mother was horrified. I wish I had listened to her. My baby would be alive. Don't do it, she had no backup and gave woefully inadequate care, did not acknowledge her limitations ... told me my baby and I were fine based on intermittent Doppler use alone, did not recommend a scan, and by the time she showed up ... my baby was dead inside of me.
>
> (R52, Rigg et al., 2018b, p. 7)

> I was misled to believe that homebirth was safe, and that there was no difference between a registered midwife and a formerly registered midwife ... It was the worst experience of my life and resulted in the death of my baby.
>
> (R67, Rigg et al., 2018b, p. 7)

UBWs can present as experienced and skillful in providing more than simple support. They can also misrepresent the risks of a woman's situation, to create a false sense of safety and security for women. This is evidenced by the comments from women in our study whose babies died, and additionally during the high-profile case involving the ex-registered midwife who attended women as a UBW during a homebirth. One mother, who gave evidence at the coroner's hearing, said she trusted and believed that the UBW was experienced and specialised in breech births. The coroner concluded the mother 'did not feel any danger to her child or to herself' (Schapel, 2012). This exemplifies the dangers and problems that can arise when an ex-registered midwife becomes a UBW. Following this inquest, the UBW was placed under covert surveillance and subsequently charged with manslaughter. As discussed above, the UBW was recently acquitted at trial.

While UBWs may have well-meaning intentions, unlike registered midwives, they are not required to adhere to any professional standards or codes of practice.

> My birth worker was negligent. Registered midwives are held to account for the care or lack of care they provide. Birth workers are not. There is no protection or safeguards for women and their families when using a birth worker.
>
> (R16, Rigg et al., 2018b, p. 7)

Safe midwifery practice can be ignored to the detriment of the woman and her baby and the battle to secure a legitimate, medically supported homebirth choice for women becomes even more difficult as a result, and cases like this cast a negative shadow on the midwifery profession as a whole. Further, anecdotally, within the freebirth and homebirth social media networks and communities, when negative outcomes occur there is a tendency to avoid open dialogue about the risks associated with freebirthing, or a UBW-supported homebirth, without medical or midwifery support. This can lead women into a false sense of security, placing them and their infants at greater risk of harm. When women cannot access their choices they feel dissatisfied, disrespected and some are traumatised. This can lead them to believe they have no other option but to choose a UBW-supported homebirth (Rigg et al., 2018b).

Conclusion

In Australia, the rise of UBW-supported birth at home is strongly linked to women's prior experiences with mainstream care, which were reported as negative, traumatising and lacking in support for the woman's choice either to have a normal birth or birth at home with midwives who can provide this service. Lack of access to this choice, and inflexibility with care options, can result in women feeling they have no other choice but to seek an alternative care provider outside the system, which is an unsafe scenario. The risk for negative outcomes occurring in childbirth is an ever-present possibility irrespective of mode and place of birth. There is, however, sufficient evidence globally to support the view that homebirth is as safe as a hospital birth providing appropriately trained, qualified and experienced midwives and medical support services are available to support this choice for women with a low-risk pregnancy. Overregulating midwifery practice has resulted in loss of midwife autonomy and a shift in the focus of care from women-centred to medical institution-centred care. This is problematic, as institutionalised, highly risk-averse care practices generate power imbalances and a one-size-fits-all approach to care that is inflexible towards women. If changes do not occur, no amount of legislation will prevent UBW practice from expanding.

Our research is not about idealising UBWs or suggesting UBW-supported homebirth is an optimal, safe or ideal choice. The women who lost their babies are testament to this. Our research found that UBWs practice in ways that midwives should be able to practice but are prevented from doing so by highly restrictive regulations. They provide a humanistic approach to care that is focused on empowerment of women, their choices and normal birth. UBWs believe home is the optimal place for birth to happen and most women (except for the three whose babies died) in my study were highly satisfied with their care experience, having felt loved, respected and embowered.

The way forward

- Birth and birth care practices need to be humanised by making these practices less medicalised and more flexible to improve women's experience of hospital care
- Homebirth needs to be fully supported as a viable option for all women with appropriate medical and transport services put in place
- Policy-makers and the professions need to listen to women and change the way mainstream service models are funded, managed and provided to women
- Midwives must be acknowledged as an independent profession separate from nursing and enabled to practise autonomously, to their full scope of practice
- UBWs and midwives need to work together to ensure safety for women and their infants
- The system needs to develop pathways to formal midwifery training for UBWs and support the recognition of significant skills that could be used to enhance midwifery practice, as many midwives have lost these basic midwifery skills

Notes

1 A publicly funded homebirth programme is a midwifery model of care provided through the public hospital system and caters to women who are at low obstetric and medical risk. Midwives working within this model are employed by the public hospital and the midwives' hospital employer provides their professional indemnity insurance. Women's ability to access this model is limited and assessed against strict medical selection criteria and women must remain low-risk throughout their childbirth experience.

2 Medicare is the universal healthcare system that funds primary healthcare through the Department of Human Services for Australian citizens and permanent residents. Eligible citizens can claim a rebate for treatments from medical practitioners, eligible midwives, nurse practitioners and allied health professionals who have been issued a Medicare provider number, and can also obtain free treatment in public hospitals (Australia Government, 2019).

3 The Pharmaceuticals Benefits Scheme (PBS) is a scheme that is part of the Australian Government's National Medicines Policy, and is available to anyone who holds a Medicare card. It provides access to subsidised medicines and sometimes free medications if individuals have reached their PBS safety net threshold (Australian Government Department of Health, 2019 , Rigg et al., 2018b).

4 The Australian National Law is the umbrella term used to describe Health Practitioner Regulation National Laws that are in force in each state and territory.

References

Australian Government Department of Health. (2019) *PBS: The Pharmaceutical Benefits Scheme* [Online]. Canberra: Commonwealth of Australia. Retrieved from: www.pbs.gov.au/info/about-the-pbs - What_is_the_PBS [accessed 18 February 2019].

Barclay, L., Brodie, P., Lane, K., Reiger, K. & Tracy, S. (2003) *The Australian Midwifery Action Project (AMAP)*. Sydney: Centre for Family Health and Midwifery: University of Technology.

Barrett, L. (2013) *About me* [Online]. Homebirth: A Midwife Mutiny … Turning a ripple into a wave. Retrieved from: www.homebirth.net.au/about-me [accessed 25 January 2016].

Dahlen, H. (2012) Pushing home birth underground raises safety concerns. *The Conversation*. Online: The Conversation.

Government of South Australia. (2013) Proposal to protect midwifery practice in South Australia: Consultation paper.

Health Care Complaints Commission. (2012) *Code of conduct for unregistered health practitioners*. Sydney, NSW: Health Care Complaints Commission.

Hunt, N. (2014) Police investigating homebirth advocate Lisa Barrett over deaths of five newborn babies. *Sunday Mail (SA)*.

Keedle, H., Schmied, V., Burns, E. & Hannah, D. (2013) Women's reasons for, and experiences of, choosing a homebirth following a caesarean section. *Women and Birth*, *26*, S9.

Mamamia News. (2012) Homebirths killed three babies. It's official. *Mamamia News*.

Nursing and Midwifery Board of Australia. (2016) *Registration standard: Professional Indemnity insurance arrangements*. Melbourne: NMBA.

Organisation for Economic Cooperation and Development. (2018) *Health at a glance: Europe 2018 state of health EU cycle*. Paris: OECD Publishing.

Rigg, E., Schmied, V., Peters, K., & Dahlen, H. (2015) Not addressing the root cause: An analysis of submissions made to the South Australian Government on a Proposal to Protect Midwifery Practice. *Women Birth*, *28*, 121–128.

Rigg, E., Schmied, V., Peters, K., & Dahlen, H. (2017) Why do women choose an unregulated birth worker to birth at home in Australia: A qualitative study. *BMC Pregnancy and Birth*, *17*, 14.

Rigg, E., Schmied, V., Peters, K., & Dahlen, D. (2018a) The role, practice and training of unregulated birth workers: A qualitative study. *Women and Birth, 788***,** 11.

Rigg, E., Schmied, V., Peters, K., & Dahlen, H. (2018b) A survey of women in Australia who chose the care of unregulated birthworkers for a birth at home. *Women & Birth*, *901*, 11.

Royal Australian and New Zealand College of Obstetricians and Gynaecologists (RANCOG). (2017) *Home births*. Melbourne: RANCOG.

Schapel, A. E. (2012) Findings of inquest. In: Coroner's Court. Retrieved from: www.courts.sa.gov.au/CoronersFindings/Pages/Findings-for-2012.aspx. Government of South Australia.

South Australian Government. (2013) Health Practitioner Regulation National Law (South Australia) (Restricted Birthing Practices) Amendment Act 2013. No. 26 of 2013 assented to 21.11.2013. Adelaide: South Australian Government.

Tully, S. (2013) Statement for public release: Order prohibiting you Lisa Jane Barrett, from providing specified Health Services in South Australia persuent to section 56C (2) of the Health Commission Services Complaints Act 2004 (the Act). South Australia: HCSCC.

United Nations. (2015) *Universal Declaration on Human Rights*. Geneva: UN.

Vanstone, J. (2019) R v. Barrett (No 3) [2019] SASC 93 Reasons for the Verdicts of The Honourable Justice Vanstone 4 June 2019. South Australia Supreme Court of South Australia.

World Health Organisation (2018) *WHO recommendations. Intrapartum care for a positive childbirth experience*. Geneva: WHO.

6 Identifying the poisonous gases seeping into the coal mine

What women seek to avoid in choosing to give birth at home

Heather Sassine and Hannah Dahlen

> Women are not only concerned about the interventions per se but about the loss of control and involvement in decision-making that they associated with intervention in hospital.
>
> (Heather Sassine)

About the authors

While studying Chinese Medicine, I (Heather Sassine) stumbled onto the midwifery section of the university library and had my view of childbirth turned on its head. I believed that hospital birth was safer than homebirth and I was confused when research did not always reflect this. In fact, for some women, it showed the opposite was true.

I trained to be a doula, but I became frustrated with the lack of informed consent and coercion I witnessed on a regular basis. While I knew homebirth wasn't for everyone, I felt if women had *all* the information (rather than the information care providers want them to have so they make the choices providers wanted them to make) they would make very different choices.

I became a midwife and practised as a homebirth midwife with a private group practice in Sydney before leaving midwifery practice to spend time growing, birthing and nurturing two little boys. With so many women unable to find a midwife (or being aware that having a known midwife was an option) and rail-roaded into accepting choices they didn't want, I felt so lucky to be able to choose my midwife, be able to afford to pay her, to know she would support my choices and to ultimately have two beautiful, normal homebirths. With all my privilege, knowledge and confidence in my choices, I still adjusted my dates (both times!) so I had an extra week – to protect myself and my midwife in case I went over 42 weeks. My hope is that the NHBS helps the decision-makers see that overregulation is not making childbirth safer, it is forcing women to withhold information, attempt to manipulate or leave the system all together. I hope all women (not just white, educated, wealthy women living in urban areas) have access to continuity of midwifery care in the venue of their choice.

I (Hannah Dahlen) was Heather's supervisor for her Honours thesis and I have already described my story earlier in the book.

Introduction

When Megan Markel, Her Royal Highness Meghan, Duchess of Sussex, talked about a homebirth recently with her first baby, much was made of the decision in mainstream news reports. A prominent UK obstetrician, Timothy Draycott, reportedly mocked the Duchess' birth choices at the American College of Obstetricians and Gynecologists annual conference saying, 'Megan Markle has decided she's going to have a doula and a willow tree … let's see how that goes' (DeGraaf, 2019). We hope the Duchess was blissfully unaware of this going on around her and that she was surrounded by a supportive team that respected her choices. However, it is not what women seek that is often behind the choice to have a homebirth, but what they are seeking to avoid.

The majority of women who plan a homebirth in Australia hire a privately practising midwife (PPM). Access to homebirth with a registered midwife is limited due to cost, availability of PPMs, increasing regulation and restrictions placed on PPMs and the small number of publicly funded programmes nationally available (14 in total) with strict eligibility criteria. As you will have read in Chapter 5, there are concerns about how the increasing regulations and restrictions in Australia, aimed at improving safety, are limiting midwives' scope of practice and increasingly removing the option of a midwife-attended homebirth.

Research shows that women choose homebirth for many positive reasons, such as continuous care from a known midwife, belief in the natural process, the desire to have family present and a desire for a comfortable, familiar and private environment (Boucher, Bennett, McFarlin, & Freeze, 2009; Ashley & Weaver, 2012a, 2012b; Bernhard, Zielinski, Ackerson, & English, 2014). Avoidance of medical intervention and previous negative experiences are also commonly cited influences, particularly among women who have had a previous hospital birth (Ashley & Weaver, 2012a, 2012b; Bernhard et al., 2014). Studies have shown that medical intervention in childbirth may be associated with dissatisfaction with the childbirth experience (Janssen, Carty, & Reime, 2006; Cheyney, 2008; Boucher et al., 2009; Christiaens & Bracke, 2009). While avoidance of medical intervention appears to be a major motivation for women choosing homebirth, the particular interventions which women seek to avoid are less clear.

What women seek to avoid by choosing a homebirth

We undertook a literature review to explore which interventions women are avoiding when choosing to give birth at home. The search covered the period from January 2004 to September 2016 and resulted in 22 papers meeting

Table 6.1 Interventions and interferences reported in the literature

Main interventions	*Other interventions*	*Interferences*
Caesarean section	Antenatal screening	Time restrictions
Medical pain relief	Blood pressure monitoring	Change of shifts/staff
Instrumental birth	Medications for the newborn	Bright lights
Induction and augmentation of labour	Intravenous drips	Strangers at the birth/lack of privacy
Foetal monitoring	Medications (unspecified)	Interference with the baby
Vaginal examinations		Drive to hospital
		Restriction of movement
		Noise
		Frequent interruptions

all of the inclusion criteria. This review of the literature revealed the main interventions and interferences that women were avoiding in choosing to give birth at home, which we set out in Table 6.1.

Caesarean section

Twelve of the studies included in this review cited avoidance of caesarean section as a reason for choosing homebirth (Cheyney, 2008; Lindgren, Rådestad, Christensson, Wally-Bystrom, & Hildingsson, 2010; Jackson, Dahlen, & Schmied, 2012; Laurel Merg & Carmoney, 2012; McCutcheon & Brown, 2012; Murray-Davis et al., 2012; Lothian, 2013; Regan & McElroy, 2013; Bernhard et al., 2014; Lessa, Tyrrell, Alves, & Rodrigues, 2014; Keedle, Schmied, Burns, & Dahlen, 2015; Sweeney & O'Connell, 2015). Cheyney (2008) found that women choosing homebirth were concerned about the rising caesarean rate and the cascade of intervention that often precedes it:

> I was not going to be like all of my friends. You know the story … They go overdue by a couple of days, go in for an induction that doesn't work, and they end up with a C-section. Then they're in too much pain and too depressed to nurse [breastfeed], so they have to find a support group to process their feelings of victimization. I didn't know much, but I knew I didn't want that.
>
> (2008, p. 257)

Nine further studies reported that women felt this cascade of intervention, culminating in caesarean section, increased risks for themselves and for their babies (Lindgren et al., 2010; Jackson et al., 2012; McCutcheon & Brown, 2012; Murray-Davis et al., 2012; Murray-Davis, McDonald, Rietsma, Coubrough, & Hutton, 2014; Regan & McElroy, 2013; Catling et al., 2014; Keedle et al., 2015).

A common theme found throughout the studies was that by choosing to give birth at home, women avoided the time restrictions they felt would be placed on them in hospital (Andrews, 2004a; Cheyney, 2008; Laurel Merg & Carmoney, 2012; McCutcheon & Brown, 2012; Murray-Davis et al., 2014). While not a medical intervention in itself, women associated these time limits with increased medical intervention and caesarean section in particular. In one study this was also linked to issues of litigation (McCutcheon & Brown, 2012):

> they give you a certain amount of time and I know they get worried because of litigation these days … so they'd much rather whip you in and do a c-section.
>
> (McCutcheon & Brown, 2012, p. 26)

Bernhard et al. (2014) and Lindgren et al. (2010) reported lack of options as a reason some women chose to give birth at home. In one case, a woman with a history of precipitous births was told a caesarean section was her only option (Lindgren et al., 2010). Another woman wanted to avoid the lack of choice she experienced in hospital during a previous birth where she was offered an epidural or a caesarean, when she wanted neither (Bernhard et al., 2014).

Medication for pain relief

Thirteen of the studies in this review cited avoidance of pain relief medication as a contributing factor in the choice to give birth at home (Longworth, Ratcliff, & Boulton, 2001; Andrews, 2004a; Cheyney, 2008; Lindgren et al., 2010; Catling-Paull, Dahlen, & Homer, 2011; Jackson et al., 2012; Jouhki, 2012; Lothian, 2013; Regan & McElroy, 2013; Bernhard et al., 2014; Catling, Dahlen, & Homer, 2014; Lessa et al., 2014; Murray-Davis et al., 2014). As with caesarean section, women were concerned about increased risks to themselves and their baby from pain relief medication (Lindgren et al., 2010; Jackson et al., 2012; Lothian, 2013; Regan & McElroy, 2013). These perceived risks were associated with the medication itself, for example, the effects of an epidural, as well as concern for the increased risks related to the cascade of intervention:

> Having an epidural might seem an easy way but as far as I know it also has a negative effect and increases the risk for an instrumental delivery or caesarean section.
>
> (Lindgren et al., 2010, p. 167)

In the three papers that cite instrumental birth as an intervention that women are avoiding, it is mentioned in conjunction with epidurals and the cascade of intervention (Lindgren et al., 2010; Jackson et al., 2012; Lothian, 2013).

Some studies reported that women did not want to be offered pain relief medication as an option (Longworth et al., 2001; Cheyney, 2008; Lindgren et al., 2010; Catling-Paull et al., 2011; Catling et al., 2014), preferring to find natural ways to cope with the pain:

> It's so easy to use equipment or drugs just because they are there. When you are at home, you have to use your capacity to find ways to cope with pain.
>
> (Lindgren et al., 2010, p. 167)

Women felt that the relaxed atmosphere at home, and the freedom to move around and choose their own birth positions, meant that the pain was easier to manage, rendering medical pain relief unnecessary (Andrews, 2004b; Lindgren et al., 2010; Jouhki, 2012; Murray-Davis et al., 2012).

Bernhard et al. (2014), Lothian (2013) and Catling et al. (2014) reported that some women wanted to avoid being pressured by hospital staff to accept pain medication. Women's perception as reported by Regan and McElroy (2013) was that many interventions were done for the convenience of the staff and the institution rather than for the benefit of the woman or her baby:

> During my research about when and why epidurals came to be, I learned they make it easier for the doctor. The same thing is true with positioning in labor.
>
> (Regan & McElroy, 2013, p. 245)

Lothian (2013) and Cheyney (2008) reported that women associated pain relief medication with a loss of control and autonomy and the perception that something special would be taken away from them:

> I'll take the pain, the power, the pleasure, the intimacy of an unmedicated birth over an epidural any day. I didn't want a sterile, white-washed, 'Oprah on the television in the background' birth, thank you very much!
>
> (Cheyney, 2008, p. 264)

This perception of unmedicated labour as an essential part of the special experience of labour and birth was not necessarily shared by hospital care providers (Lothian, 2013):

> So I asked [my obstetrician] about epidurals and she looked at me and said, 'You'd have novocaine for a root canal wouldn't you?' I thought, 'She doesn't get that this is bringing a new life into the world.'
>
> (Lothian, 2013, p. 269)

Induction and augmentation of labour

Seven of the studies included in the review cited induction or augmentation of labour as an intervention women were avoiding in choosing homebirth (Viisainen, 2001; Cheyney, 2008; Jackson et al., 2012; Lothian, 2013; Regan & McElroy, 2013; Bernhard et al., 2014; Keedle et al., 2015). Bernhard et al. (2014) and Viisainen (2001) reported that women felt pressured into interventions based on the timetable and agenda of the hospital:

> You know there is the threat that if the baby is not born by a certain date I will be induced … I do not want that; I want my babies born naturally.
>
> (Viisainen, 2001, p. 1115)

Women were also concerned about induction or augmentation leading to further interventions (Cheyney, 2008; Jackson et al., 2012; Bernhard et al., 2014). This had occurred for some women in previous births:

> I seriously feel that if they hadn't started the syntocinon and just let me do what I needed to do then she would have rotated but the syntocinon forced her into a bad position and just pushed her there and held her there so she couldn't turn and I ended up with a caesarean.
>
> (Jackson et al., 2012, p. 565)

Throughout the literature, women choosing homebirth frequently expressed faith in their body's ability to labour and give birth naturally if given the time:

> Why are you putting stuff in my body to make things go faster? My body knows how to give birth.
>
> (Lothian, 2013, p. 269)

Foetal monitoring and vaginal examinations

Continuous electronic monitoring of the foetal heart rate and vaginal examinations were cited in six studies as interventions women were trying to avoid (Viisainen, 2001; Boucher et al., 2009; Symon, Winter, Donnan, & Kirkham, 2010; Miller & Shriver, 2012; Bernhard et al., 2014; Keedle et al., 2015). Bernhard et al. (2014) reported that women felt that, in hospital, the focus was on monitors and their cervix rather than on them as an individual and that this communicated a lack of respect:

> I felt like an exam animal or something. I mean you've got your feet in the air, the shifts change, you've got people all the time peeking at you … sticking their fingers in places … poking you with things. It was just so out of my realm of normal.
>
> (Bernhard et al., 2014, p. 163)

These interventions were often mentioned in the literature together with other routine hospital interventions that women felt could be avoided by staying at home to give birth:

> No: monitors, IVs, drugs, laying on my back, family pushed away, baby taken away, baby given sugar water.
>
> (Boucher et al., 2009)

Women expressed faith that their body could give birth without these interventions (Boucher et al., 2009; Miller & Shriver, 2012; Bernhard et al., 2014) which were of questionable safety (Viisainen, 2001) and a potential cause of unnecessary concern:

> I just can't see going to the hospital for a birth. No way. Why? So a doctor can stick his hands in me and put a monitor in the baby and tell me why I should be worried? [rolls her eyes].
>
> (Miller & Shriver, 2012, p. 714)

As shown in Table 6.1, there are many other interventions and interferences that women are also trying to avoid by choosing to have a baby at home.

The National Homebirth Survey (NHBS)

Based on our literature review, we undertook a survey, in Australia, of women who had had a homebirth or sought a homebirth. Of the 1413 women who completed the survey, the majority said they would prefer to give birth at home with a registered midwife. If, however, a midwife was not available, more than half (56%) said they would birth elect to freebirth or find an unregistered birthworker to support them at home. Only 24% of women said that they would plan a hospital or birth centre birth.

Several women said they would lie or withhold information about their health history in order to access a hospital-based programme:

> I would likely lie to services and not disclose my previous miscarriages or complications in order to qualify if necessary.
>
> (Participant 64)

Others would book through the hospital system but plan to 'accidentally' have the baby at home:

> If I could not find an unregistered midwife to support me, I would go to a hospital for prenatal care then, provided everything was going well, 'accidentally' birth my baby at home.
>
> (Participant 766)

Women also included options like travelling elsewhere to access a registered midwife who would attend to them at home, or finding unregistered midwives or 'midwife friends' still willing to attend their homebirth 'underground'. Four women said they wouldn't have another baby if they were unable to access a registered midwife to attend their homebirth.

Fifty-three percent of women reported at least one risk factor during pregnancy or a previous birth which, if screened, would disqualify them from accessing a publicly funded homebirth programme in Australia. Risk factors cited included a previous caesarean section (11%), being over 42 weeks gestation (10%) and having a BMI over 35 or >100 kg (10%). Worryingly, the women most likely to be unable to find a midwife to support their homebirth are also more likely to have a freebirth or use an unregulated birthworker. Midwives are also most likely to be reported to the regulatory body in Australia for supporting a VBAC (see Chapter 11).

In the NHBS survey, women also reported choosing to give birth at home to avoid specific medical interventions such as induction of labour, forceps and episiotomy. Women were also avoiding time pressure, the hospital environment, the risk agenda of the hospital, hospital policies and coercion. Homebirth was chosen to enhance access to continuity of midwifery care (93% of women) and uninterrupted skin-to-skin contact with their baby (see Table 6.2).

Women who experienced a homebirth reported that they felt comfortable asking questions and that the midwife respected their opinion and personal preferences. By contrast, women who experienced a hospital birth were more likely to report feeling coerced into accepting options proposed by their care provider and less likely to feel they had enough time during prenatal visits.

Women's previous hospital experiences were reported as traumatic by 49% of the women surveyed, with 9% reporting that a diagnosis of PTSD followed their traumatic hospital birth. In contrast, only 6% of women considered their homebirth experience to be traumatic and 1% reported having a diagnosis of PTSD. The majority of these women, however, associated the trauma with how they were treated when transferred in labour to hospital.

Discussion

Both the literature review and the NHBS showed that avoidance of intervention during labour and birth was a common motivator for women to choose homebirth. Women are aware of the increase in intervention rates in hospitals and are concerned about the effects of the cascade of intervention for themselves, their babies and their futures as mothers.

There were some differences between the literature and the NHBS findings. In the literature review, the most commonly mentioned intervention that women reported avoiding was caesarean section. By contrast, in the NHBS, induction, forceps and episiotomy were most commonly cited as

Table 6.2 Interventions and other factors women were avoiding in choosing homebirth

For my most recent homebirth I was choosing to avoid the following:	*% Agree (completely or strongly)*	*% Disagree (completely or strongly)*
Induction	89	3
Forceps	88	2
Episiotomy	87	3
Cardiotocography (CTG)	84	3
Artificial rupture of membranes (ARM)	83	3
Pain-relieving drugs	80	4
Primary caesarean	78	6
Antibiotics	75	6
Vaginal examinations (VEs)	67	4
Routine group b Streptococcus testing	64	10
Repeat caesarean	60	35
Routine ultrasound	51	12
Other factors women are avoiding when choosing a homebirth	*% Agree (completely or strongly)*	*% Disagree (completely or strongly)*
Time pressure	92	2
A hospital environment that does not support normal birth	90	2
Risk agenda of the hospital	88	2
Hospital policies	86	2
Hospital staff that do not support normal birth	86	2
Added risk in hospital	83	2
Hospital staff/strangers	83	2
Coercion	82	4
Lack of informed consent	81	3
Repeat of negative hospital experience	61	13

the interventions women wanted to avoid. This difference may reflect recent changes in maternity care in Australia, where caesarean section rates are levelling out but induction, forceps and episiotomy rates are rising. It may also be the way we phrased the question, as we divided caesarean section into several subgroups (elective, emergency).

Caesarean rates have been rising globally and rates of caesarean section in Australia are among the highest in the world at 33% (Australian Institute of Health and Welfare, 2016; Betrán et al., 2016), with some hospitals reporting rates as high as 47.4% (Bureau of Health Information, 2014). Rates of caesarean section in Australia have risen from an average of 18.5% in 1990 to 33% in 2014, and research indicates that this increase is not attributed to increased obstetric risk or women's choice (Miller, Prosser, & Thompson, 2012; Betrán et al., 2016). Worldwide, caesarean section rates have increased from 6% in 1990 to 19% in 2014 (FIGO, 2018). High rates of medical intervention in labour and childbirth are associated with postnatal depression and PTSD (Olde, van der Hart, Kleber, & van Son, 2006; Andersen, Melvaer, Videbech, Lamont, & Joergensen, 2012; Simpson, Schmied, Dickson, & Dahlen, 2018), interference with mother–baby bonding and reduced breastfeeding rates (Torvaldsen, Roberts, Simpson, & Thomson, 2006; Wiklund, Norman, Uvnäs-Moberg, Ransjö-Arvidson, & Andolf, 2009; Bai, Wu, & Tarrant, 2013). The results of this literature review and survey indicate that women are concerned about the iatrogenic risks associated with giving birth in hospital and consider giving birth at home to be safer for them and their babies (Boucher et al., 2009; Jackson et al., 2012; Lothian, 2013; Keedle et al., 2015).

Throughout the studies included in this review and the NHBS results, women were not only concerned about the interventions per se, but about the loss of control and involvement in decision-making that they associated with interventions in hospital. There is support for their concerns. A study in Queensland found that up to 60% of women felt they were not informed about a procedure and as many as 34% felt they were not involved in decision-making (Thompson & Miller, 2014). This loss of control and involvement in their own care is associated with birth trauma and postnatal depression (Olde et al., 2006; Elmir, Schmied, Wilkes, & Jackson, 2010). Elmir et al. (2010) found that women who had high-intervention, traumatic births reported feeling invisible, subjected to authoritative decision-making and being denied adequate information regarding procedures and interventions. In both the literature review and the NHBS, women felt many hospital interventions were performed for institutional convenience and that the focus was on monitors or disparate body parts rather than on women as individuals. In choosing to homebirth, women reported greater control, individualised care and involvement in decision-making (Viisainen, 2001; Andrews, 2004b; Cheyney, 2008; Boucher et al., 2009). These factors lead to greater birth satisfaction and reduced rates of postnatal depression (Fair & Morrison, 2012; Meyer, 2013).

The review and NHBS also showed that women associate physiological birth and a satisfying birth experience with a positive transition to motherhood and a stronger relationship with their baby. Women feel that it is not just medical interventions that can impact negatively on the mother–baby dyad, but also more subtle interferences that can affect the normal progress of labour and mother–infant bonding. These interferences include the drive to hospital, time restrictions, lack of privacy, change of staff, restriction of movement, frequent interruptions, separation from their baby, bright lights and noise.

Many women will continue to choose to give birth at home and research shows it is a safe option for healthy, low-risk women (de Jonge et al., 2009, 2015; Janssen et al., 2009; Brocklehurst et al., 2011; Halfdansdottir, Smarason, Olafsdottir, Hildingsson, & Sveinsdottir, 2015). However, literature from this review and NHBS, combined with rising rates of freebirth and high-risk homebirth, reveals that many women are fleeing a hospital-dominated maternity care system that is not meeting their needs (Dahlen, Jackson, & Stevens, 2011). Improved access to home-like birth environments, continuity of midwifery care and publicly funded homebirth programmes would provide more options for women and could encourage more women to engage with maternity services.

As noted above, the NHBS recorded a vast difference in the rates of trauma reported for a homebirth, when compared with a hospital birth. In homebirth, 6% said their experience was traumatic and 1% reported a diagnosis of PTSD, whereas in hospital 49% reported traumatic experiences and 9% were diagnosed with PTSD. In relation to trauma arising from homebirth, of the women who left comments, almost half reported that it was their home-to-hospital transfer and subsequent care in hospital which they found traumatic, either because of a change in venue or treatment by hospital staff. A study by Stramrood et al. (2011) found that planned homebirths were associated with fewer PTSD symptoms, with slightly higher rates of PTSD in women who transferred to hospital.

While birth trauma and PTSD are associated with increased intervention in childbirth and mode of birth, studies indicate that the quality of interpersonal relationships is more influential (Moyzakitis, 2004; Thomson & Downe, 2008, 2010; Elmir et al., 2010). In particular, women are more likely to report a traumatic birth or display PTSD symptoms if they experience a loss of control over decision-making or feel unsupported or abandoned by care providers (Moyzakitis, 2004; Elmir et al., 2010, Ford & Ayers, 2011; Harris & Ayers, 2012; O'Donovan et al., 2014). In Reed et al.'s (2017) study into birth trauma and care-provider interactions, women reported feeling dismissed, violated and abused, and said that care providers used lies and threats to coerce them into accepting interventions. Similar findings were reported in a study on women who had a homebirth after caesarean (see Chapter 7), with women feeling ignored, intimidated and bullied in the hospital and ultimately fleeing the system and choosing to give birth at home (Keedle et al., 2015).

The link between birth trauma and feelings of loss of control and involvement in decision-making (Elmir et al., 2010), could, at least in part, explain why comparatively fewer women in the NHBS reported their homebirth as traumatic. Between 93% and 95% of women reported that their homebirth care provider involved them in decision-making, gave them information and time to consider their options and respected their choices, as compared with 21–23% of hospital-based care providers who reportedly did the same. Only 5% experienced feeling coerced into accepting options suggested by their homebirth care provider, compared to 48% for their hospital-based care provider. Research into women's reasons for choosing a private midwife in Western Australia found that women were seeking a deep relationship of mutual trust and respect with their midwife and to feel safe and in control (Davison, Hauck, Bayes, Kuliukas, & Wood, 2015).

Birth trauma interferes negatively with mother–baby bonding and can lead women to consider harming themselves or their baby (Elmir et al., 2010; Fenech & Thomson, 2014). Maternal suicide is the leading cause of maternal death in Australia (Humphrey et al., 2015). This research provides valuable information indicating that women are fleeing a traumatising system and seeking a better experience in choosing homebirth and continuity of midwifery care, where they are significantly less likely to experience their birth as traumatic and, in some cases, may even find it healing (Laurel Merg & Carmoney, 2012; Keedle et al., 2015).

Conclusion

Women who choose to give birth at home often do so to avoid medical interventions. The literature indicates that women are not only avoiding the interventions themselves but the sequelae of negative effects that occur when the process of normal birth is disturbed for themselves and their baby. Women are not only seeking to avoid clinical examinations, medical procedures, medical technology or administration of medications, they are also avoiding a range of interferences that they feel hinders the normal progress of labour and birth. Women associate medical intervention in hospital with a loss of control. They seek greater involvement in decision-making and compassionate care which acknowledges the needs of the individual over the needs of the institution. The NHBS shows that the majority of women with risk factors would plan a freebirth at home if they cannot access a midwife. Women who plan homebirth are not only avoiding specific medical interventions and interferences associated with a hospital birth, they are also accessing continuity of care with a known midwife and a safe and familiar environment to support their physiological birth.

The way forward

- Excessive regulation of midwives attending homebirth will only increase risk as women are pushed to freebirth
- A system which supports women's right to choose homebirth while also protecting the midwives who support them needs to be established
- Hospital visiting rights for PPMs will provide continuity in case of transfer, allow women with risk factors to have the support of a PPM in any setting and likely improve communication and relations between hospital staff and PPMs
- Regular education of hospital midwives and obstetricians on ethical ways to present information and how to support women who make choices outside of guidelines may be beneficial
- More home-like birth units in the hospital – combined with access to PPMs – may lead more women with risk factors to choose hospital birth

References

Andersen, L. B., Melvaer, L. B., Videbech, P., Lamont, R. F., & Joergensen, J. S. (2012) Risk factors for developing post-traumatic stress disorder following childbirth: A systematic review. *Acta Obstetricia et Gynecologica Scandinavica, 91*, 1261–72. Retrieved from: www.ncbi.nlm.nih.gov/pubmed/22670573.

Andrews, A. (2004a) Home birth experience 1: Decision and expectation. *British Journal of Midwifery, 12*, 518–523.

Andrews, A. (2004b) Home birth experience 2: Births/postnatal reflections. *British Journal of Midwifery, 12*, 552–557.

Ashley, S. & Weaver, J. (2012a) Factors influencing multiparous women who choose a home birth: A literature review. *British Journal of Midwifery, 20*, 646–652.

Ashley, S. & Weaver, J. (2012b) Factors influencing multiparous women to choose a home birth: An exploratory study. *British Journal of Midwifery, 20*, 710–715.

Australian Institute of Health and Welfare. (2016) *Australia's mothers and babies 2014*. Canberra: AIHW. Retrieved from: www.aihw.gov.au/WorkArea/DownloadAsset.aspx?id=60129557657.

Bai, D. L., Wu, K. M., & Tarrant, M. (2013) Association between intrapartum interventions and breastfeeding duration. *Journal of Midwifery & Women's Health, 58*, 25–32. Retrieved from: www.ncbi.nlm.nih.gov/pubmed/23317341.

Bernhard, C., Zielinski, R., Ackerson, K., & English, J. (2014) Home birth after hospital birth: Women's choices and reflections. *Journal of Midwifery & Women's Health, 59*, 160–166. Retrieved from: www.ncbi.nlm.nih.gov/pubmed/24612335.

Betrán, A. P., Ye, J., Moller, A. B., Zhang, J., Gülmezoglu, A. M., & Torloni, M. R. (2016) The increasing trend in caesarean section rates: Global, regional and national estimates: 1990–2014. *PLoS ONE, 11*(2), e0148343. Retrieved from: www.ncbi.nlm.nih.gov/pubmed/26849801.

Boucher, D., Bennett, C., McFarlin, B., & Freeze, R. (2009) Staying home to give birth: Why women in the United States choose home birth. *Journal of Midwifery & Women's Health, 54*, 119–126. Retrieved from: http://ezproxy.uws.edu.au/login?url=http://search.ebscohost.com/login.aspx?direct=true&db=rzh&AN=2010228690&site=ehost-live&scope=site.

Brocklehurst, P., Hardy, P., Hollowell, J., Linsell, L., Macfarlane, A., McCourt, C. … Stewart, M. (2011) Perinatal and maternal outcomes by planned place of birth for healthy women with low risk pregnancies: The birthplace in England national prospective cohort study. *BMJ (Clinical Research Edition), 343*, d7400. Retrieved from: www.bmj.com.ezproxy.uws.edu.au/content/343/bmj.d7400.

Bureau of Health Information. (2014) Healthcare in focus 2013: How well does NSW measure up? Publication No. 140119. Retrieved from: www.bhi.nsw.gov.au/__data/assets/pdf_file/0008/216971/Main-report_HealthcareInFocus-2013.pdf.

Catling, C., Dahlen, H., & Homer, C. S. E. (2014) The influences on women who choose publicly-funded home birth in Australia. *Midwifery, 30*, 892–898.

Catling-Paull, C., Dahlen, H., & Homer, C. S. E. (2011) Multiparous women's confidence to have a publicly-funded homebirth: A qualitative study. *Women and Birth: Journal of the Australian College of Midwives, 24*(3), 122–128. Retrieved from: www.sciencedirect.com/science/article/pii/S1871519210000648.

Cheyney, M. J. (2008) Homebirth as systems-challenging praxis: Knowledge, power, and intimacy in the birthplace. *Qualitative Health Research, 18*, 254–267. Retrieved from: http://qhr.sagepub.com/content/18/2/254.abstract.

Christiaens, W. & Bracke, P. (2009) Place of birth and satisfaction with childbirth in Belgium and the Netherlands. *Midwifery*, *25*(2), e11–19. Retrieved from: www.sciencedirect.com/science/article/pii/S0266613807000381.

Dahlen, H., Jackson, M., & Stevens, J. (2011) Homebirth, freebirth and doulas: Casualty and consequences of a broken maternity system. *Women and Birth: Journal of the Australian College of Midwives*, *24*, 47–50. Retrieved from: www.sciencedirect.com/science/article/pii/S187151921000082X.

Davison, C., Hauck, Y. L., Bayes, S. J., Kuliukas, L. J., & Wood, J. (2015) The relationship is everything: Women's reasons for choosing a privately practising midwife in Western Australia. *Midwifery*, *31*, 772–778.

De Graaf, M. (2019). World's top obstetricians laugh about Meghan Markle's home birth plan at global summit – but others say the duchess is right to confront dangers of childbirth for black women in the UK. *Daily Mail*, 5 May 2019. Retrieved from: www.dailymail.co.uk/health/article-6994943/amp/Meghan-Markle-sparks-debate-global-obstetrics-summit.html

Elmir, R., Schmied, V., Wilkes, L., & Jackson, D. (2010) Women's perceptions and experiences of a traumatic birth: A meta-ethnography. *Journal of Advanced Nursing*, *66*, 2142–2153. Retrieved from: www.ncbi.nlm.nih.gov/pubmed/20636467.

Fair, C. D. & Morrison, T. E. (2012) The relationship between prenatal control, expectations, experienced control, and birth satisfaction among primiparous women. *Midwifery*, *28*, 39–44. Retrieved from: www.sciencedirect.com/science/article/pii/S0266613810001749.

Fenech, G. & Thomson, G. (2014) Tormented by ghosts from their past: A meta-synthesis to explore the psychosocial implications of a traumatic birth on maternal well-being. *Midwifery*, *30*, 185–193. Retrieved from: www.sciencedirect.com.ezproxy.uws.edu.au/science/article/pii/S0266613813003513.

FIGO. (2018) FIGO position paper: How to stop the caesarean section epidemic. *Lancet*, *392*, 1286–1287.

Ford, E. & Ayers, S. (2011) Support during birth interacts with prior trauma and birth intervention to predict postnatal post-traumatic stress symptoms. *Psychology & Health*, *26*, 1553–1570. Retrieved from: www.tandfonline.com/doi/abs/10.1080/08870446.2010.533770.

Halfdansdottir, B., Smarason, A. Kr., Olafsdottir, O. A., Hildingsson, I., & Sveinsdottir, A. (2015) Outcome of planned home and hospital births among low-risk women in Iceland in 2005–2009: A retrospective cohort study. *Birth (Berkeley, California)*, *42*(1). Retrieved from: www.ncbi.nlm.nih.gov/pubmed/25613161.

Harris, R. & Ayers, S. (2012) What makes labour and birth traumatic? A survey of intrapartum 'hotspots'. *Psychology & Health*, *27*, 1166–1177. Retrieved from: www.tandfonline.com/doi/abs/10.1080/08870446.2011.649755.

Humphrey, M. D., Bonelli, R., Chugtai, A., Macaldowie, A., Harris, K., & Chambers, G. M. (2015) Maternal deaths in Australia 2008–2012. Maternal Deaths Series no. 5. Cat. no. PER 70. Retrieved from: www.aihw.gov.au/publication-detail/?id=60129551119.

Jackson, M., Dahlen, H., & Schmied, V. (2012) Birthing outside the system: Perceptions of risk amongst Australian women who have freebirths and high risk homebirths. *Midwifery*, *28*, 561–567. Retrieved from: www.sciencedirect.com/science/article/pii/S0266613811001811.

Janssen, P., Saxell, L., Page, L. A., Klein, M. C., Liston, R. M., & Lee, S. K. (2009) Outcomes of planned home birth with registered midwife versus planned hospital birth with midwife or physician. *Canadian Medical Association Journal*, *181*, pp. 377–383. Retrieved from: www.pubmedcentral.nih.gov/articlerender.fcgi?artid=2742137&tool=pmcentrez&rendertype=abstract.

Janssen, P. A., Carty, E. A., & Reime, B. (2006) Satisfaction with planned place of birth among midwifery clients in British Columbia. *Journal of Midwifery & Women's Health*, *51*(2), 91–97.

de Jonge, A., van der Goes, B. Y., Ravelli, A. C. J., Amelink-Verburg, M. P., Mol, B. W., Nijhuis, J. G. … Buitendijk, S. E. (2009) Perinatal mortality and morbidity in a nationwide cohort of 529,688 low-risk planned home and hospital births. *British Journal of Obstetrics and Gynaecology*, *116*, 1177–1184. Retrieved from: www.ncbi.nlm.nih.gov/pubmed/19624439.

de Jonge, A., Geerts, C. C., van der Goes, B. Y., Mol, B. W., Buitendijk, S. E., & Nijhuis, J. G. (2015) Perinatal mortality and morbidity up to 28 days after birth among 743 070 low-risk planned home and hospital births: A cohort study based on three merged national perinatal databases. *British Journal of Obstetrics & Gynaecology*, *122*, 720–728. Retrieved from: https://obgyn.onlinelibrary.wiley.com/doi/full/10.1111/1471-0528.13935.

Jouhki, M.-R. (2012) Choosing homebirth – The women's perspective. *Women and Birth*, *25*(4), e56–61. Retrieved from: www.sciencedirect.com/science/article/pii/S1871519211002393.

Keedle, H., Schmied, V., Burns, E., & Dahlen, H. G. (2015) Women's reasons for, and experiences of, choosing a homebirth following a caesarean section. *BMC Pregnancy and Childbirth*, *15*, 206. Retrieved from: www.biomedcentral.com/1471–2393/15/206.

Laurel Merg, A. & Carmoney, P. (2012) Phenomenological experiences: Homebirth after hospital birth. *International Journal of Childbirth Education*, *27*(4), 70–75. Retrieved from: http://ezproxy.uws.edu.au/login?url=http://search.ebscohost.com/login.aspx?direct=true&db=rzh&AN=2011705073&site=ehost-live&scope=site.

Lessa, H. F., Tyrrell, M. A. R., Alves, V. H., & Rodrigues, D. P. (2014) Social relations and the option for planned home birth: An institutional ethnographic study. *Online Brazilian Journal of Nursing*, *13*, 239–249.

Lindgren, H., Rådestad, I. J., Christensson, K., Wally-Bystrom, K., & Hildingsson, I. M. (2010) Perceptions of risk and risk management among 735 women who opted for a home birth. *Midwifery*, *26*, 163–172. Retrieved from: www.sciencedirect.com/science/article/pii/S0266613808000491.

Longworth, L., Ratcliffe, J., & Boulton, M. (2001) Investigating women's preferences for intrapartum care: Home versus hospital births. *Health and Social Care in the Community*, *9*, 404–413.

Lothian, J. A. (2013) Being safe: Making the decision to have a planned home birth in the United States. *Journal of Clinical Ethics*, *24*, pp. 266–275.

McCutcheon, R. & Brown, D. (2012) A qualitative exploration of women's experiences and reflections upon giving birth at home. *Evidence Based Midwifery*, *10*, 23–28.

Meyer, S. (2013) Control in childbirth: A concept analysis and synthesis. *Journal of Advanced Nursing*, *69*, 218–228. Retrieved from: www.ncbi.nlm.nih.gov/pubmed/22671134.

Miller, A. C. & Shriver, T. E. (2012) Women's childbirth preferences and practices in the United States. *Social Science & Medicine (1982)*, *75*, 709–716. Retrieved from: www.sciencedirect.com/science/article/pii/S0277953612003516.

Miller, Y. D., Prosser, S. J., & Thompson, R. (2012) Going public: Do risk and choice explain differences in caesarean birth rates between public and private places of birth in Australia? *Midwifery*, *28*, 627–635. Retrieved from: www.sciencedirect.com/science/article/pii/S0266613812001039.

Moyzakitis, W. (2004) Exploring women's descriptions of distress and/or trauma in childbirth from a feminist perspective. *Evidence Based Midwifery*, *2*(1), 8–14. Retrieved from: http://search.ebscohost.com.ezproxy.liv.ac.uk/login.aspx?direct=true&db=jlh&AN=106549211&site=ehost-live&scope=site.

Murray-Davis, B., McNiven, P., McDonald, H., Malott, A., Elarar, L., & Hutton, E. (2012) Why home birth? A qualitative study exploring women's decision making about place of birth in two Canadian provinces. *Midwifery*, *28*, 576–581. Retrieved from: www.sciencedirect.com/science/article/pii/S0266613812000216.

Murray-Davis, B., McDonald, H., Rietsma, A., Coubrough, C., & Hutton, E. (2014) Deciding on home or hospital birth: Results of the Ontario choice of birthplace survey. *Midwifery*, *30*, 869–876. Retrieved from: www.sciencedirect.com/science/article/pii/S0266613814000229.

O'Donovan, A., Alcorn, K. L., Patrick, J. C., Creedy, D. K., Dawe, S., & Devilly, G. J. (2014) Predicting posttraumatic stress disorder after childbirth. *Midwifery*, *30*, 935–941.

Olde, E., van der Hart, O., Kleber, R., & van Son, M. (2006) Posttraumatic stress following childbirth: A review. *Clinical Psychology Review*, *26*, 1–16. Retrieved from: www.sciencedirect.com/science/article/pii/S0272735805000991.

Reed, R., Sharman, R., & Inglis, C. (2017) Women's descriptions of childbirth trauma relating to care provider actions and interactions. *BMC Pregnancy and Childbirth*, *17*(1), 21. Retrieved from: http://bmcpregnancychildbirth.biomedcentral.com/articles/10.1186/s12884–016–1197–0.

Regan, M. & McElroy, K. (2013) Women's perceptions of childbirth risk and place of birth. *Journal of Clinical Ethics*, *24*, 239–252.

Simpson, M., Schmied, V., Dickson, C., & Dahlen, H. G. (2018) Postnatal post-traumatic stress: An integrative review. *Women and Birth*, *31*, 367–379.

Stramrood, C. A., Paarlberg, K. M., Huis In 't Veld, E. M. J., Berger, L. W. A. R., Vingerhoets, A. J. J. M., Weijmar Schultz, W. C. M., & van Pampus, M. G. (2011) Posttraumatic stress following childbirth in homelike and hospital settings. *Journal of Psychosomatic Obstetrics & Gynaecology*, *32*(2), 88–97.

Sweeney, S. & O'Connell, R. (2015) Puts the magic back into life: Fathers' experience of planned home birth. *Women and Birth*, *28*, 148–153. Retrieved from: http://dx.doi.org/10.1016/j.wombi.2014.12.001.

Symon, A., Winter, C., Donnan, P. T., & Kirkham, M. (2010) Examining autonomy's boundaries: A follow-up review of perinatal mortality cases in UK independent midwifery. *Birth*, *37*, 280–287. Retrieved from: www.ncbi.nlm.nih.gov/pubmed/21083719.

Thompson, R. & Miller, Y. D. (2014) Birth control: To what extent do women report being informed and involved in decisions about pregnancy and birth procedures? *BMC Pregnancy and Childbirth*, *14*(1), 62. Retrieved from: www.pubmedcentral.nih.gov/articlerender.fcgi?artid=3923734&tool=pmcentrez&rendertype=abstract.

Thomson, G. & Downe, S. (2008) Widening the trauma discourse: The link between childbirth and experiences of abuse. *Journal of Psychosomatic Obstetrics & Gynecology*, *29*, 268–273. Retrieved from: www.tandfonline.com/doi/full/10.1080/01674820802545453.

Thomson, G. M. & Downe, S. (2010). Changing the future to change the past: Women's experiences of a positive birth following a traumatic birth experience. *Journal of Reproductive and Infant Psychology*, *28*, 102–112. Retrieved from: www.tandfonline.com/doi/full/10.1080/02646830903295000.

Torvaldsen, S., Roberts, C. L., Simpson, J. M., Thomson, J. F., & Ellwood, D. A. (2006) Intrapartum epidural analgesia and breastfeeding: A prospective cohort study. *International Breastfeeding Journal*, *1*, 24. Retrieved from: www.pubmedcentral.nih.gov/articlerender.fcgi?artid=1702531&tool=pmcentrez&rendertype=abstract.

Viisainen, K. (2001) Negotiating control and meaning: home birth as a self-constructed choice in Finland. *Social Science & Medicine*, *52*, 1109–1121. Retrieved from: www.sciencedirect.com/science/article/pii/S0277953600002069.

Wiklund, I., Norman, M., Uvnäs-Moberg, K., Ransjö-Arvidson, A.-B., & Andolf, E. (2009) Epidural analgesia: Breast-feeding success and related factors. *Midwifery*, *25*(2), e31–38. Retrieved from: www.sciencedirect.com/science/article/pii/S0266613807000915.

7 The journey of homebirth after caesarean (HBAC)

Fighting the system or birthing in peace

Hazel Keedle with Sarah O'Connor

> This [HBAC] was the healing, empowering experience I so desperately hoped for. I've never felt stronger or prouder to be me.
>
> (Sarah O'Connor)

About the authors

I (Hazel) became interested in the topic of VBAC following my own journey of an unnecessary caesarean and then being pregnant again very quickly. With a less than a six-month gap between the caesarean and conception of the subsequent pregnancy I was at a greater uterine rupture risk (Stamilio, 2007), but I was determined to have a VBAC. I had a fight on my hands, but as a midwife I had access to research and made an educated decision to choose a VBAC. Even during my labour, in a hospital that knew me as a midwife, I had to fight the looming deadline of the knife and my daughter was born vaginally exactly at the time I was told I would be wheeled into theatres. My recovery was amazing, both physically and emotionally, but it sparked something in me. I wanted to know if the fight was just something I experienced as a 'difficult woman' or something all women planning a VBAC were experiencing. Within a couple of years, I was on my VBAC research journey, first exploring women's experience of having a homebirth after caesarean (HBAC) for my Master of Philosophy and then women's antenatal experiences of planning a VBAC in Australia for my PhD.

To illustrate the VBAC journey, I approached Sarah O'Connor, who shared her recent birth story on a VBAC social media group. Sarah agreed to write her birth stories for this chapter. Sarah experienced many interventions and different births and her birth stories will ring true for so many women currently experiencing the Australian maternity system.

Vaginal birth after caesarean (VBAC)

After a woman has had a caesarean she has different options for her next birth. For most women, a vaginal birth after caesarean (VBAC) is a safe option for both herself and her baby, with the other option being a repeat caesarean. Research suggests there is a range of 60–80% of women who plan a VBAC and have a VBAC, with the remainder of women having a repeat caesarean (Gardner, Henry, Thou, Davis, & Miller, 2014). Actual rates of women having a VBAC worldwide vary widely. In Australia 14% of women had a VBAC in 2016 (AIHW, 2018). Across Europe, VBAC rates vary from 20% to 55% (EURO-PERISTAT Project, 2013; Lundgren, van Limbeek, Vehvilainen-Julkunen, & Nilsson, 2015). In the USA, the national average VBAC rate in 2016 was 12% (Martin, Hamilton, Oserman, Driscoll, & Drake, 2018). In comparison, though, a US study found 45% of women out of 3006 surveyed with a previous caesarean planned to have a VBAC for their next birth (Attanasio, Kozhimannil, & Kjerulff, 2019).

VBAC is an important contemporary health issue as caesarean section rates increase globally. The *Lancet* series on optimising caesarean section use identified an international doubling of caesarean rates since the year 2000 with an estimated 29.7 million caesareans worldwide in 2015 (Boerma et al., 2018). Rising caesarean rates are linked with poorer outcomes for both mother and baby, are associated with higher risk of severe acute maternal morbidity and impact long-term health (Clark, 2011; Sandall et al., 2018; Korb et al., 2019). Caesarean sections are costly to health services (Fawsitt et al., 2013; Fobelets et al., 2018). Yet, repeat caesarean is the main reason women have a caesarean in Australia (AIHW, 2018). VBAC does come with some unique health issues, due to the previous caesarean. Very rarely, the site of the previous caesarean in the wall of the uterus can open partially or fully and lead to a uterine rupture and if not identified early can lead to maternal shock and haemorrhage and foetal death (Guiliano et al., 2014). The uterine rupture rate is around one in 200 women (Motomura et al., 2017). Hysterectomy and perinatal mortality rates related to uterine rupture are very low. A recent European study found rates of 2.2 and 3.2 per 10,000 during labour for a VBAC (Vandenberghe et al., 2019). Uterine rupture rates do increase with shorter interpregnancy rates and with the use of pharmacological induction methods, such as prostaglandin pessaries and synthetic oxytocin infusions (Stamilio, 2007; Dekker, 2010).

The research I have undertaken focused on the experiences of women planning a VBAC. The first study interviewed 11 women who had a HBAC (Keedle, Schmied, Burns, & Dahlen, 2015). Following this, I went on to publish a meta-ethnography of 20 qualitative studies on women's experiences of VBAC entitled 'The journey from pain to power' (Keedle, Schmied, Burns, & Dahlen, 2018). A meta-ethnography uses a methodological process to synthesis and analyse qualitative studies around a topic and develops new interpretations of the data (Noblit, 1988). We found that women planning a VBAC go on a unique journey from the previous, often traumatic, caesarean to their triumphant VBAC. Along the journey women experience a range of highs and lows that can impact decision-making around their choice of healthcare providers and their planned birth location. The journey to having a VBAC can be daunting, lonely and traumatising.

Identifying the journey became the basis for the qualitative study, the four factors to having a VBAC, with 11 women being followed during their VBAC journey (Keedle, Schmied, Burns, & Dahlen, 2019). This chapter will explore the reasons why some women plan a VBAC at home (sometimes referred to as an HBAC) and then discuss the factors that are important for women planning a VBAC that may help engage women back into the healthcare system.

The VBAC journey

Our meta-ethnography of 20 qualitative studies on women's experiences of VBAC entitled 'The journey from pain to power' found that the start of the journey was the experience of having a caesarean (Keedle et al., 2018). Having a caesarean was often a frightening experience, heightened by women's fear for their baby and themselves. Women often experienced poor treatment in the operating theatre and felt objectified and disrespected by theatre staff and ignored as conversations occurred above them. Following the caesarean section, women felt a sense of failure and loss for not having achieved a vaginal birth and confusion about their inability to have a vaginal birth. These feelings could extend to issues with bonding and/or breastfeeding their baby that they felt resulted from experiencing major abdominal surgery. This negative experience stays with the woman and becomes the starting point for the journey towards another pregnancy.

Introducing Sarah's story

Sarah's first birth was an induction of labour and the day started with a very painful internal vaginal examination.

> As the obstetrician began the procedure, he inserted his finger and the instrument and simultaneously a contraction began to build. Suddenly the room was spinning, the pain I felt was nothing like I'd ever experienced. His finger and the instrument had become stuck in my cervix. I lay there screaming 'stop, stop, stop' while he apologised explaining he was stuck and could not stop. He and the midwife both had a horrified look on their faces while I lay there helplessly screaming through it. Finally, as the contraction was ending my cervix released his finger and the instrument and out gushed the amniotic fluid.
>
> I was not coping and begged for pain relief. I was offered nitrous gas and oxygen and soon enough was begging for an epidural. Once administered the epidural only took to one side, leaving me fully numb down one side and feeling everything on the other. The syntocinon

> infusion began and things intensified. I was stuck on the bed for the rest of my labour. I remember feeling afraid and out of control. After a 12-hour active labour, I gave birth to my first baby, my son Levi Hugh. He was a healthy 7.5 lbs. I needed no stitches, there was no need for any type of assisted instrumental delivery on paper my birth story sounded 'normal' it sounded successful, not near as bad as some I'd heard, so why did I feel so traumatised?
>
> The impression left on me was that labour was torture. I thought I was prepared because I'd done the childbirth classes the hospital offered, I did the birth suite tour, I read a book on pregnancy and babies and I lapped up glossy pregnancy magazines. With the knowledge I now have I know I was not at all prepared and I feel sad for the young naive woman I was.
>
> After the birth I remember feeling overwhelmed with love and joy for my baby boy. I told myself it was all OK because he was of course worth it. I focused on him and whenever thoughts of his birth entered my head, I pushed them away. I'd heard the horror stories before and now I had my very own.

Now with a history of a traumatic birth, Sarah went into her second pregnancy fearful of vaginal birth. When her baby was breech she was hoping that the baby didn't turn.

> I wanted the caesarean section the second I heard it was possible that I could avoid another vaginal birth. At every appointment when they'd check my baby's position, I was so happy to hear that she was still breech. The procedure itself was a daunting thought, I didn't like the idea of having a scar but that was outweighed by my fear of another vaginal birth. I felt caesarean section (CS) was the best choice and was thrilled I didn't have to birth vaginally.
>
> The day came, I was excited and nervous at the same time. The procedure went well, my daughter Addison Bridget was born, a healthy baby girl, my smallest at 7.1 lbs. She had sustained an injury during the procedure, a small cut on her hip where the obstetrician sliced her when he made the CS incision. This really broke my heart knowing she'd been injured. He apologised and kind of brushed it off. They stuck some butterfly clips on it to help it heal (she still has a scar). I came out of the CS feeling OK, but as the numbness wore off the pain hit. I struggled just to pick my baby up. I could hardly do simple things like walk to the bathroom or stand in the shower. The painkillers they gave me made me foggy and these first precious days with my baby are a blurry memory to me. We stayed 5 nights in hospital before we could finally head home. I remember I struggled to walk to the car, every step was agony.

Sarah's daughter had a difficult start in life, contracting septicaemia and meningitis in her first few weeks of life.

I beat myself up thinking if I'd had her vaginally maybe this wouldn't have happened. My baby girl fought hard, she was in excellent care and she recovered. Her immune system seemed to be compromised from this rough start, and in her first 2 years of life she was often sick and had other hospital admissions.

The first step in the VBAC journey is information gathering

The first step along the VBAC journey for women is information gathering. In both the meta-ethnography and the HBAC study this stage of the journey involved internet searching and reading as much as possible about VBAC, as well as finding relevant social media groups for VBAC (Keedle et al., 2015, 2018). Information sources identified were blogs, websites and social media sites alongside scholarly journal articles. During this period of knowledge-seeking women had the opportunity to reflect on their previous caesarean, in the light of new information. Often women would learn about the cascade of intervention and identify with other women who shared their traumatic caesarean stories, finding similarities with their own experiences. This period of reflection, whether before or during the following pregnancy, would help arm women with knowledge on their choices and preferences for the subsequent birth and would often increase their understanding on why they craved a vaginal birth experience.

Sarah reflects this information gathering in her story. She approached the birth of her third child differently.

> By now I'd come across some positive VBAC stories on social media. It really sparked my interest. As soon as I found out I was pregnant I joined a support group on Facebook for VBAC women. I wasn't sure to begin with what my birth options would be, but I was very curious to learn as much as I could. I wanted to give my baby the best possible start and felt vaginal birth was best for his health even if I was still afraid of vaginal birth.
>
> Through this group of VBAC women I found so much support and great advice. They shared their successful VBAC birth stories, evidence-based articles, information on human rights in child birth (before this I wasn't even aware I could say no to certain things in a hospital). It was invaluable to me and for the first time I started to feel positively about vaginal birth. I started believing in my body and my baby and our ability to have a positive birth.

Fight the fight, give up the fight or leave the fight

With this increased knowledge women faced their first obstacle, which was explaining their choices and wishes to healthcare professionals in the antenatal appointments. Many women reported hostility and disparaging comments, especially when discussing birth plans or when trying to negotiate different interventions for labour and birth. Negotiating care and interventions was like two different worlds colliding into each other. One world was that of the woman, with her personal experience of having a caesarean, her increased knowledge about VBAC and her desire to not repeat the previous experience by avoiding the interventions that may have contributed to it in the first place. The other world was that of the healthcare professional(s) with their risk-based language and policies and guidelines. The result of the collisions between these two and the inflexibility of the healthcare system influenced the rest of the journey. The woman had some choices to make: fight the fight, give up the fight or leave the fight.

Choosing to fight the fight and plan a VBAC within the hospital system can be challenging. Many hospitals, especially in regional and rural Australia, don't offer VBAC as a birthing option, with women either opting to stay local and have an elective caesarean or having to travel in labour to a hospital further away. Sarah also found this to be an issue, which she found out when visiting her GP.

> I found the journey to a VBAC wasn't going to be without challenges. When seeing a GP to refer me for my antenatal care I was told the local hospital wouldn't take me if I planned to VBAC and would only take me if I agreed to a planned CS. My only option was to go to a tertiary hospital 35 minutes away, that was VBAC friendly. It may have been a VBAC 'friendly' hospital but a lot of the care providers I encountered seemed to be biased, favouring repeat CS. I would see someone different at every appointment and majority of the time I would be lectured about all the risks of a VBAC and encouraged to book a CS.

Sarah also experienced healthcare professionals using the size of the baby to persuade her into agreeing to a repeat caesarean.

> My pregnancy was healthy, and towards the end I started measuring largely. I was referred for an ultrasound and told I had a large baby and a lot of amniotic fluid. I was told I was borderline polyhydramnios. At my 36-week appointment I was being pressured by an obstetrician to book in a CS because of the risk of rupture, then it became about the risk of a big baby, then the risk of cord prolapse due to polyhydromnios. I explained I'd done my own research and was happy to continue with my plans to VBAC. I held my ground, which wasn't easy. I felt so much pressure at my next few appointments. I continued to refuse scheduling a CS and I had to sign a waiver saying I was going against their advice.

After agreeing to an induction of labour at 39 weeks due to decreased foetal movements and irregular contractions Sarah found herself on the bed on her back after having an injection of pethidine and experienced a difficult birth.

> I remember pushing his head out and then some time went by and he wasn't coming down. Suddenly there was an element of fear in the room as more people entered, then a panicked obstetrician I'd never met ran in and started yelling at everyone to push my legs back further. I have a blurry memory of maybe six or seven people standing over me, my legs pushed up as far as they'd go and everyone telling me to push, push, push! The obstetrician then manually assisted me to deliver my baby boy Kyle James, a healthy 9.1 lbs (4.1 kg). It felt like it had been a serious emergency but really, I don't know. I wasn't all that with it because of the pethidine and I never had any type of debriefing with the hospital. It felt like it was quite brutal to my body and I had flash backs of it for a while after the birth.

The option of leaving the fight to have a VBAC can lead some women to explore different birthing options and find the option of homebirth. Homebirth potentially eliminates the need to continue negotiating and fighting about interventions and care options. If available and affordable some women find a privately practising midwife (PPM) and others find an unregulated birth worker (UBW) or choose to freebirth without assistance (Jackson, Dahlen, & Schmied, 2012; Keedle et al., 2015; Rigg, Schmied, Peters, & Dahlen, 2018).

Two years after her hospital VBAC, Sarah was pregnant with her fourth baby.

> This time around I wanted things to be very different. I wanted continuous care with a trusted provider who supported me. I wanted less trauma and believed the best way to achieve that was with an unmedicated physiological birth. After everything I'd experienced and all I'd learned I trusted that I could birth this way. I didn't want any intervention unless there was a true need for it, I didn't want any drugs, I didn't want to have limitations because of hospital policy. I didn't want to be surrounded by strangers and machines in a clinical setting. I wanted to do the best I could to have a positive birth and I believed it was possible. I looked at all my options and had lots of conversations with my husband and we concluded that for us a homebirth supported by independent midwives was the best way to facilitate that.

Homebirth after caesarean (HBAC)

In the HBAC study we undertook, 12 women were interviewed on their experiences of planning and having a VBAC at home (Keedle et al., 2015). The overarching theme of this qualitative study was 'it's never happening again'. Most of the women in the study found a PPM who provided continuity of care throughout pregnancy, labour and birth and the postnatal period. Unlike the difficult negotiations in the hospital system the women reported feeling they were in a partnership with their midwife and they were encouraged to make their own decisions. They felt more in control.

Relationships developed with their midwife were based on trust and friendship and appointments were longer and focused on more than physical examinations. Women described how their midwife provided emotional support and debriefing services and this was also identified in a focus group with PPMs. Midwives in the focus group highlighted the respectful partnership based on equality that was the foundation of their care (Keedle, 2015).

Women did need to be aware of who they told about planning a HBAC and they would use 'selective telling' with friends, family and healthcare professionals as a deliberate act of self-preservation. By not telling they were protecting themselves from criticism, negativity and judgement. Women in the HBAC study also gained knowledge and friendship when 'gathering support' from other women in the homebirth community, both online and locally and by learning alternate ways of experiences labour. Even though this was her fourth pregnancy, it was Sarah's first planned homebirth.

> In preparation for this birth I read countless homebirth stories and watched numerous homebirth videos online. I joined a homebirth group on Facebook where I found lots of great stories and supportive women to connect with. I read so many books I lost count. My husband came with me to birth preparation workshops, one of them being birth with confidence by Rhea Dempsey and it was brilliant! We did a hypnobirthing class and regularly practised the techniques. We felt prepared and excited and so hopeful that this would be the positive birth experience we wanted.

With support from her midwives and a lot of patience, Sarah went into labour naturally at 42 weeks gestation. After a slow build-up of surges throughout the day and night Sarah called her midwife over early the next day. Here is Sarah's account of the birth of her fourth baby, born on 6 December 2018.

> At 6:30 a.m. my midwife arrived. We were in a happy excited bubble of love. We had our wedding playlist on and I remember singing all the songs in between surges and really having a great time. Daniel was lovingly helping me work through surges with lots of affection and the soft touch massage we learnt in our hypnobirthing classes. Every surge I focused on relaxing my body and opening while I did the breathing techniques and visualisations we'd practised.
>
> The pool was so relaxing, my surges spaced out again and I was able to rest and went into my own zone. I remember occasionally still singing along to the music. I remember looking up into my husband's eyes and telling him I loved him and kissing. I remember looking at my birth affirmations on the wall and then I'd zone out again and go deeply into my own little world.

My midwife was checking in on me and baby, she was so gentle and quiet that I hardly even noticed, but I sensed her presence with me. Every check she would quietly assure me baby's heart rate is perfect, all is well. After some time in the pool she asked if I'd like to hop out and maybe have some time on the toilet. I liked that idea and realised I hadn't urinated for a while and had been drinking a lot of water.

At about 10:00 a.m. I got out of the pool and things went up another level. I sat on the toilet and I couldn't go but I remained there for a few surges. Things were building up, surges were very intense, and I needed to keep changing what I was doing. Both of my midwives were so helpful and had so many suggestions and tried different things to help me through. My second midwife used the rebozo on me in between surges as I leaned forward, a technique called shake the apple tree. At another point she set up the rebozo hanging from a door and encouraged me to hang from it and move up and down.

My midwives were incredible, they talked me through these intense surges and encouraged me to let my body open and visualise my baby tucking her chin and moving down. I found these words so helpful, but I quickly moved from the rebozo[1] back to Daniel's arms. I remember at some points I was really hanging all my weight off him and he held me up as I swayed and moved up and down, dragging and pulling on him. His strength was incredible; I adore him for this!

My midwives continued encouraging me and using soft touch massage. Things got so intense, I remember a few times saying help me, that I couldn't do it anymore, everyone worked to reassure me. I asked my baby 'Please baby come on mummy needs you to come now.' I was experiencing pain and pressure in my lower tummy and pelvis that was different to anything I'd ever felt. I couldn't tell when a surge was starting or ending and I felt like something wasn't right. My midwife suggested a catheter may help as I'd been unable to urinate earlier and maybe it would help to empty my bladder. I was willing to try it and felt desperate for some form of relief.

I moved to my bed for a cervical check before the catheter could be done and I was very open (I don't know numbers) with a cervical lip. Then suddenly something changed my surges became pushing surges. 'I think I'm pushing' I yelled out. It all seemed so fast. I was happy for another quick check which revealed sure enough baby was right there, I put my fingers inside and could feel her head, and the waters were still intact. I remember wanting my waters broken at some point thinking it would help but my midwives encouraged me to keep going and that they would break on their own or that I could even pop them with my nails if I wanted to. They remained intact and I roared as my baby's head moved down the birth canal.

I could feel my body pushing with each surge like an incredible expulsion feeling, the foetal ejection reflex! I think it was at this point my waters broke. I was still laying on my bed on my back and my midwife suggested I get on all fours and I remember saying 'I can't', and with that my midwife assured me that I could do it and I'm so glad she did! The next minute I was on all fours and roaring through another surge.

I could feel this incredible power forcing my baby down with each surge. I reached down to feel her come. Slowly my body opened and stretched, and her head began to come through. I roared and roared. I felt her firm wet head slowly filling up my open hand. Her head finally came all the way through and for a moment she rested in my hand. I will never forget that incredible overwhelming feeling of love, strength and amazement, my baby's head in my hands between two worlds. Then there was a bit of a pause and I knew she was a little stuck.

I'd wanted to catch her but I needed to support myself and I just knew she wasn't coming that easily. Nothing needed to be said, I just knew and I was OK and trusted everything was alright. My previous hospital VBAC had shoulder dystocia so I knew what this was. We were in good hands, the room was quieter and I said 'come on my baby, come on'. I focused on relaxing and opening and breathing/roaring through this while my midwife manually but very gently helped us. Finally, her slippery body slid out and my midwife passed her through my legs. 11:28 a.m. she arrived.

I remember the instant relief; I looked down at her in so much awe and wonder. I knelt up and picked up my baby. I remember my second midwife saying blow on your babies face a little and as I did she let out some cries and she was perfect. I held her to me saying 'Oh my baby, oh look at you, we did it darling, oh we did it'. I was so proud, relieved and in awe! I relished in this moment looking at her and talking to her. I announced her name 'Alannah Marika' then I felt a gush of warmth and wetness between my legs and the midwives helped me turn over and to lie back on my bed and they examined my loss and rubbed my fundus. All was fine. Everything worked out so beautifully. I am so, so proud and elated and in love with my gorgeous not-so-little 9.36 lb baby girl Alannah Marika, my biggest baby. She came when she was ready. I'm so glad I trusted my body and baby and waited for her to pick her own birthday. We worked hard together, and it was a beautiful outcome.

This was the healing, empowering experience I'd so desperately hoped for. I've never felt stronger or prouder to be me.

In the HBAC study I asked all the women how they felt after their HBAC and they would pause, take a deep intake of breath and respond with 'I felt like Superwoman!', 'Elated', 'Healed' and 'One of the best moments of my life'. What had often been a choice made from frustration with the hospital system became a turning moment in these women's lives. They felt they could take on the world, and win, in bodies that were no longer broken and not to be trusted but strong and capable and powerful (Figure 7.1).

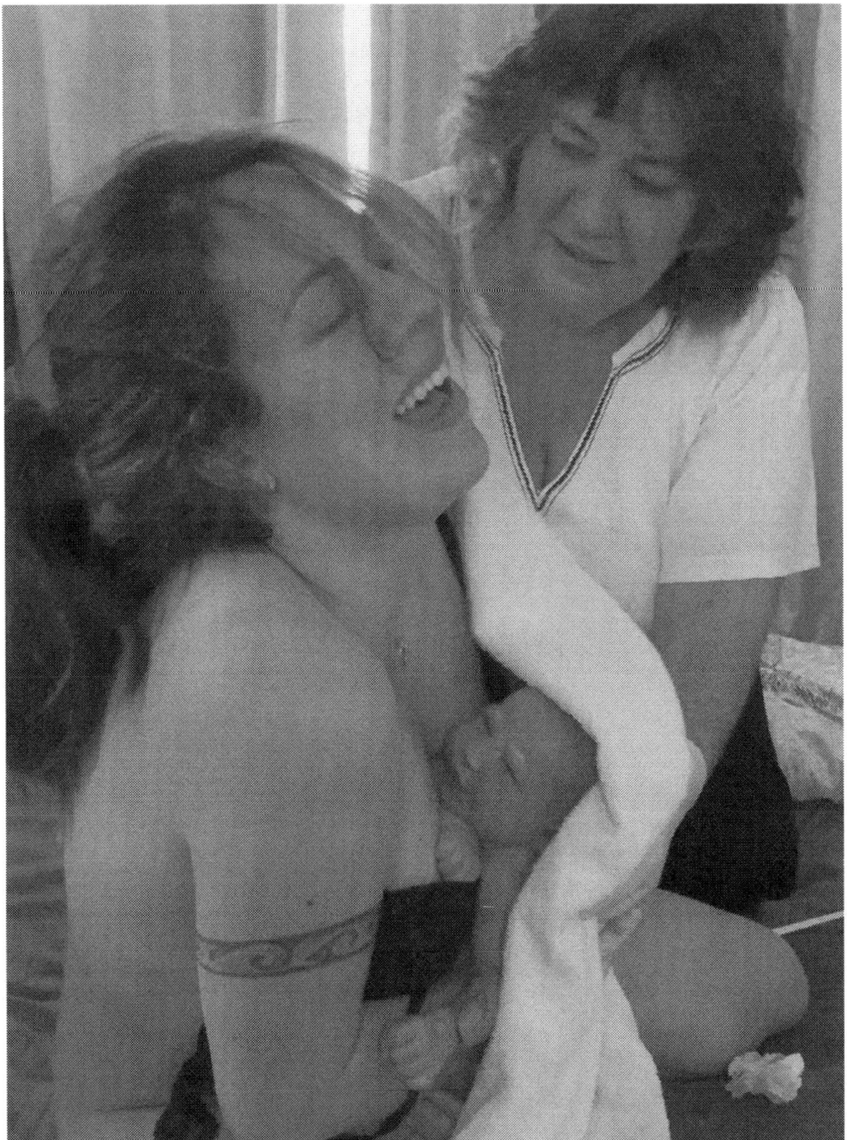

Figure 7.1 Sarah's VBAC

After doing this study and listening to the amazing stories of women I felt both assured and committed to women having the option of HBAC in the increasingly legislated and controlled arena of homebirth, where I also worked as a PPM, but also frustrated and disappointed that most women planning a

VBAC in the hospital system have a fight on their hands. I wanted to explore the journeys that women across models of maternity care and birth location had and learn how those journeys influenced their decisions and experiences of planning a VBAC in Australia. My hope was that by learning about these journeys, from the women experiencing them, we as researchers and clinicians can make their journeys better and more women can feel like Sarah did after her empowering HBAC.

Alongside my PhD supervisor team, I designed a study that would allow women to do a voice or video recording following every antenatal appointment during their pregnancy. I wanted to get those moments when women reflect on what went on in the appointment, who said what and what that meant through their perspective. The 'myVBACapp' study followed 11 women through their pregnancies and followed them all up with interviews six weeks after the birth. Data collection took nine months and altogether 53 recordings and 11 interviews were collected (Keedle et al., 2019).

The four factors that influence how women feel about their birth after a previous caesarean

To analyse the data, I used narrative analysis which allowed me to keep each of the women's stories intact, rather than mixing it all up and coming out with themes. The stories were so rich and informative that I loved reading and re-reading them and making notes as I compared one story to another. Through the expanse of stories and notes four factors became clear, factors that each of the women had experienced on a continuum. These are control, confidence, relationship and active labour. The four factors are interdependent and have a cumulative effect with positive feelings associated with higher levels of the factors and negative feelings with lower levels of the factors.

Control

The factor 'having control' relates to how in control the woman felt during the pregnancy, labour and birth and immediate postbirth period. Feeling a loss of control is a common theme for women who have had a traumatic birth (Elmir, 2010; Simpson, Schmied, Dickson, & Dahlen, 2018) and can be seen in Sarah's story, especially in the birth where she had an induction of labour. Potentially it is difficult to remain in control during an induction of labour, especially if synthetic oxytocin is required and the external locus of control remains with the clinicians titrating the infusion and monitoring the foetal heart rate. In these pregnancies Sarah felt she had a low level of control and this contributed to the negative feelings she had after the births. Conversely, in her planned HBAC she displayed high feelings of control, she was able to choose her midwives and choose how and where she laboured and birthed. These higher feelings of control influenced her positive feelings after her birth.

Confidence

The same works with 'having confidence'. This relates to the confidence the woman has in her own ability to have a VBAC and her confidence in her healthcare professionals' feelings in her ability to have a VBAC. Examples of this include how doctors were encouraging Sarah to have a repeat caesarean instead of a VBAC, resulting in Sarah probably doubting their confidence in her own ability. Consistent and continuous exposure to negative language from clinicians can chip away at women's own self-confidence and result in women becoming passive and compliant to an unwanted repeat caesarean. On the other end of the confidence continuum, women with high levels of self-confidence in their ability to birth vaginally being cared for by clinicians who also believe in their ability have more positive feelings after the birth.

Relationship

The relationship women develop with their healthcare provider understandably influences women's experiences and their feelings after their pregnancy and birthing journey. Midwifery continuity of care has been repeatedly shown to increase maternal satisfaction and decrease intervention rates (McLachlan et al., 2008; Tracy et al., 2013; Sandall, Soltani, Gates, Shennan, & Devane, 2016) and the 'myVBACapp' study supported those findings. Some women developed a good relationship with a private obstetrician, although the appointments were less chatty and there was less access to them outside of appointment times. Continuity of care alone didn't mean that a good relationship developed; one woman found her doctor that she saw throughout her pregnancy and labour wouldn't remember her or her birth wishes, and she continuously had to explain her reasons for wanting a VBAC. A good relationship is based on equity and respect, with both parties invested in the same goal and women who experienced this during their journey of planning a VBAC reported more positive feelings compared to women who had a poor or complete lack of relationship with a healthcare provider.

Staying active in labour

Women spend their VBAC journey preparing for the onset of labour and birth and the importance of how women feel and are treated during this time cannot be underestimated. The expectations, hopes and fears are all tested, and women go into labour carrying the burden of their previous experiences and, for some, the memories of trauma. Staying active in labour and having freedom of movement increases the probability of a normal birth (Prosser, Barnett, & Miller, 2018) and is preferred by many women (Hall, Foster, Yount, & Jennings, 2018). As in Sarah's journey, she had prepared for her HBAC by accessing alternate birth preparation courses and resources and she was supported and encouraged to use them during her labour. Her midwives also had tricks up their sleeves to assist Sarah in her goal by using the Mexican Rebozo and suggesting different positions in labour and birth. Sarah remained active in both her body and active in her ability to feel that her chosen support team and her environment were there to nurture and keep her and her baby safe. This is in stark comparison to her previous births where she had little control and a lot of interventions that limited her movement, with clinicians she didn't know and an environment not familiar to her.

In the 'myVBACapp' study, women who remained active during labour, with limited or no interventions, expressed more positive feelings after their birthing journey, regardless of mode of birth. One woman who had continuity of care felt in control and had high confidence in her birthing ability and was active throughout her labour, but requested a caesarean when the baby didn't descend when she was in second stage, and had positive feelings after her journey as she feels that she had the best chance possible to have a VBAC and she felt supported during the whole experience. Indeed, as in Sarah's case, for her first VBAC, her journey wasn't supported, she had no positive relationships with clinicians, a lack of control towards the end of pregnancy and during labour and unable to remain active during transition and birth due to the impact of interventions and she felt proud but disappointed with her VBAC journey.

Women seeking alternatives to the hospital system are increasingly in a position of not having access to midwife-supported care. Publicly funded homebirth programmes and birth centres rarely accept women planning a VBAC and access to PPMs is subject to location and accessibility (Rigg et al., 2018). This can lead women to plan a birth 'outside the system', without the presence of a health professional (Jackson et al., 2012; Rigg et al., 2018).

International guidelines have recently been changing to become less-restrictive for women who want a VBAC. In 2017 the American College of Obstetricians (ACOG) released their VBAC practice summary. Recommendations were given recognising women with a history of two previous caesareans, women pregnant with twins, women needing an external cephalic version for breech presentation and women needing an induction of labour to be 'considered candidates' for planning a VBAC (ACOG, 2017). The National Institute for Health and Care Excellence (NICE) in the UK recently updated their intrapartum care guidelines discouraging routine insertion of intravenous cannulas in labour and discouraging amniotomy while supporting informed choice for options of pain relief, including labour and birth in water (NICE, 2019). The guidelines initially included offering continuous electronic foetal monitoring (CTG) only to women planning a VBAC who are using oxytocin for delay in first or second stage of labour and/or if performing an amniotomy, but these were quickly withdrawn and replaced with recommending all women planning a VBAC should be continually monitored in labour (NICE, 2011, 2019). It is a disappointment that a change supported and wanted by women could be removed so quickly under pressure apparently from the obstetric lobby without an opportunity for open discussion and consultation from women and professionals. Considering 1:10 women having a homebirth in Australia have a HBAC, many of them to avoid these very same routine interventions, it appears to have been a missed opportunity.

It is hoped that the positive changes will, in time, affect current Australian guidelines and encourage healthcare practitioners to be less-restrictive in their attitudes and treatments of women planning a VBAC.

Conclusion

Having a positive birthing experience is more than just a one-day event. Women remember their birthing experiences for the rest of their lives and for many it is the first time they encounter healthcare providers and the hospital environment. Having a negative, even traumatic, birthing experience could impact the woman psychologically, emotionally, physically and socially. Planning a VBAC, being supported in the journey and having an active, positive birth can potentially provide healing from a previous traumatic birth and veer women towards a motherhood journey full of pride and power.

The way forward

- Respect women's knowledge
- Listen to women's wishes
- Be positive with women planning a VBAC
- Be willing to negotiate on policies and guidelines and document the reasons why
- Don't give uneducated or inflated threats, women can and will find out the truth and will lose any respect they had in you

Note

1 Rebozo – a long wool or linen scarf covering the shoulders and head, worn by Latin American women. Can be used during labour to wrap around the abdomen/hips to aid with movement.

References

ACOG. (2017) *Practice Bulletin No. 184 Vaginal Birth after Cesarean Delivery*. Retrieved from: www.acog.org/Womens-Health/Vaginal-Birth-After-Cesarean-VBAC

AIHW. (2018) *Australia's mothers and babies 2016 – In brief*. Australian Institute of Health and Welfare. Retrieved from: www.aihw.gov.au/reports/mothers-babies/australias-mothers-babies-2016-in-brief/contents/table-of-contents.

Attanasio, L. B., Kozhimannil, K. B., & Kjerulff, K. H. (2019). Women's preference for vaginal birth after a first delivery by cesarean. *Birth*, *46*, 51–60. doi:10.1111/birt.12386

Boerma, T., Ronsmans, C., Melesse, D. Y., Barros, A. J. D., Barros, F. C., Juan, L., … Temmerman, M. (2018). Global epidemiology of use of and disparities in caesarean sections. *The Lancet, 392*(10155), 1341–1348. doi:10.1016/s0140-6736(18)31928-7

Clark, E. A. S., & Silver, R. M. (2011). Long-term maternal morbidity associated with repeat cesarean delivery. *American Journal of Obstetrics and Gynecology, 205*(6), S2–S10.

Dekker, G. A., Chan, A., Luke, C.G., Priest, K., Riley, M., Halliday, J., … Cornes, S. (2010). Risk of uterine rupture in Australian women attempting vaginal birth after one prior caesarean section: A retrospective population-based cohort study. *British Journal of Obstetrics and Gynaecology, 117*, 1358–1365.

Elmir, R., Schmied, V., Wilkes, L., & Jackson, D. (2010). Women's perception and experiences of a traumatic birth: A meta-ethnography. *Journal of Advanced Nursing*, 66, 2142–2153.

EURO-PERISTAT Project, w. S., EUROCAT. (2013). *European Perinatal Health Report: The health and care of pregnant women and their babies in 2010*. Retrieved from: www.europeristat.com/reports/european-perinatal-health-report-2010.html

Fawsitt, C. G., Bourke, J., Greene, R. A., Everard, C. M., Murphy, A., & Lutomski, J. E. (2013). At what price? A cost-effectiveness analysis comparing trial of labour after previous caesarean versus elective repeat caesarean delivery. *PLoS ONE, 8*(3), e58577. doi:10.1371/journal.pone.0058577

Fobelets, M., Beeckman, K., Faron, G., Daly, D., Begley, C., & Putman, K. (2018). Vaginal birth after caesarean versus elective repeat caesarean delivery after one previous caesarean section: A cost-effectiveness analysis in four European countries. *BMC Pregnancy Childbirth, 18*(1), 92. doi:10.1186/s12884-018-1720-6

Gardner, K., Henry, A., Thou, S., Davis, G., & Miller, T. (2014). Improving VBAC rates: The combined impact of two management strategies. *Australian and New Zealand Journal of Obstetrics & Gynaecology, 54*, 327–332. doi:10.1111/ajo.12229

Guiliano, M., Closset, E., Therby, D., LeGoueff, F., Deruelle, P., & Subtil, D. (2014). Signs, symptoms and complications of complete and partial uterine ruptures during pregnancy and delivery. *European Journal of Obstetrics, Gynecology and Reproductive Biology, 179C*, 130–134. doi:10.1016/j.ejogrb.2014.05.004

Hall, P. J., Foster, J. W., Yount, K. M., & Jennings, B. M. (2018). Keeping it together and falling apart: Women's dynamic experience of birth. *Midwifery, 58*, 130–136. doi:10.1016/j.midw.2017.12.006

Jackson, M., Dahlen, H., & Schmied, V. (2012). Birthing outside the system: Perceptions of risk amongst Australian women who have freebirths and high risk homebirths. *Midwifery, 28*, 561–567. doi:10.1016/j.midw.2011.11.002

Keedle, H. (2015). Women's reasons for and experiences of having a homebirth following a previous caesarean experience. Master's of Nursing Honours, Western Sydney University, Sydney. Retrieved from: http://hdl.handle.net/1959.7/uws:34598

Keedle, H., Schmied, V., Burns, E., & Dahlen, H. G. (2015). Women's reasons for, and experiences of, choosing a homebirth following a caesarean section. *BMC Pregnancy Childbirth, 15*(1), 206. doi:10.1186/s12884-015-0639-4

Keedle, H., Schmied, V., Burns, E., & Dahlen, H. (2018). The journey from pain to power: A meta-ethnography on women's experiences of vaginal birth after caesarean. *Women and Birth, 31*(1), 69–79.

Keedle, H., Schmied, V., Burns, E., & Dahlen, H. G. (2019). A narrative analysis of women's experiences of planning a vaginal birth after caesarean (VBAC) in Australia using critical feminist theory. *BMC Pregnancy Childbirth, 19*(1), 142. doi:10.1186/s12884–019–2297–4

Korb, D., Goffinet, F., Seco, A., Chevret, S., Deneux-Tharaux, C., & Group, E. S. (2019). Risk of severe maternal morbidity associated with cesarean delivery and the role of maternal age: A population-based propensity score analysis. *Canadian Medical Association Journal, 191*(13), E352–E360. doi:10.1503/cmaj.181067

Lundgren, I., van Limbeek, E., Vehvilainen-Julkunen, K., & Nilsson, C. (2015). Clinicians' views of factors of importance for improving the rate of VBAC (vaginal birth after caesarean section): A qualitative study from countries with high VBAC rates. *BMC Pregnancy Childbirth, 15*(1). doi:10.1186/s12884–015–0629–6

Martin, J. A., Hamilton, B., Oserman, M., Driscoll, A., & Drake, P. (2018). *Births: Final data for 2016* (1). Retrieved from www.ncbi.nlm.nih.gov/pubmed/29775434.

McLachlan, H. L., Forster, D. A., Davey, M. A., Lumley, J., Farrell, T., Oats, J., … Biro, M. A. (2008). COSMOS: Comparing Standard Maternity care with one-to-one midwifery support: A randomised controlled trial. *BMC Pregnancy Childbirth, 8*, 35. doi:10.1186/1471–2393–8-35

Motomura, K., Ganchimeg, T., Nagata, C., Ota, E., Vogel, J., Betran, A., … Mori, R. (2017). Incidence and outcomes of uterine rupture among women with prior caesarean section: WHO Multicountry Survey on Maternal and Newborn Health. *Scientific Reports (Nature Publisher Group), 7*, 44093. doi:10.1038/srep44093

NICE. (2011). *Caesarean section.* Retrieved from: www.nice.org.uk/guidance/cg132

NICE. (2019). *Intrapartum care for women with existing medical conditions or obstetric complications and their babies.* Retrieved from: www.nice.org.uk/guidance/ng121

Noblit, G., & Hare, R. (1988). *Meta-ethnography: Synthesizing qualitative studies.* Newbury Park, CA: Sage Publications, Inc.

Prosser, S. J., Barnett, A. G., & Miller, Y. D. (2018). Factors promoting or inhibiting normal birth. *BMC Pregnancy Childbirth, 18*(1), 241. doi:10.1186/s12884–018–1871–5

Rigg, E. C., Schmied, V., Peters, K., & Dahlen, H. G. (2018). A survey of women in Australia who choose the care of unregulated birthworkers for a birth at home. *Women and Birth.* doi:https://doi.org/10.1016/j.wombi.2018.11.007

Sandall, J., Soltani, H., Gates, S., Shennan, A., & Devane, D. (2016). Midwife-led continuity models versus other models of care for childbearing women. *Cochrane Database of Systematic Reviews*, 2016(4).

Sandall, J., Tribe, R. M., Avery, L., Mola, G., Visser, G. H. A., Homer, C. S. E., … Temmerman, M. (2018). Short-term and long-term effects of caesarean section on the health of women and children. *The Lancet, 392*(10155), 1349–1357. doi:https://doi.org/10.1016/S0140–6736(18)31930–5

Simpson, M., Schmied, V., Dickson, C., & Dahlen, H. G. (2018). Postnatal post-traumatic stress: An integrative review. *Women and Birth, 31*, 367–379. doi:https://doi.org/10.1016/j.wombi.2017.12.003

Stamilio, D. M., Defranco, E., Pare E., Odibo A., Peipert J., Allsworth J., … Macones, G. (2007). Short interpregnancy interval. *Obstetrics and gynecology, 110*, 1075–1082.

Tracy, S. K., Hartz, D. L., Tracy, M. B., Allen, J., Forti, A., Hall, B., … Kildea, S. (2013). Caseload midwifery care versus standard maternity care for women of any risk: M@NGO, a randomised controlled trial. *The Lancet, 382*(9906), 1723–1732. doi:10.1016/s0140–6736(13)61406–3

Vandenberghe, G., Bloemenkamp, K., Berlage, S., Colmorn, L., Deneux-Tharaux, C., Gissler, M., … Oberaigner, W. (2019). The International Network of Obstetric Survey Systems study of uterine rupture: A descriptive multi-country population-based study. *British Journal of Obstetrics & Gynaecology, 126*, 370–381.

8 Seeking control over birth in the Middle East

Suha Hussein and Virginia Schmied

Fatima gave birth without any sound but her eyes were filled with tears and something in her eyes told me she was broken.

(Suha Hussein)

About the authors

I (Suha Hussein) am a Jordanian woman and a midwife. I have given birth to five beautiful children – three girls and two boys aged between eight months and eight years. I am also a midwife trained in Jordan, but I have not worked as a midwife for some time. Three of my children, including my first child, were born in Australia and two were born in Jordan. I only ever wanted two children, as I thought that was enough. I wanted to do things with my life in addition to being a mother. This has not changed. While I love my five children, I did not plan to stay at home caring for children. I aimed to achieve other things in my life, although this is not typical for Jordanian women. I am passionate about changing birth practices in Jordan. I want my daughters to be able to enjoy and remember positively their birth experience. I embarked on my research journey seven years ago, when I bravely attended Western Sydney University to ask about my options for undertaking further study. There, I met Virginia and Hannah and they hatched a plan for me to undertake a literature review related to changing routine use of episiotomy. Following this, I gained entry to my Master's Honours degree, where I focused on Jordanian health professionals' attitudes and practices related to episiotomy. It was the negative attitudes of health professionals, including midwives, towards women that motivated me to undertake my doctoral research about women's experiences of birth and strategies for change.

I (Virginia Schmied) am one of Suha's PhD supervisors, along with Hannah Dahlen. My biography appears in the introduction to the book.

Introduction

> It's normal, birthing at home is what you do, with your family and [a] Daya.
>
> (Siham, Suha's mother, reflecting on birth at home)

> Where were you? I was calling out for you [the staff] to come and help me.
>
> (Siham, speaking about Suha's birth in a public hospital)

> But I told them I would not be knocked out – that was not happening to me.
>
> (Suha, birthing in a private hospital in Jordan in 2015)

The statements above reflect the rapid change that has occurred over the last three to four decades in birth practices and the place of birth in Jordan and in other Middle Eastern countries (Cindoglu & Sayan-Cengiz, 2010). Traditionally, women in Jordan birthed at home supported by Dayas (traditional midwives). This practice continued until the late 1980s and early 1990s. In Jordan today, almost all women give birth in a public hospital, but increasingly, women who can afford it are choosing a private hospital. Overwhelmingly, women report their birth experiences in Middle Eastern countries as dehumanising and disrespectful (Hatamleh, Sinclair, Kernohan, & Bunting, 2013; Mohammad, Alafi, Mohammad, Gamble, & Creedy, 2014; Jahlan, Plummer, & McIntyre, 2016; Hussein, Dahlen, Ogunsiji, & Schmied, 2018). Most women give birth without family present, in crowded spaces with no privacy (El-Nemer, Downe, & Small, 2006; Cindoglu & Sayan-Cengiz, 2010; Mohammad et al., 2014). Today, public hospitals have limited options for medicated or non-medicated pain relief. Instead, as one woman in our recent study said, 'women suffer'.

In this chapter, Suha Hussein (first author) talks with Virginia Schmied (second author) about birth in Jordan and in Australia. Suha describes her mother's birth experiences and her own experience, particularly her first three births. Suha reflects on the impact of her observations as a student midwife and later as a registered midwife working in Jordan. Throughout the chapter, we refer to other research as well as to participants in Suha's doctoral work to demonstrate how, in a relatively short period of time, birth in Jordan has become a dehumanising and traumatic experience and one for which some women seek sedation as the best option. In the last section of the chapter, we look at what happens when either a woman seeks, or a health professional tries to implement, a supported birth experience. We draw on the experience of one Jordanian-American woman who sought to birth 'outside of the system' and the consequences arising from her endeavour. In the conclusion, we consider what needs to happen for birth to become more humane, not just in Jordan or other Middle Eastern countries, but also in high-income countries like Australia.

Change in birth place over time

Virginia: There appear to have been quite rapid changes in the way women birth in Jordan, what has your mother told you about her birth experiences?

Suha: Before I had my first child, my mother had said little to me and my sisters about pregnancy and birth. It was never discussed. There was only the expectation that girls become mothers; that being their main or only role in life. When I became pregnant with my first child, I asked her about her experiences. What she said worried me, so I decided I would have an epidural if I needed it; no question about that. Even though my mother did not advocate this, I decided I was not going to suffer like she did in a public hospital.

My mother, Siham, was the eldest girl in her family. She has two sisters and three brothers. My grandmother passed away when my mother was 10 years old. Although my grandfather married another woman to take care of the children, my mother actually assumed care of her younger siblings, despite her young age. As is expected of a mother in Jordan, she made many sacrifices for her family. My mother lived with her father and her stepmother until she completed high school. Then, at the age of 17, she married a relatively young man who lived in another city. She left her family to live with her parents-in-law. Her husband (my father) was away most of the time working outside the country. She had her first baby at the age of 18 with no support from her family or her husband. Her mother-in-law and sisters-in-law attended the birth. Over the ensuing years my mother gave birth to more children. Throughout this time, no one really close to her gave her any advice about labour and birth.

My mother had ten children; eight girls and two boys. Her first baby was born in 1979 at home and the last baby was born in 2000 in a public hospital. She had five children at home and another five in hospital. My mother said she preferred giving birth at home because she was comfortable, it was familiar, clean and she was surrounded by family (her in-laws and her children). She said that, in contrast to giving birth in a public hospital, birthing at home was private, with only the Daya and people close to you (family) attending the birth. The Daya stayed with her for the duration of birth, from the start of contractions until delivery. The midwife also encouraged the use of herbs and oil for perineal massage. She recalls being able to eat, drink and move while birthing at home. My mother said:

> I preferred it at home and because at that time it was normal, everyone did it. It was just the norm of giving birth at home and not going to the hospital. Also because the midwife was the same one, so it was normal. I was used to it.

However, what was considered 'normal' was beginning to change. In 1982, after her first two births at home, she had me (her third baby) in a public hospital. She said that her labour with me was different. She had laboured for several days with irregular mild contractions until the family eventually convinced her to go to the hospital to try to bring her labour on. Once in hospital, she was put into the labour room with two other labouring women, and then, the midwife left her. Her contractions were initially weak but as soon as they ruptured her membranes, the contractions got progressively stronger. She was left alone that whole night, with strong contractions and no pain relief. When her contractions became very strong, she started screaming out to the midwives and doctors to attend her: 'Come on, I am giving birth very soon'. No one came. My mother delivered her baby by herself. The staff came into the room when they heard the baby crying. My mother said, 'Where were you, I was calling out for you to come and help me?' The midwives did not respond.

After this first experience of a hospital birth, my mother decided that, next time, she would insist on a homebirth. She managed to have three more births at home after me. In the late 1980s and 1990s, however, through the course of her last four pregnancies, she found it harder to find a Daya to attend her at home. There were no newly trained midwives providing homebirth services. Many of the existing Dayas had become too old to practise or had died. Unfortunately for my mother, her husband and family insisted she attend hospital to give birth.

My mother described her births in hospital as frightening. Even before having me in hospital, she heard stories about women having their feet tied to the bed. She said that, 'the other old women used to scare me with their stories' such that my mother much preferred to give birth at home. I asked her why she did not continue birthing with a midwife at home. She told me that because practices were changing, it was considered 'safer' and everyone was doing the same. It was also harder to get a midwife at home.

In my current doctoral research, the statement 'It is what you do, you go to hospital for birth' reflects the experience of many women birthing in a public hospital. But my mother did not want to go for two reasons: first, she had birthed at home and saw no benefit in attending hospital, and second, she was scared of what would happen to her in hospital. She had not liked her first experience in a hospital. Since that time she had heard many scary stories regarding birthing in hospitals. My mother said the midwives in hospitals were 'careless', leaving her alone in a labour room without any covering until she was fully dilated. She was not offered pain relief or olive oil for massaging the perineal area during birth. She said, 'I was not allowed to eat or drink and even to move around while I was in the hospital to give birth. I was stuck on my back the whole time and that was hard on me because I was used to walking around when birthing at home'. My mother said that she was 'not the type to make a fuss or scream during birth. [She] accepted all the procedures and followed instructions of health staff because [she] trusted the health professionals as they know the best for [her] and the baby'. So while this was not my mother's preference, she did not disrupt or argue with advice. She did what she was told to do.

Despite having a number of hospital births, my mother continued to view labour pain as normal, something women put up with and she did not see the need for pain relief, 'It is something women do, I am not the only woman that gives birth, we all do. Everyone is the same. So why not be strong and handle the pain'.

Shaping birth expectations

Virginia: What motivated you to study midwifery and how did this experience influence your birth decisions?

Suha: I decided to become a midwife because I had a strong feeling inside me that I wanted to help people when they were not well or vulnerable, especially women. I preferred to become a midwife because helping woman to give birth is a happy event in a family. It is not a disease that brings grief to the person and the family, so I chose to study midwifery and I am enjoying my career.

As a midwifery student, and as a midwife working in a public hospital in Jordan, I did not like what I saw. I was shocked by the way women were treated. The staff in the birthing unit often denied women any kind of pain relief, whether pharmacological or non-pharmacological. Just like my mother described, there is no privacy and medical students examine you without asking your permission. You cannot have your own female doctor, or your own room, and women birth without family present, in crowded spaces with no privacy among strangers. But what saddened me most and what staff have also told me in my research is that the medical professionals treat women as if they are uneducated and weak and they get angry with women for not cooperating with them (Hussein, Dahlen, Duff, & Schmied, 2016).

One event stands out in my memory. It was my worst experience as a midwife. Fatima (pseudonym) was having her first baby and when we admitted her, she was very distressed by the labour pain she was experiencing. She begged the staff to give her pain relief, but they ignored her at first. Eventually the midwife in charge gave her a pethidine injection. When the pethidine wore off, the woman started to scream again, very loudly. As a student I did not know how to help her, but the staff members started verbally abusing her, telling her it was her own fault for getting pregnant and even for having sex with her husband. It seemed their goal was to humiliate her in front of the other labouring women in the room. As the pain got stronger, and she began to scream more, the staff began shouting and slapping her legs to stop her screaming. When she refused to accede to their instructions, the staff brought her husband in to force her to follow

> instructions. Her husband asked his wife to calm down and stop screaming, but she was not listening to anyone. After a while, her husband slapped her face and told her to shut up. Finally, Fatima gave birth without a sound but something in her eyes, filled with tears, told me she was broken.
>
> This experience had a profound impact on me. I always ask myself: why I did not stop them, why did I watch and not act?

What we know about birth in Jordan and the Middle East today

The literature reporting women's birth experiences, in Jordan and in other Middle Eastern countries, supports my mother's experience and my experience as both a student and as a registered midwife. We have recently published a synthesis of studies exploring women's experiences of birth in Jordan and the Middle Eastern countries, demonstrating that in these settings many women experience childbirth as abusive, disrespectful and dehumanised (Hussein et al., 2018). In our synthesis of 12 studies conducted in Jordan, Lebanon, Egypt, Saudi Arabia, United Arab of Emirates and Qatar we identified an overarching theme, 'dehumanised childbirth', which reflected the negative impact on women of their encounters with healthcare providers and the maternity care system. This overarching theme comprised five subthemes: (1) 'feeling mistreated'; (2) 'technocratic care'; (3) 'intrusion by others'; (4) 'feeling ignored and alone'; and (5) 'lack of information from health professionals'. Women felt mistreated partly because they lacked privacy, felt exposed and were treated poorly during labour and birth. Women described specific acts of physical and verbal abuse during childbirth, such as: 'the use of force from health care providers to open their legs during vaginal examination and during birth' (El-Nemer et al., 2006, p. 84). In one study, one woman describes her distress: 'I was scared and cried as the nurse pinched and hit my thigh [which] in a funny way forced me to breastfeed my baby, but I did not like the way the nurse treated me' (Jahlan et al., 2016, p. 16). Our synthesis also found that there was limited rapport between women and health professionals, that women lack information about the facilities they birth in or the procedures that will be used on them, and women do not always give their consent for procedures. Typically, women labour on their backs, with no access to a support person or any privacy, and with limited support from health professionals. Participants in the studies included in this review also described a tense atmosphere in the labour and birth room. El-Nemer et al. (2006, p. 85) describes this dynamic well:

> The five medical students came to the room. The senior doctor on the morning shift asked them to examine the case and give him a report about each one. But what happened was completely inhuman. Instead of a student examining a woman and giving a report about her, each one examined all the women … If someone got a different report from the others he would go back to examine the woman again to be sure of his examination … It was like a queue, when one finished with the woman,

> the other one took his turn. Suddenly the five women were screaming and crying at the same time.

To understand this experience better, particularly in relation to how practices can change, Suha's doctoral research examined the experiences of women across generations. As noted at the start, it was not that long ago that women gave birth at home in Jordan. Older women, or experienced mothers, speak positively about their experience of birth at home while recent mothers (women who had a baby in the past ten years in Jordan) are less positive. The following quotes illustrate the distress that new mothers feel about the abuse or mistreatment they received in a Jordanian public hospital:

> Everything was opened, there were no doors in the labour room, people coming in and out, no privacy at all.
>
> (Mouna)

> I went in crying, I did not expect what happened to me, it was new to me. Especially when you see all the other women in front of you, all giving birth in the same room.
>
> (Lubna)

> (They) slapped my thigh because I loosened up and the baby was coming out and told me 'why you get pregnant and why did you open your legs to your husband', so no one dared to talk and ask for anything.
>
> (Rawan)

These experiences contrast with reports from experienced mothers (like my mother):

> The midwife at home gives me more privacy and care, I had been at home with myself no one with me.
>
> (Sabah)

> She used to be patient with me not like in the [public] hospital they would leave you alone in the room. Staying with one person the whole time during birth is better.
>
> (Fadia)

> I felt comfortable staying at home and my family around me, I had kind people around me. I was comfortable with my surroundings.
>
> (Amena)

Interestingly, in reviewing this literature of Middle Eastern women's experiences of birth, we did not come across any studies that reported a homebirth experience as resulting in birth trauma. This warrants further examination.

My first birth was traumatic

Virginia: Suha, your own birth stories are different to many Jordanian women as you gave birth to three children in Australia and two in Jordan. Can you tell us about your first birth in Australia, because you describe this birth as traumatic and it had a profound influence on you?

Suha: Yes, my first birth was very traumatic. When I was pregnant with my first child in 2010, I was living in Australia. I was very anxious because of what I had witnessed in Jordan and what my mother had told me, I had no idea about the degree of labour pain I will go through. However, I believed that my experience in Australia would be different from birth in Jordan.

I was overdue by 12 days. Hospital staff tried to induce my labour with prostin (prostaglandin gel), but after three unsuccessful attempts, they decided to break the water. I had an IV drip of syntocinon inserted into my arm, but no one ever asked my permission. I discovered the drip when I read the label and then asked the midwife, 'Why did you put the syntocinon in the drip without taking my permission?' She replied that the doctor ordered it. I was so angry. I said, 'You have to ask me before that, you shouldn't do that'. The midwife seemed surprised at how upset I was and said, 'Oh, okay, okay, I'm sorry'.

Shortly after, the pain became very strong and I could not cope with it, so the midwife gave me 'gas' to manage the pain. The gas worked in the beginning but it also made me confused. At one point, I remember the midwife letting midwifery students examine me internally, while I was confused with the gas. I shouted, 'How could you do that? You didn't ask my permission!'

After another hour, the pain became unbearable. I began to feel that I had come to a place that I could not escape. I knew there was nowhere to run from the pain. I would have done anything for the pain to go away. After *24 hours* of lying there, induced and in pain, I asked the midwife for an epidural, but she said the anaesthetist was busy with an operation. She suggested that I have some pethidine instead. I refused and started screaming and demanding an epidural. Finally, I was given an epidural. I was in so much pain, I struggled while the anaesthetist was trying to insert the epidural needle, but I liked the feeling when it was working.

During the second stage of labour, my baby's heart rate dropped during a contraction, so the doctor decided to perform an episiotomy and used the vacuum to get my baby out quickly. When she was born, I did not want to have her or give skin to skin. I just wanted to be left alone. I felt like my body was very sensitive to any touch. I did not want anyone to even touch me, I felt like the baby was the one who was responsible for the pain I went through and for everything I experienced during my labour. So I preferred to not even give my baby a hug after coming into the world.

The midwife was trying to support me to birth naturally without using any pain relief. She did not ask me what I wanted; she decided that by herself. I felt like I was a puppet and she moved the strings as she wanted. I had wanted to enjoy my birth experience, but I did not enjoy it at all. I had nightmares for months, where I felt the contractions and heard the foetal monitor. Sometimes I would wake up, terrified, in the middle of pushing and realise it was just a dream. I thanked God for that. I still resent everything about my first birth, even after eight years. The experience was so distressing, I did not want to get pregnant again. When I became pregnant with my second child, I was shattered.

Taking control: 'a redemptive birth'[1]

Virginia: I am sorry that you had that experience in Australia, it seems sometimes, birth in Australia is possibly no better than birth in a public hospital in Jordan. Please tell us about your second birth.

Suha: My second baby was also born in Australia in 2011. I planned to not repeat the first birth experience. I was overdue by five days but, this time, I went into labour naturally. By the time I arrived in hospital, my cervix was 5 cm dilated. I asked the midwife to organise an epidural and inform the anaesthetist to be ready. I told her not to trick me by telling me that the doctor is busy with an operation. She was surprised, but said nothing. I did not want to be traumatised again – having an epidural was my way of protecting myself from the same traumatic experience. The midwives still tried to convince me not to have an epidural, and to try the gas or pethidine. I refused and said I wanted a pain-free labour. I was adamant about an epidural. When I refused to listen to any other options, they obliged.

This birth was very different. I felt like I had control and, when my son was born, I was very happy to have him skin-to-skin with me, and I immediately started breastfeeding him. He is the only one of my children that I put skin-to-skin straight away. It was a different feeling and till today, he is very precious to me. He is the child I feel closest to.

Negotiating birth options in a private Jordanian Hospital

Virginia: After the birth of your first two children, you returned to Jordan to live and you agreed with your husband to have another baby. Given your experience working in Jordan and having studied episiotomy practices in Jordan for your Master's, what were your thoughts about having a baby in Jordan?

Suha: My third baby was born in Jordan in 2015. I knew this was going to be a different experience to birthing in Australia. Even though my first birth was so traumatic, I knew the only option for me in Jordan was to give birth in a private hospital. There I hoped I would be able to avoid the abuse and humiliation that dominates birth in public hospitals in Jordan. I wanted to protect myself and my baby from this.

I knew that in a private hospital I would have access to an epidural and my own female doctor. I went to a famous private hospital where I paid a lot of money to have my own room. Even in the private hospital, you can be put in a room with two or more women in a room, depending on your insurance or financial outlay. As a midwife, I had witnessed health professionals administering midazolam in private facilities. This creates a physical state known as 'Twilight Sleep' (discussed below). I saw women who, while under the influence of these drugs, were treated appallingly. I saw women with their legs tied up, the staff slapping their thighs or making fun of them, and then recounting jokes to them about their behaviours during 'Twilight Sleep'. I refused to be in that position.

Virginia: We digress here to talk about twilight sleep. As Suha has just described, she refused to be knocked out during her labour. The epidural was welcomed, but she did not want to be anaesthetised.

Twilight Sleep in the Middle East

Anaesthesia during childbirth became popular in the nineteenth century after Queen Victoria used ether during her labour and birth (Leavitt, 1980). Around 1915, however, another type of anaesthetic became the choice for childbirth – 'Twilight Sleep', as it was called by German doctors who were using it in their clinics (Sandelowski, 1984). Twilight Sleep was induced by giving women a combination of morphine to dull the pain and scopolamine to dull the memory of the childbirth experiences. It was presented as a miracle discovery as women were reportedly able to sleep through their birth. Unfortunately, although the women did not remember having birthing pain, they were still experiencing pain (Leavitt, 1980; Hairston, 1996). The combination of the two drugs made many women lose control during labour. Some were described as 'going crazy' or mad. To manage this behaviour and ensure women did not hurt themselves or staff, the women were restrained or tied to the bed. Soon, doctors required that women be put into specially designed beds, like a crib to contain them (Bauer, 1989; Caton, Fröhlich, & Euliano, 2002; Barnett, 2005).

This new German method of so-called painless childbirth attracted many wealthy women at first. It was promoted as a new form of freedom, an attempt for women to gain control over their birthing experience. Women started to advocate for Twilight Sleep, asserting that it was their right to choose a painless birthing experience. The Twilight Sleep Association was established to advocate for the drugs. Association leaders included feminists who represented the ideals of the women's movement (Leavitt, 1980; Hairston, 1996).

Initially, American doctors were suspicious of the practice and aware of the dangers to infants and mothers alike (Leavitt, 1980). However, they soon embraced it, particularly when it became known that wealthy American women, otherwise their customers, were travelling to Germany to give birth (Bauer, 1989; Skowronski, 2015).

Twilight Sleep remained a common practice for decades, despite ongoing debate as to whether the drugs used were safe for mother and baby (Caton et al., 2002). Just one year after Twilight Sleep was introduced in the USA, prominent supporter Francis Carmody died giving birth to her third baby while under the influence of the Twilight Sleep drugs (Hairston, 1996). In addition and over time, many women began to recall their painful birth experiences and health professionals began to speak out about the inhumane treatment women endured during Twilight Sleep. The practice fell out of favour and, by the early 1970s, it was no longer routine for women to be anaesthetised to the point of unconsciousness (Leavitt, 1980).

The era of Twilight Sleep is now recognised as one of the darkest periods in history for birthing women (Leavitt, 1980). The era contrasts with the contemporary emphasis on being awake, aware and in control during the birthing experience (Barnett, 2005). Fortunately, Twilight Sleep is no longer used in the Western world (Skowronski, 2015). It has, unfortunately, become a common practice in the Middle East, deployed as a means to attract financially able women seeking to avoid inhumane practices in the public sector. Arguably, Twilight Seep in the private sector has become an extreme choice in order to avoid the trauma of modern birthing practices in Jordan. In many Western countries, a comparative strategy is the maternal request for an elective caesarean section. Instead of leaving the system, however, women in Jordan are seeking to escape the memory of the birth by rendering themselves unconscious during delivery. They are escaping the system mentally, albeit not physically.

We now return to Suha's birth in a private hospital in Jordan.

'But at the end they knocked me out'

Suha: The birth I planned at an expensive private hospital to gain control over what would happen to me did not go as I hoped. I had my own room, but my husband was denied entry, which made him shout at the staff because he wanted to be with me. The midwife said, 'you and your husband are both behaving like it is your first baby'. The midwife then called my doctor and said, 'she's not really in pain, so just take your time to come in to the hospital'. By the time my doctor arrived, I was fully dilated. The doctor blamed the midwife for not telling her the truth.

I had an epidural about an hour before my doctor's arrival. The anaesthetist was not well-trained. The epidural only numbed my left side, even after she administered more pain relief. The doctor offered me Twilight Sleep, but I refused. I wanted to be awake for my birth. When I was shouting a lot, apparently unable to handle the pain, my doctor whispered to the midwife to knock me out without asking me first. While I was asleep, the doctor vacuumed the baby out and gave me an episiotomy. I woke up with no understanding of what happened to me. It was not a nice feeling; I was confused for at least 30 minutes after waking up. I could not remember anything and I did not ask about the baby. After an hour, I realised the baby was not with me in the same room. I asked the midwife, who told me the baby was in the nursery. Once again, I felt disconnected from my baby.

I still ask myself, how does a midwife with five children experience such different and difficult birth experiences? Despite what happened and how I feel about my first birth, I at least had family around to support me in Australia. The staff were kinder and patient, they respected me as a Muslim woman. For example, when a male doctor came to examine me, he asked for both my and my husband's permission beforehand. In Australia, I was given privacy and everything seemed clean. In Jordan, on the other hand, I liked the idea that, in a private hospital, they give you pain relief and you do not have to suffer pain.

What options are possible for women to achieve a positive birth experience in Jordan?

We ask ourselves what it will take to improve the birthing experiences of women in Jordan and other Middle Eastern countries. What has to happen for women to be free from abuse by health professionals, and control by doctors and the health system?

Seeking an alternative to hospital birth in Jordan

Virginia: How can birth for women in Jordan be different? What would happen if women resisted the dominant medical approach to birth?

Suha: I have started discussing options with other like-minded midwives, but most feel defeated about changing the system. In my Master's research, midwives told me: 'It is not worth arguing against the doctors, it will always go against you'.

> I will not risk trouble and have to come in front of physicians, as they will accuse me of being a trouble-maker.
>
> (Hussein et al., 2016, p. 325)

> They will take your action as a personal criticism and they will consider that you are trying to correct them or challenge their decisions. This makes them more aggressive.
>
> (Hussein et al., 2016, p. 326)

Like these midwives, it had never occurred to me to seek an alternative option for birth and, in my midwifery training, I had not come across women seeking homebirth or demanding better care from the public health system. Soon after starting my PhD, I was contacted by a Jordanian-American woman, Suzanne. She wrote about her birth experience, and her desire to find something different for her labour and birth. Suzanne published her story in *Midwifery Today* with the intention of shedding light on birth in Jordan, for mothers and activists alike (Dwaik, 2013).

Suzanne advocated for the introduction of evidence-based and humane birth in Jordan. She is passionate about reviving respectful, sensitive birth practices as a rite of passage and empowerment for women. She lived in the USA until the age of 17, after which she returned to Jordan with her family. She studied nursing in a Jordanian university, until she became pregnant with her first baby. She attended the university clinic for antenatal check-ups and chose to birth at the university hospital. She realised the hospital was worse than she expected; she became concerned about the lack of evidence-based practices and services, information and psychological support (Dwaik, 2013).

In her effort to find the best place for her baby to be born, she conducted research on birthing options in Jordan. She formed the conclusion that there were three potential options for birth: (a) a biomedical approach with doctors in hospital; (b) a Daya (if one can be found) to support a homebirth; or (c) an unassisted birth. She chose to birth at home, but her choice was rejected by her husband and family because of perceived danger to the baby. Her family insisted that birthing in hospital was the only safe place for her and the baby. Suzanne started to look for other alternatives. In the end, she chose an unassisted birth, but she kept her decision to do this from her husband, her family and in-laws. Suzanne described her decision:

> My pregnancy was a battle to find truth myself, to be allowed to follow it and to find someone to help me reach it. Passively accepting to be violated, humiliated and abused again, along with my baby, was a cruel, ruthless request from those around me. Having refused to flow into the system trustingly and naively, my desperate search for alternative options began.
>
> (Dwaik, 2013, p. 2)

Suzanne's labour began in the early morning. She wanted to stay at home as long as possible, hoping to give birth alone without any assistance. She laboured for 13 hours by herself without telling her husband or her family and even managed to hide it from her mother-in-law who visited her the same day. In the evening, her husband returned home and realised, from looking at her face, that she was in pain. With that realisation, she was taken to the 'battlefield' (hospital). Once there, she tried to give birth naturally without interventions. She faced a lot of opposition from the health staff. She said:

> When the OB came in furious, I realized I had to put down my weapons and accept that I was in their hospital, a battlefield I could not win in. He got his equipment ready without a word or a look. I was already conquered, so why speak to me? I was reduced to below human, so why look at me? I asked meekly how many stitches he would do. He sneered it was none of my business how he worked. I shot back, 'How is it none of my business? This is my body!'
>
> (Dwaik, 2013, p. 6)

Suzanne's story demonstrates the challenges of attempting change. She encountered, in childbirth, one of the most pervasive problems in Middle Eastern countries, the patriarchal domination of women and the dominant position of men. Suzanne was put in her place, in the same way that I was put in my place during my birth in the private hospital in Jordan; indeed, I was sedated to put me in my place – to control me.

My Master's research (Hussein et al., 2016) showed that doctors dominated maternity care practices and directed policy related to maternity care in Jordanian hospitals. In this highly medical context, it was also evident that health professionals – doctors and midwives alike – viewed women in a disparaging way, believing that they lacked knowledge regarding the birth process (Hussein et al., 2016). Health professionals in Jordan blamed women for the mistreatment the women suffered in labour and birth, asserting that it was because the women were uninformed and uncooperative:

> They do not follow our instructions during birth, which means the process of birth does not go well.
>
> (Hussein et al., 2016, p. 127)

> It is hard to deal with an uncooperative woman during birth as we expect many complications associated with the process of birth.
>
> (Hussein et al., 2016, p. 127)

> Being scared with no knowledge makes it easier for physicians to think and decide instead of the pregnant woman.
>
> (Hussein et al., 2016, p. 126)

Health professionals rocking the boat

Virginia: Suha, can you tell us what would happen if a midwife or other health professional tried to make changes to birthing practice in Jordan?

Suha: Change is very difficult. I can answer this by using an example from my own midwifery training. When I was training to be a midwife in one of the public hospitals in Jordan, one of the university midwifery educators who had recently graduated from a UK university was strongly opposed to routine episiotomy. She got in trouble because a woman in her care sustained a severe cervical tear that needed suturing under general anaesthesia. The educator had not followed the system's rules and no one would support her opposition to routine episiotomy, even though, in this case, an episiotomy would have not prevented a cervical tear. The hospital staff lodged a complaint with the university administration and, as a consequence, the educator was given a written notification regarding her practice. The incident is now held up as an example or a lesson for anyone trying to break the rules or make a change in childbirth practice. In my Master's research, the midwife participants still recalled this event and referred to it in their interviews (Hussein et al., 2016). The midwives reported that it was always better to go with the flow, and not to rock the boat.

Taking small steps

Suha: In the final phase of my doctoral research, I formed a small group of like-minded midwives and others who want change in Jordan. The purpose of this participatory action group is for us to envision how change can occur and how to propose small steps or actions that may be possible. At the first meeting of this group, the participants were pessimistic that change could occur and stated: 'They will not listen, you need hundreds of woman to speak up and a lot of energy to walk that path' (Laila) and 'We have no say, no matter what we do, no matter what noise we make' (Souad).

These sentiments illustrate the challenges of making change. In this first meeting, the participants discussed what is arguably the most pervasive problem: the patriarchal domination of women in Middle Eastern countries. However, in this meeting as in other related research (Shin, 2004; Foureur et al., 2010; Jenkins, Josey, & Kruske, 2014; Aksoy & Komurcu, 2018), it was suggested that women's privacy can be protected by ensuring women are covered, even just by a sheet and using screens when the door is opened. Most importantly, health professionals require training in how to provide compassionate care to labouring women (Oweis & Abushaikha, 2004; Oweis, 2009; Kridli, Ilori, & Goeth, 2012; Mohammad et al., 2014). In my Master's study, participants also suggested increasing the opportunity for prenatal education classes and improving the quality of information given to women, ensuring it is evidence-based and culturally sensitive.

What will I tell my daughters?

Virginia: Suha, you have had difficult birth experiences and you were traumatised by your first birth, what will you tell your daughters about birth?

Suha: I have thought about this a lot, and I already talk with Salma, my eldest, about birth. My mother and I always argue about the best way to birth. My mum used to say our bodies can handle the pain of labour, and we should not resort to taking medication straight away. She used to say, 'try and keep busy so you forget the pain. Go out, clean the house, talk to a friend so you can forget the pain'. But I think, why should I stay in pain when there is a solution to take away the pain? My mother always tells me that 'It [labour pain] is something women do, I am not the only woman that gives birth, we all do, so why not to be a strong woman and handle the pain'.

I want Salma to be a strong and an independent woman. I encourage her to finish her university degree and have a career. Sometimes, she asks me about falling in love with someone and giving birth to babies. I have tried to explain it to her but in a way that suits her age. In the future, I will be the first person to tell her everything and it will be the truth, as I will not let anyone else assume this role in my daughter's life. I also acknowledge, however, that what is true for me may not be the same for my daughters and I have to be careful not to pass my trauma on to the next generation.

I wish my daughters an easy labour and birth and I hope they enjoy their birth experiences as much as they possibly can.

Conclusion

In this chapter, we explored the changing context of birth in Jordan and the Middle East. This chapter illustrated how birth has changed – moving from home to public hospitals and now for some women with sufficient financial resources, to private hospitals that offer anaesthesia or sedation in labour. Birth has moved from being in a place of comfort and care, to a place where women are violated and their need for respect, support, medicated or non-medicated pain relief and privacy during birth, is disregarded. Unfortunately, to escape this, women are turning to private hospitals where they have the option purchase some privacy, some continuity and sedation to give birth. This disrespect for women is deeply embedded in a maternity system dominated by medicine and associated patriarchal cultural practices and beliefs (Hatamleh et al., 2013; Hussein et al., 2018). But this chapter also demonstrates that it is not only in the Middle East that women's needs are disregarded. We have a global problem when it comes to humanised care and listening to women, and we need to work together to fix this now so future generations do not face what we endured.

The way forward

- In labour and birth, women want support and care from family and caring professionals, they want privacy and most of all women want to be respected and treated with dignity
- Women want to have access to medicated and non-medicated pain relief during labour and birth
- Women require information that is evidence-based and culturally sensitive
- There is an urgent need for staff training in compassionate and respectful maternity care in the Middle East and elsewhere
- Listening and learning from women's birth stories may assist health professionals to be more compassionate

Note

1 The term 'redemptive birth' was first used by Gill Thomson.

References

Aksoy, S. & Komurcu, N. (2018). Privacy in perinatal services: A qualitative study. *IOSR Journal of Nursing and Health Science*, *7*(5), 64–73.

Barnett, R. (2005). A horse named 'Twilight Sleep': The language of obstetric anaesthesia in 20th century Britain. *International Journal of Obstetric Anesthesia, 14*, 310–315.

Bauer, D. M. (1989). Twilight Sleep: Edith Wharton's brave new politics. *Arizona Quarterly: A Journal of American Literature, Culture, and Theory, 45*, 49–71.

Caton, D., Frölich, M. A., & Euliano, T. Y. (2002). Anesthesia for childbirth: Controversy and change. *American Journal of Obstetrics and Gynecology, 186*, S25–S30.

Cindoglu, D. & Sayan-Cengiz, F. (2010). Medicalization discourse and modernity: Contested meanings over childbirth in contemporary Turkey. *Health Care for Women International, 31*, 221–243.

Dwaik, S. (2013). Birth and rebirth: A Jordanian-American experience. *Midwifery Today with International Midwife*, *2013*(108), 25–31.

El-Nemer, A., Downe, S., & Small, N. (2006). 'She would help me from the heart': An ethnography of Egyptian women in labour. *Social Science & Medicine, 62*, 81–92.

Foureur, M., Davis, D., Fenwick, J., Leap, N., Iedema, R., Forbes, I., & Homer, C. S. (2010). The relationship between birth unit design and safe, satisfying birth: Developing a hypothetical model. *Midwifery, 26*, 520–525.

Hairston, A. H. (1996). The debate over twilight sleep: Women influencing their medicine. *Journal of Women's Health, 5*, 489–499.

Hatamleh, R., Sinclair, M., Kernohan, G., & Bunting, B. (2013). Birth memories of Jordanian women: Findings from qualitative data. *Journal of Research in Nursing, 18*, 235–244.

Hussein, S. A. A. A., Dahlen, H. G., Duff, M., & Schmied, V. (2016) The barriers and facilitators to evidence-based episiotomy practice in Jordan. *Women and Birth, 29*, 321–329.

Hussein, S. A., Dahlen, H. G., Ogunsiji, O., & Schmied, V. (2018). Women's experiences of childbirth in Middle Eastern countries: A narrative review. *Midwifery, 59*, 100–111.

Jahlan, I., Plummer, V., & McIntyre, M. (2016). What women have to say about giving birth in Saudi Arabia. *Middle East Journal of Nursing, 10*, 10–18.

Jenkins, B., Josey, N., & Kruske, S. (2014). BirthSpace: An evidence-based guide to birth environment design. Queensland Centre for Mothers and Babies, The University of Queensland, St Lucia.

Kridli, S. A.-O., Ilori, O. M., & Goeth, J. (2012). Health beliefs and practices of Qatari women: A qualitative study. *Avicenna*, *2012*(1).

Leavitt, J. W. (1980). Birthing and anesthesia: The debate over twilight sleep. *Signs: Journal of Women in Culture and Society, 6*, 147–164.

Mohammad, K., Alafi, K., Mohammad, A., Gamble, J., & Creedy, D. (2014). Jordanian women's dissatisfaction with childbirth care. *International Nursing Review, 61*, 278–284.

Oweis, A. (2009) Jordanian mother's report of their childbirth experience: Findings from a questionnaire survey. *International Journal of Nursing Practice, 15*, 525–533.

Oweis, A. & Abushaikha, L. (2004). Jordanian pregnant women's expectations of their first childbirth experience. *International Journal of Nursing Practice, 10*, 264–271.

Sandelowski, M. (1984). *Pain, pleasure, and American childbirth: From the twilight sleep to the Read method, 1914–1960*. New York, NY: Praeger.

Shin, J. H. (2004). Hospital birthing room design: A study of mothers' perception of hominess. *Journal of Interior Design, 30*, 23–36.

Skowronski, G. (2015). Pain relief in childbirth: Changing historical and feminist perspectives. *Anaesthesia and Intensive Care, 43*, 25–28.

9 Why South Asian women make extreme choices in childbirth

Kaveri Mayra and Bashi Kumar-Hazard

> … she will have to listen to a lot of comments if she is poor … if someone is rich or from a better income society, then staff behave very patiently and respectful maternity care comes out of them. They know how to do it … it just depends on whether you are worthy.
>
> (Midwife from Rajasthan)

About the authors

I (Kaveri Mayra) am an Indian researcher qualified in midwifery, nursing and public health. I have over 12 years' research experience in nursing and midwifery workforce policies and maternal healthcare provision, mainly in India. Having seen mistreatment during childbirth early on as a student midwife and witnessed a lack of leadership in nursing and midwifery decision-making power, I began researching and advocating for women. I am a global speaker on disrespect and abuse during childbirth, nursing and midwifery governance, workforce policies and welfare, and the gender-based challenges underlying all these issues. I am currently pursuing my PhD on Obstetric Violence at the University of Southampton, UK.

You have already read some of my (Bashi Kumar-Hazard) story in the introduction to this book. In 2017, in my role as a Director on the Board of Human Rights in Childbirth, I helped organise the first international human rights conference on childbirth in India. My family is from Telengana and Tamil Nadu. I tell more of my story in this chapter.

Introduction

For decades, South Asian women have received the attention of global health experts for an unenviable reason: we are more likely to die in childbirth, both in our low-income native countries and in the middle- to high-income countries to which we immigrate or seek refuge (Manzoor, 2011). In relation to India, Nepal and Bangladesh, global health experts have long assumed that incentivising women to attend facilities for pregnancy and childbirth would automatically reverse the trend in maternal mortality rates. Approximately two decades ago, India initiated such a change, with Nepal and Bangladesh in close pursuit. Traditional birthing systems within villages and communities were disrupted, virtually overnight, by programmes designed to do away with traditional birth attendants (TBAs), while using monetary incentives to encourage women to birth in institutions. While the number of women seeking institutional care was initially hailed as a victory by global health advocates and the World Health Organisation (WHO), the outcomes were not as promising as expected, with few questions asked about the quality of care women would receive once at these facilities (Das, Hammer, & Leonard, 2008; Das & Hammer, 2014). Fewer questions still were asked about the sustainability of using short-term financial incentives to compel or coerce women into birthing in facilities that were located days away from their homes, were poorly resourced, did not have the recommended ratio of human resources for health services, lacked fresh water, toilets or pain medication, and resulted in significant out-of-pocket personal costs for the woman and her family. Finally, the shift to facility-based maternity healthcare coincided with a sharp increase in reports of mistreatment of women during childbirth and indications that the mistreatment was likely to pose a major deterrent to accessing healthcare in subsequent pregnancies (Freedman, 2016).

In middle- to high-income countries to which South Asian women immigrate, maternal mortality and morbidity remains a pressing but largely undisclosed issue. To put it simply, women of South Asian (and African) descent are significantly more likely to die in childbirth as compared with their white counterparts in middle- to high-income countries (WHO, 2016). This is despite giving birth in high-resource settings and being subjected to greater intervention in childbirth (Merry, Small, Blonde, & Gagnon, 2013). The paucity of research in this field and the failure of governments to publicise this information is not surprising. Governments in receiving countries like the USA, UK, Canada, Australia and New Zealand struggle to acknowledge, let alone address, both the direct and systemic forms of racism that is prevalent in their cultures. Discrimination, including systemic racism, is rarely acknowledged and, if alleged, is responded to with defensiveness, denial and aggression (Di Angelo, 2010). In healthcare systems developed by predominantly white male cultures, systemically practised racial profiling and the resulting discriminatory bias that women face is rarely recognised.

In this chapter, we discuss the stories told by South Asian-born women to understand their experiences in a variety of healthcare settings and subsequent choices in pregnancy and childbirth. We explore the impact of disrespectful and abusive treatment during institutionalised childbirth in private and public facilities. From the perspective of the woman, attending a facility known to abuse and disrespect women is seen as much of an extreme birth choice as the decision to refuse to give birth in the facility. The choices that women make, from both the women's perspectives as care seeker and midwives' perspectives as primary care provider, are based on their perceptions of safety, including safety from discrimination and abuse during childbirth. Financial incentives are unlikely to address any perceived qualitative shortcomings in the provision of maternity healthcare.

Our interviews and discussions with South Asian women revealed a further and significant dimension as yet unexplored in the research around disrespect and abuse in facility-based childbirth. Tropes and generalisations about South Asian women, such as being associated with poverty, lower socio-economic status, limited intellectual capacity and poor health, are negatively influencing care-provider attitudes in *both* country of birth and in the countries to which South Asian women emigrate. This profiling is often mislabelled as 'high-risk' in high- to middle-income countries, with or without factual basis. In both the countries of birth and the countries to which they immigrate, these 'high-risk' women are seen as unnecessarily increasing the burden of care and the potential risks to care provider.

To illuminate these experiences, we discuss an Indian midwife and researcher's experiences and interactions with women and midwives in the states of Rajasthan, Odisha, Madhya Pradesh, Bihar and West Bengal, with first-person narratives of South Asian women in South India (Maharashtra, Tamil Nadu) and Australia. We show how, in both India and Australia, discrimination quickly transforms into abuse and disrespect of South Asian women, especially when care providers report feeling under pressure for having to care for higher-risk women. In both country settings, the greater the vulnerability of the woman, the greater the abuse and disrespect she is likely to face within the health facility at the hands of the dominant group.

On becoming a midwife

Kaveri Mayra

> 'Lift your sari and lie down', he instructed. She held my hand, stepped on the tiny stool to climb the narrow tall labour table. The doctor, male, lifts her sari roughly to expose her from waist down while muttering 'checking', but stops right before starting a vaginal examination. He looks at her pubic hair and comments, 'how does your husband want to do anything with you with the jungle you have grown there!' He chuckles, as do the two staff members standing there. I freeze and she quietly covers her face with her pallu (a part of her saree). The staff nurse sees me and says, 'Eh, the doctor is just joking!'

I was a student nurse-midwife, just 19 years of age, taking care of this woman in a public tertiary-level hospital in a major metropolitan city in India. What I observed that day was the sexual and verbal abuse, humiliating exposure and unprofessional treatment of a woman through the duration of her birthing experience. I was at the bottom of the medical hierarchy. When I complained, the nurse in charge did not do anything about it and my supervisor could only offer advice; that I should learn to never engage in the dehumanising practice I had observed in the labour room that day. I realised that, for all their teachings, the nursing and midwifery teachers were themselves not sufficiently elevated in the workplace hierarchy to be able to effect any systemic or meaningful change in practice or workplace culture. No matter what level we rose to as nurses and midwives in education, teaching or clinical practice, we were all powerless!

Since that day, my passion for midwifery turned to listening to women's birth stories and to understanding how quality of care can be improved. Over the next few years of my education and training, I regularly saw women being abused at facilities. I saw how this behaviour was being normalised. I felt like the process of desensitising myself to the pain and suffering of women who were being abused while giving birth was a core element of my nurse-midwifery education. No one reacted when care providers hit, pinched, slapped or made derisive and disparaging comments at a woman. Over the next 12 years, I continued to observe, understand and advocate against disrespect and abuse during childbirth, at a significant personal cost to me. My biggest challenge in my research work has been the fact that women are not used to anyone even caring enough to ask them questions about how they felt when they were mistreated. In some cases, poor care around childbirth, including the mistreatment of women, was seen as a standard component in the provision of care and something women just learn to endure. It is justified on the basis that the women are at least receiving some care, or that it was their fault they were treated a certain way. In other cases, the women are taken aback by my questions and don't know how to respond. They share only what is considered extreme to them, and much of that gets lost in not having the language to express their pain or not knowing what to expect in the first place.

Mistreatment from the perspective of midwives

In the analysis of the secondary data of a qualitative study I conducted in 2018 as part of my PhD, midwives shared their own experiences of evidencing the mistreatment of women and their understanding of what drives mistreatment at birth. The in-depth interviews were conducted in the following States: Bihar (three), Odisha (three), Rajasthan (six), Madhya Pradesh (one) and West Bengal (five). Eight nursing and midwifery leaders were interviewed at the national level in India.

Midwives expressed a disconnect between their training and philosophy on the one hand and their lived realities practising as nurse-midwives on the other. Midwives believe that 'respectfulness is a philosophy of life' (Odisha) and that it is a woman's right to birth the way she wants. A participant from West Bengal explains, 'if she wants to sit and deliver then she should or if she wants to stand because of pain, listen to her and provide care so her experience of childbirth is good. It is her right.' However, in their lived experience, they see women endure disrespect and abuse during childbirth, including verbal, physical and sexual abuse, lack of privacy and mistreatment owing to poor physical infrastructure or policy environment:

> ... nakedness is a common sight [in the labour room].
>
> (West Bengal)

> ... so you did it [had sex] out of fun then, but it is not that fun now?
>
> (Rajasthan)

> I have seen doctors hitting women on vulva with artery forceps.
>
> (India)

> They get irritated because everyone just comes and does a per vagina (PV) examination. Sometimes five doctors come together ... all five students by turn do PV on the same woman while the doctor checks in too. Ten PVs are done on average on every woman ... every primi gets an episiotomy.
>
> (Bihar)

> ... everyone gets induced.
>
> (Rajasthan)

The midwives I interviewed recognised that some of their own behaviours amounted to mistreatment. Some took the view that their practices were justified, such as the occasional raising of the voice:

> ... sometimes we have to shout so that she will listen to us and push. It is for her own good. Delivery is done well that way.
>
> (Rajasthan)

Some acknowledged that mistreatment of women during childbirth in a healthcare facility is an issue that women might not face during homebirths:

> ... there isn't much difference between the care provider and woman giving birth, culturally. In homebirths, the dai is from the same caste. Cleaning is part of their work ... provider is more respectful at home.
>
> (India)

Midwives perceived prevailing negative attitudes towards women as one of the driving factors underpinning disrespectful care around childbirth, even if perpetrated by other women. The nurse-midwives in India are often victims of a medical hierarchy that precludes them from having any decision-making power, as they are supervised by a male medical officer who often lacks compassion and is a bully towards them and the birthing women. This lack of compassion, together with top-down decision-making power and control, creates a culture of abuse, initiated at the top and ending in the treatment of the care-seeking woman perceived as being at the bottom of the social hierarchy. This is facilitated by insensitive healthcare policies that do not allow for, let alone encourage, respectful care. In addition to the gender discrimination, a woman's characteristics or vulnerabilities such as education, age, parity, religion, socio-economic status and physical appearance (including colour of skin) are all factors which affect how she will be treated during childbirth. The greater the vulnerability, the higher the incidence of mistreatment:

> … she will have to listen to a lot of comments if she is poor … if someone is rich or from a better income society, then staff behaves very patiently and respectful maternity care comes out of them. They know how to do it … it just depends on whether you are worthy.
>
> (Rajasthan)

> They come with skin diseases sometimes. No one wants to touch them. They have to hear a lot of comments. Low socio-economic status is a factor. We don't care if one has shaved or not. Many mothers come after trimming. Looks like they have come straight from the parlour, freshly waxed. They get good care; we like touching them.
>
> (West Bengal)

Mistreated midwives

The poor treatment of midwives as a feminised workforce in India has been widely discussed in academic literature. Midwives report work-related burnout, bullying at work, poor leadership and poor working conditions that impact on the provision of care (Deery, 2008; Hall, 2013; Sadler, Ruiz-Berdun, & Rojas, 2016). Midwives are denied decision-making capacity at any level, from practising at the local primary care centre to policy formulation and implementation of nursing and midwifery practice standards in India. The midwives I interviewed reported that they rarely received appropriate supervision or guidance from someone who understood the daily challenges they faced:

> The confidence of staff breaks as soon as they see a crowd [of women, patients and their family members]. They worry how to provide care to so many.
>
> (Rajasthan)

> Doctors grab the opportunity saying we are not capable. They don't give nurses and midwives the opportunity. We can handle policy making and governance but need to be supported.
>
> (Madhya Pradesh)

> … more power, be strengthened, more leadership qualities. [Midwives need to] be involved in decision making. They are the people [who provide care] when women need. If you strengthen midwives, then they will strengthen the nation.
>
> (Odisha)

Even midwives who birthed at their own facility were not spared the mistreatment and disrespect, even when they knew what to expect:

> … nurses did not behave properly … she was listening to foetal heart sound (FHS) and I refused asking 'why are you listening to FHS when I am in pain, can't you wait till the contraction is over?' I complained to the nursing superintendent. She saw my name and realised who I am … she called the staff and said 'where have you learnt midwifery, don't you know she is a teacher?' She apologised and then everyone cooperated.
>
> (Bihar)

Why accessing facility-based maternity healthcare is the extreme choice in childbirth

Policy-makers' belief that childbirth is safest within a health facility dramatically transformed birthing practices in India. In a country where 27 million babies are born every year (36 every minute), the impact of a birthing culture on the female population can be profound and enduring. In 2005, Janani Suraksha Yojana (JSY) was launched under the National Health Mission (NHM), under which women received an incentive of 1400 rupees to deliver in a healthcare facility (Randive, Sebastian, De Costa, & Lindholm, 2014). By 2016, India's institutional delivery rate had increased to 80%: National Family Health Survey #4 (Government of India, 2011, 2015). More than triple the number of women 'chose' to birth in a publicly funded healthcare facility. This did not, however, reduce the maternal mortality at the same rate (130:100,000 currently and 172 in 2015). Negative reports about the JSY scheme quickly emerged, with concerns that facilities were inadequately prepared and under-resourced in the face of the sudden workload increase.

The push towards facility-based births failed to take into account the underlying discrimination that the women of India face as part of their everyday and lived experiences. Behavioural attitudes towards women within facilities reflect the value placed on, and the social status afforded to, women in any given society. In the fourth National Family Health Survey, a large-scale Indian national survey conducted in 2016, 27% of women reported being married before turning 18, 8% were pregnant or mothers by the ages 15–19 years at time of survey, 53% were anaemic, 5% reported being beaten during their pregnancy and 31% experienced spousal and domestic violence (NFHS #4; Government of India, 2015). Further reports of female feticide, female infanticide, son preference, daughter aversion, honour killings, domestic violence and violence during pregnancy provide ample examples of the limited value placed on women and girls at different stages of their life in India. An overwhelming proportion of India's women are treated as modern slaves and forced into subordinate roles in a conservative, male-dominated society preoccupied with social traditionalism, and this includes a nursing dependent midwifery profession (Mayra, 2019; Mayra, Matthews, Padmadas, & Sandall, 2019).

Studies have now confirmed that women are often disrespected and abused during childbirth in India when a woman is at her most vulnerable (Bhattacharya et al., 2013; Patel, Makadia, & Kedia, 2015; Chattopadhyay, Mishar, & Jacob, 2018; Mayra & Kumar, 2017; Mayra, 2019; Raj et al., 2017; Madhiwala, Ghoshal, Mavani, & Roy, 2018; Rao et al., 2019). Research suggests that obstetric violence leads to post-traumatic stress disorder in women (Kitzinger, 2006; Beck, Driscoll, & Watson, 2013; Olza, 2013) and tokophobia (Slade, Balling, Sheen, & Houghton, 2019). In the long run, mistreatment in childbirth will likely affect any progress towards improving maternity healthcare generally in a country (Bohren, 2015; Nayak & Kumar, 2018; Sen, Reddy, & Uyer, 2018). A woman's birthing experience impacts whether she will seek maternity healthcare for her future births or avoid care-seeking even during complications (Matthews, Ramakrishna, Mahendra, Kilaru, & Ganapathy, 2005; Bhattacharya, 2013; Jha, Larsson, Christensson, & Svanberg, 2017; Mayra & Kumar, 2017), or lead to women choosing planned caesarean section for future births (Eide, Morken, & Baeroe, 2019). As a result, the reality in India today is that opting to birth in a facility may in fact be the extreme choice for women who prioritise privacy, dignity and respectfulness in the provision of maternity care. Women who have been abused during childbirth often do not have the language to express how they feel about what happened to them. Their narratives are similar to the narratives of rape victims, as both feel 'tethered', 'forcibly exposed', with 'sexual organs on display' and 'stripped off' (Kitzinger, 2006). Women's expectations determine the quality of care and increase the accountability of care providers and policy-makers. The lack of awareness among women in relation to their rights, choices and entitlements, and the lack of awareness among care providers and policy-makers in terms of what women want and need, feeds into poor-quality care.

Maternal healthcare needs to be designed and implemented through the lens of women's human rights. Freedman (2003) discusses the essential role that constructive accountability holds in implementing a rights-based approach to the planning and provision of maternal health care. Through its acceptance of the Universal Declaration of Human Rights (1947), India is obliged to protect women's dignity and right to equality in childbirth. Disrespect and abuse during childbirth constitutes a violation of at least six of the 30 articles enshrined in the Declaration (Mayra, 2019; Mayra et al., 2019). All countries have yet to pursue a rights-based approach to the planning and provision of maternal healthcare, and India has been no exception to this rule.

It is difficult to determine whether, in India, women are in fact making informed choices to give birth in a particular health facility given the limited information available to them about individual care-provider preferences, a facility's policies on childbirth practices and the intrapartum care being provided to the women in the absence of the doctor. The choice of birth place is more likely determined by reference to family pressures, financial pressures and fear than on factors that prioritise or support a woman's human rights in childbirth. While it can be difficult to determine the choices relevant to women in a society where women are denied even basic freedoms in life, there are some preferences which clearly emerge from the research. For example, women have expressed a desire to have their husbands as birth companions; to provide support and protect them from care-provider aggression and violence (Mayra & Kumar, 2017). Their choices have yet to be acknowledged, let alone supported, in India.

Lastly, a shared understanding of what constitutes a safe and ideal choice in birthing for women in India has yet to be addressed. As long as the women who are giving birth, the nurse-midwives who are at the frontline of intrapartum care provisions, the doctors who manage and oversee the provision of care and manage complications and the administrators who develop maternal healthcare policies carry vastly different ideas of what an ideal birthing scenario is, it will be challenging for governments to ensure a safe, respectful, culturally appropriate and satisfying birthing experience for women. For as long as these ideas remain in conflict, all the choices women make will be extreme choices, as they currently do not have any option of safe birth in India.

On becoming a mother

Bashi Kumar-Hazard

> I was rushed to the nearest hospital during a precipitous labour. Between contractions, I saw the ambulance officer look meaningfully at the hospital midwife during handover and say, 'Homebirth gone wrong …' and I saw the midwife roll her eyes. His claim was false, but neither of them thought I was human enough to ask me directly. The midwife took over, put me on another trolley and tried to make me lie down on my back. I felt the urge to push, I could feel my baby coming, so I tried to stand up. The midwife was preoccupied with strapping me to a CTG monitor, without even asking for permission. She was frustrated by my movements. After a few more attempts to keep me down, her team lost patience and flipped me onto my back, hard, and told me to stay there unless I wanted to kill my baby. I remember looking at the midwife and thinking 'How strange – I can feel my baby, I know what he's doing. How could you even presume to speak for him?' Once I was strapped onto the trolley, the team started running, wheeling me to the theatre. 'Wait!' I said, 'Why are you

> moving me? Where is my husband?' No one answered me. A young registrar whispered to me 'Don't worry about it. You'll be ok. Just sign this form'. I could barely keep up with the preparations that were happening around me without my consent, and she kept waving this paper in my face. I became really irritated, and I said, 'No! Take that away – I am not signing anything, I'm a lawyer.' For a moment, no one moved. Then, all hell broke loose. I was pushed into the theatre, strapped down and my legs were put in stirrups. Bright lights were positioned onto my face. I could hear my husband banging on the other side of the theatre door, demanding entry. A strange man appeared, stood over me and pointed at my face. 'Let's all get a grip here', he said, 'You need a reality check'. It was the obstetrician. He stood between my legs, crossed his arms as my baby crowned and glared aggressively at me. 'Don't cut me', I said. 'Oh, don't worry', he said, 'you are making your own fine mess down here – all by yourself'. He looks around at the rest of the team and sneers loudly, 'This is a fourth degree, for sure'. The staff grinned back, some chuckling maniacally as if they had just won the lottery. I heard my husband shouting again – saying he was going to call the police if they didn't let him into the room. My private midwife magically appeared by my side and starts whispering in my ear. It seems the plan was to put me under general anaesthetic without my consent and perform a caesarean section. No one factored in that I was educated, had hired a private midwife and I had a white husband. They didn't care. I was a sub-human host to the real prize – a live baby.
>
> After pushing as hard as I could to avoid a forced caesarean section, I hear my baby cry out. My arms and body immediately ache and crave contact with him, but I cannot reach for him because I am strapped down. My private midwife deftly scoops him up onto my belly. I am overwhelmed when I see him – the crazy, unnecessary flap and chaos that is going on around me fades away for a few moments. Then, I hear a snap. 'Please, please don't clamp the cord!' I say. 'Too late', the obstetrician replies churlishly. 'Well take it off – look the cord is still pulsing; my baby needs it!' He looks down at me with absolute contempt, 'No, he doesn't'. My midwife says, softly, 'You could just cut the clamp'. He glares at her, crosses his arms like a petulant child and says loudly, 'I can't. I don't have the right equipment'. 'Please!', I say, 'I am begging you, take it off!' He storms out of the theatre, demanding that my private midwife follow. Meanwhile, the hospital midwives are staring at my baby, who is doing the breast crawl. They declare that in their 20 years of service each as hospital midwives, they have never witnessed a baby doing the breast crawl. That was the moment when I decided that I needed to get the hell out of that crazy institution, as soon as I was physically able to move.

I am an Indian woman and a first-generation migrant. I was giving birth to my third child in one of the wealthiest publicly funded teaching hospitals in the

Lower North Shore of Sydney, Australia. The obstetrician in question was, at that time, a senior lecturer in obstetrics at the University of Sydney, the oldest and most prestigious school of medicine in the country. He was angry with me for refusing a caesarean section and he made sure that his team sympathised with him – at my expense. When he stormed out of the room, the obstetrician left me strapped to the table with a young registrar who didn't know what to do and an anaesthetist who had the physique, and the aggressive disposition, of a man on bodybuilding steroids. The registrar was incompetent and, for the most part, unsupervised. The anaesthetist stood over my husband who, by this time, was holding my newborn baby and shouted at him for his apparent 'insubordination', that is, for demanding to be reunited with me. When I heard that, I started crying again, and begged him to stop shouting over my newborn baby, who was hiding his little face in my husband's chest in distress. But this aggression-infused anaesthetist was too self-absorbed to even realise that he was shouting so aggressively over a newborn baby, until the theatre nurse intervened and stopped him. She then turned to me and told me I only had myself to blame. As an afterthought, she pushed a bowl in my face and asked if I wanted to eat my placenta. After 20 minutes of this lunacy, I asked one of the staff members to call the obstetrician back – my legs were cramping badly in the stirrups, I was in so much pain and six staff members were literally standing around waiting for the obstetrician to actually do his job. My request was ignored. In the obstetrician's worldview, threatening to report my private midwife to the authorities was obviously a far more pressing and important task than just doing the job he was being paid to do. For the next three months, I lost all sensation in my right foot. I cared for two young children and nursed a newborn with crutches, all because my treating obstetrician had had a temper tantrum about my right to decide what happened to my body and baby, and left me in the stirrups for too long.

I had already undergone two traumatic caesarean sections for my previous births as I have described in the introduction to this book. I was being punished for choosing to VBAC and engaging private midwives. It occurred to me, as I was lying there watching these hostilities unfold at me and my family, that no amount of resources could correct the underlying disrespect, racism and misogyny that is so embedded in maternity healthcare in Australia. This was business as usual for the hospital team. They lacked the self-awareness or the humility to see how easily triggered they were, how they used a self-imagined crisis to dehumanise me and to use hubris, abuse, racism and aggression to punish me and anyone associated with me, with absolute impunity. There were no attempts to conceal the abuse. There was no acknowledgement of the abusive behaviour or the racial profiling. If anything, the team were openly congratulating each other for the way they 'handled' their self-created crisis and the way in which they put me, and my midwife, in our 'rightful' place – as subservient and subordinate to them. I watched them channel a dangerous culture of concealing incompetence with arrogance, aggression and blame, directed at me and my newborn baby. As a team going on the offensive against me, it didn't matter if important facts were overlooked, if they were terrorising or bullying me to the point where I was weeping in fear, or if no one ever asked for my name or made eye contact with me. As a team, they could turn to machines and resources to feign competence and cohesion and distract themselves from the simple task of engaging with me as a human being. As the leader of the team, the obstetrician could feign superiority and authority, like the leader of a gang of bullies. The relationship and trust between me and my midwife was perceived as a threat to his authority and control. He managed his discomfort by engaging in a form of emotional violence that women know only too well – he threatened my midwife for associating with me and he abused me.

I resolved, as I held my baby and walked out of that hospital, to make it my life's work to understand why pregnant women of colour have become the targets of such abuse and what we could do to protect all women from abuse and disrespect during childbirth, for good. This cannot go on.

Extreme choices – from whose perspective?

Five years later, as I, Bashi, was travelling through India as a representative of Human Rights in Childbirth and interviewing women about their childbirth experiences, I realised the scale of the problem South Asian women were facing at the hands of our care providers. As pregnant women, we are universally treated as subhuman; messy, problematic, an unwanted burden, a distasteful breeder, all over the world. It didn't matter that I lived in a different continent to the women I was working with in India. Our lived experiences in childbirth were disturbingly similar. We are not safe in healthcare facilities designed and maintained by men for their practical convenience as opposed to the needs of a mother. It mattered because we bore the brunt of that dehumanised treatment even while we are charged with the responsibility of carefully and lovingly raising the next generation of human beings.

In 2016, the Modi Government introduced its flagship social scheme, *Beti Bachao, Beti Padhao*, which, for the purposes of curbing female infanticide, focused greater effort on the move to institutionalise all childbirth in India. At the WHO PMNCH 2018 Partner's Forum in New Delhi, Women and Child Development Minister Maneka Gandhi declared that the scheme's apparent success in reducing female infanticide was due, in part, to superseding the role of traditional midwives or *dais* who, in her view, were primarily responsible for committing and concealing female infanticide, and by forcing women to register their pregnancies and deliver at health facilities. The Minister claimed to have supporting evidence from secret informants planted within villages and communities, who were paid to spy on and report women and midwives allegedly responsible for female infanticide. No evidence was presented to support these claims. The Minister appeared to not recognise that the policy would exacerbate the disempowerment of pregnant women. The process of eliminating traditional birth attendants, and spying on and policing pregnant women, will not improve already negative social attitudes towards women – the same attitudes that drive female infanticide.

Asha (name changed) was one of the casualties of this scheme. I met her when she was living with her community on the abandoned Platform Nine at Mumbai Railway Station. Asha was about 19 years of age but, as her family had never registered her birth, no one really knew for sure. Her beautiful, narrow green eyes were watchful, and she carried herself with the dignity and self-preservation of a queen. She never smiled. She lived on a blue tarpaulin sheet which doubled as a cover over the fissures in the hot concrete slab she shared with her mother, grandmother, husband and two children, and a shelter from the rain. Her grandmother was unable to walk and dependent on Asha. Her husband had a serious disability and was illiterate. He too depended on Asha. The family were situated right next to a river that was black with pollution and littered with plastic waste. Asha was due to deliver her second child, but had declined all offers to accompany her to hospital. She had her first child in a hospital. She said that hospital personnel would not touch her during her attendance because she was a street-dweller. They told her that she had lice all over her and that her feet were disgusting. She recounted how, as she climbed a set of stairs, she leaned too far forward during a contraction, nearly making contact with a doctor's knee with her face. His reaction was to quickly raise his shoe to her shoulder and push her backwards. She toppled backwards and was grabbed by her husband before she fell down a flight of stairs. She later tried to get contraception from the same facility, but gave up when they laughed at her because her husband, who couldn't read, could not fill in the form to grant consent to Asha's request. Asha tried to find a *dai* (traditional birth attendant) who could support her for a few rupees and provide post-natal care for at least two months in one of the nearby tin shacks close to her living space on Platform Nine. It meant she wouldn't have to abandon her toddler, she could remain close to her family and manage the costs. Unfortunately, when none of the *dais* would operate so close to a tertiary hospital for fear of government reprisals, Asha decided to birth on her own. The JSY payments were irrelevant to her because she needed a formal address to receive payments. Besides, she couldn't fill in the forms. She asked me for a mosquito net to protect her infants from the clouds of mosquitoes that emerge from the black, polluted river every night.

When I next saw Asha, she was holding a beautiful little baby girl in her arms. She had given birth about 100 metres from where we were standing, alone, by the black, polluted river. She was so happy and so proud of her baby girl. She asked me to take photographs of her family. They posed proudly together on that tarpaulin, like we were preparing for a studio shot. Two months later, I received news that Asha's baby girl had died from dengue fever, and that her son had gone missing while the family was struggling with illness. She was right to be concerned about those mosquitoes.

Conclusion

Quality of care is of particular significance to women vulnerable to experiencing discrimination on the basis of race, disability, poverty or gender. Vulnerable women are acutely aware that they lack the resources needed to recover from poor-quality care and are especially fearful of the consequences, particularly in resource-constrained countries. Equally, immigrant and refugee women also lack access to effective social support and resources in resource-rich countries, unless they are in crisis.

For South Asian women, birthing within the system can oftentimes be the extreme choice. Studies show traumatic experiences begin not just during birth but well before and endure well after birth. High-profile human rights cases in India have shed light on the difficulties women have with accessing healthcare, even when mortality is an issue (Jeffery & Jeffery, 2010; Kaur, 2012). Caselaw highlights the role that poverty and marginalisation play in determining the quality of care women receive. Policies may be in place, but they are either not being observed, or they are being negatively interpreted through the profiling that already affects women of colour.

In both Australia and India, healthcare facilities were designed and subsequently maintained by a predominantly male government administration and medical profession for their own convenience. This male cohort already enjoys the social recognition associated with being more affluent, informed and influential. That power and social dominance is used, in turn, to influence, maintain and oversee a workplace culture and practice for self-benefit. It is so powerful that it remains impervious to the introduction of policies or laws aimed at stemming the mistreatment women experience in facilities. This workplace culture is as far removed from the lived realities of pregnant women of colour as a white male millionaire is from understanding the life of a homeless orphan living in Afghanistan. It is a workplace culture that isn't just oblivious to the caring responsibilities, the burden of unpaid work, the poverty, the violence and the mistreatment that women of colour generally experience, it actively resists any engagement with or effort to understand those lived realities. In this space, vulnerabilities are perceived as a weakness or the result of personal failures. Care providers assume that they are of a superior status and intellect so as to permit them to dismiss a woman's requests or override her wishes. It is inevitable that when women of colour with unique, multiple and intersecting vulnerabilities present to health systems with a harmful workplace culture, they are managed as an unwanted added burden, and their personal or expressed concerns met with irritation, resistance and aggression. As women of colour are already sufficiently disempowered in both Australia and India, facility personnel make no effort to conceal their discriminatory biases or instinctive aversions towards women of colour. Many openly express their distaste, and then engage in a process of compartmentalising their distaste in order to focus on the task at hand – to extract a live baby from a subhuman, relatively distasteful object.

Rather than recognise and check their biases, however, careproviders are lauded for their 'scientific and objective' ability to focus on the task at hand, albeit by perceiving the woman in their care as simply another task that needs to be completed.

In both countries, Australia and India, skin colour affects the treatment that women receive in facilities. Darker-skinned women are associated with a lower socio-economic status and as lacking the knowledge or ability to understand simple instructions during their stay at a facility. Even in India, the darker the skin colour, the greater the propensity for the woman to be profiled as holding a lower status in the subhuman scale.

The differences between the two settings are found in the types of mistreatment deployed to control and coerce women in childbirth. In India, direct forms of abuse and disrespect were commonly perpetrated and continue to be a strong deterrent to accessing care in future pregnancies. This made the abuse and disrespect easily observable to an outsider. Interestingly, however, the women themselves were reluctant to acknowledge this mistreatment for fear of reprisals from care providers in future pregnancies. By contrast, in Australia, systemic mechanisms are used to indirectly coerce and mistreat women of colour. These mechanisms are often disguised as mandated policies and procedures. Women are groomed to seek permission in relation to their own bodily autonomy. Direct forms of abuse are transient and retrospectively justified with claims of altruism and paternalism, or by blaming the woman and her family for being non-compliant or disobedient during the provision of care. Care providers are also skilled at deploying associated state powers, such as enforcement services, child protection services and the lower courts, to facilitate coercion and control during pregnancy and childbirth. While more women report or complain of mistreatment during childbirth, there remains a strong element of learned helplessness in the way in which complaints are pursued.

It is clear that the majority of South Asian women do not know or understand their rights in pregnancy and childbirth. Health systems and health facilities have exploited this lack of awareness to their advantage, to the detriment of some of the most vulnerable groups of women. Until this dynamic is reversed, birthing in a facility will remain an extreme choice for South Asian women around the globe. Choosing to avoid these facilities can therefore be completely understood.

In the next section, Hannah Dahlen undertakes an interview with Indian obstetrician Evita Fernandez about the revolution in care that is starting to happen.

Interview with Indian obstetrician Evita Fernandez

Evita Fernandez is an obstetrician who runs the successful Fernandez hospitals in Hyderabad, India, and who experienced a recent renaissance in her thinking when it comes to birth. I (Hannah) interviewed her during the

2019 Normal Labour and Birth Conference (NLBC) where she gave a keynote address to welcome everyone to the 2020 NLBC Conference to be held in India. In 2014, I was presenting research about assessing progress in labour (along with Dr Denis Walsh) at the International Confederation of Midwives (ICM) conference in Prague when a softly spoken Indian woman dressed in a beautiful sari stood up and said the words 'I am an obstetrician from India' and spoke about why India needed midwives. Every head in the room spun in her direction. Obstetricians attending a midwifery conference is not common, let alone one advocating for midwives. After the session ended, I tried to find her but she was nowhere to be seen. Evita and I crossed paths again in India in 2017 during the Human Rights in Childbirth conference in Mumbai, but I still didn't realise who she was. I only realised in 2019, just before I conducted this interview, that the softly spoken obstetrician I was so impressed with in 2014 was Evita Fernandez!

I wanted to understand what changed the thinking of this successful private obstetrician who, with the world at her feet, had become a strong advocate for professional midwifery care and women's right to choose their birth in India.

Seeing birth in a new light

When I interviewed Evita, she told me that two things had happened in her life. Her hospital (Fernandez) had grown into a referral centre and, as a result, she was caring for women with high-risk pregnancies all the time. Low-risk mothers attending her hospitals were being regarded as a high-risk catastrophe waiting to happen. One day, Evita met a woman in the hospital lobby who said, 'You have no beds for us anymore, so where do we go? We are the fourth generation. My grandmother came here, and they tell me that there are no beds'. This made Evita think about what happens to the uncomplicated mother. She asked childbirth educator Nutan Pandit from Delhi (whose book *The Complete Childbirth Book* she recommended to mothers) to run a course for mothers. One day, Evita decided to attend the class and, to her horror, she realised she was asking women to read a book that was not in sync with the care they received when they came into the birthing room.

Evita then looked at research on maternal mortality and discovered that, in countries which invested in professional midwives as the backbone of their services, maternal mortality was substantially lower. Her interest in mortality grew because they had young mothers referred to the hospital for care, some of whom died after they arrived too late. It was a simple step, from the research and her lived experiences, to consider how to bring midwives into her hospitals.

Andy Beckingham, a public health consultant from the UK, was in Hyderabad when Evita shared her dream of starting a midwifery programme in her organisation. A few months later, he emailed, 'I'll give you one year of my life, and I'll help you write a curriculum. All I want is a room to stay, and food, no salary'. In 2011, the midwifery programme was launched, and with this new paradigm, Evita realised she and the hospital she ran needed to change their childbirth practices. The first midwife to work in Hyderabad was Becky Reed from the UK. Reed challenged Evita's infrastructure and thinking. She looked at the stirrups and said, 'What's this?' Evita, while wondering why a midwife of 22 years training was asking such a rudimentary question, replied 'It's stirrups'. Becky then asked her why they were needed at all. This was the beginning of many such questions and frank discussions.

In 2014, midwife Indie Kaur came from the UK, and brought others with her to help train Indian midwives. By 2014, Evita admits that she had had an 'epiphany'. She realised that, 'I had actually lost the plot, somewhere in my journey'.

Today, Evita feels that radical change is needed in India. Evita calls for a three-pronged attack:

1. Change our childbirth practices: by understanding the physiology of labour and encouraging birth without interventions and raising awareness about this among obstetric colleagues
2. Offering women *honest* information on their rights and preparing them for childbirth – this calls for working with professional midwives who will then take care of *all* uncomplicated pregnancies. This is the first phase of introducing professional midwifery in India, thus also reducing unnecessary caesarean sections
3. Working with the Government and policy-makers to introduce professional midwifery as a *mandatory* cadre in all hospital units offering maternity services

Evita is currently working on getting the government in India to make it mandatory for any healthcare facility that offers maternity care services to have midwives.

I asked Evita what she sees as the answer to engaging women back into our care and systems, and this is what she said:

Listen to women

The only way we can engage with women is to listen to them and ask them what they want. That's something doctors are not trained to do because there is such a strong hierarchy. Young woman are not going to take that attitude anymore, and rightly so. It's time that we, the medical fraternity, realise that we need to listen more and be humble enough to say, 'yes, we were doing it wrong, and we need to change'.

The more honest we are the more women will trust us

Right now, there's a trust deficit in the medical system with doctors. We have become commercial in our approach to care. Women don't see us looking at birth as normal. They realise that we've overmedicalised things and that some of us have very high caesarean section rates. They don't want to be a part of this. More and more women are looking for other options. As far as I know, we've only got two professional midwives who have set up birthing centres offering midwifery care in the country: (a) Priyanka Idicula (Birth Village) in Kerala and Vijaya Krishnan (Healthy Mother) in Hyderabad. These two are US-certified nurse midwives. They do an amazing job, but we need more of them in country with 25 million births annually.

At Fernandez, we have been very fortunate to have UK-certified and experienced midwives to teach, train and mentor our midwifery students to become confident, competent and skilled professional midwives.

What is the key thing in the next 10 years that we need in India?

We definitely need midwifery and direct-entry midwifery training.

We also have the untapped potential of nurses. About 150,000–200,000 auxiliary nurse-midwives have actually been catching babies (without adequate midwifery training) for years. These nurses have become extremely good technicians, and would probably do a vaginal breech birth without understanding the manoeuvres. They need updated training or development of clinical skills/knowledge in new midwifery. We could tap this potential with a specially designed curriculum and develop a workforce with midwifery skills and the right approach to birthing.

Traditional birth attendants (TBAs)

My attitude to TBAs changed when I visited an amazing non-governmental organisation (NGO) that is working with a tribal belt in Andhra Pradesh. The NGO taught the TBAs basic skills to improve childbirth practices. I met a TBA who, with such pride, explained how she changed her childbirth practices after what she'd learnt. There is much prevailing wisdom and experience in this group and women in the community trust them. They form a vital cadre in remote areas which are difficult to access even with road transport. If we develop a special training module, TBAs can effectively contribute to maternity services in the tribal belts. I am aware that their role/responsibility needs to be clearly defined, with a strong referral supporting system. But we need to stop denying that women are seeking their kind of care.

In obstetric training, TBAs are openly maligned. We are encouraged to believe they are dirty and dangerous, and therefore the cause of maternal mortality. Honestly, when I look back, I can see how unfair that was.

Do you get any attack on yourself, for what you do?

I don't get attacked, and I'm not sure why not. That said, it baffles me that, while they acknowledge what we are doing with midwives, they won't also invest in their own midwives. I think there are two practical reasons behind this: (1) limited investment in personnel; and (2) poor attitudes to midwifery staff. At Fernandez hospitals, we invest in staff, especially nurses. For reasons that are not clear, not many hospital owners believe in the same. They only want to know what it costs. The other concern is the poor treatment of staff. Midwives who train with us today are offered a good salary on completion.

I am so grateful to the British midwives who opened my mind. Indie Kaur has been amazing and has taught me so much about what channels midwives can pursue: leadership, mentorship and more.

How do we engage doctors?

To engage doctors, we need to share the success stories, data, evidence and we just need to keep on talking. Not to win wars, or arguments, but to quietly persist with improvement. And I feel, somewhere, those light bulbs will go on. But again, I come back to the women; if more women ask their doctors for options, the more it will happen. Today, there are women attending our hospital who ask to see a midwife. They don't want to see an obstetrician. I find that extremely exciting.

The challenges to rolling out midwifery in India

The challenge we have is to offer skilled midwifery care in response to the high volumes of birth in India. Approximately 25 million babies are born every year. In my hospital, we have recruited young women from more remote villages who were trained over two years in a mission hospital to provide basic nursing. We taught them to provide additional labour support, like doulas. They learned practical skills like back massage and intermittent monitoring. They recognise a foetal heart rate of 120, 110. This way, no woman is ever alone in labour, even if a midwife has to briefly step out of the room to see another woman (because we still don't have enough midwives).

The mothers report an amazing sense of comfort with our doula support. This is humanising birth care. When they return at six weeks with their babies, the women ask for the doulas, show them the baby and say, 'Thanks to you, I enjoyed my birth. Thank you for supporting me'. The doulas recently met and thanked me for making their work meaningful. So begins a whole new career path, and they are expressing a growing confidence, some even consider further study. Some of these young women may one day become midwives.

Do you have excitement and hope for the future?

Absolutely. It will happen because women will ask for these changes. There is a rising movement around birth in the urban sector in India. We've got organisations like Birth India and Bangalore Birth Network. We have groups coming up in Delhi and Tamil Nadu. We need to work together, not against each other, and I'm confident things will change.

The way forward

- The Government of India is currently developing, through a national task force, a curriculum for the implementation of publicly funded midwifery programmes and practice, in accordance with the International Confederation of Midwives practice modules and respectful maternity care
- The national task force needs a subgroup focused specifically on viewing and advising on the proposed policies and programmes through a human rights lens
- Governments of settler countries need to understand the complex mechanisms that create and reinforce structural racism, as well as the links with poorer health outcomes, so as to enable the development of training modules which simulate and support mechanisms for addressing discrimination
- Midwives and women's representatives need to be included when making any policies about women and midwifery professionals
- Respectful communication is needed within the healthcare teams to encourage healthy communication between healthcare providers and with women
- The training of midwives is vital to improve and humanise care in India

References

Beck, T. B., Driscoll, J. W., & Watson, S. (2013). What is traumatic birth and post-traumatic stress due to childbirth? In *Traumatic Childbirth* (pp. 8–26). New York, NY: Routledge.

Bhattacharya, S., Srivastava, A., & Avan, B. I. (2013). Delivery should happen soon and my pain will be reduced: Understanding women's perception of good delivery care in India. *Global Health Action, 6*. doi: 10.3402/gha.v6i0.22635

Bohren, M. A., Vogel, J. P., Hunter, E. C., Lutsiv, O., Makh, S. K., Souza, J. P., … Gulmezoglu, A. M. (2015). The mistreatment of women during childbirth in health facilities globally: A mixed-methods systematic review. *PLoS Medicine, 12*(6), e1001847.

Chattopadhyay, S., Mishra, A., & Jacob, S. (2018). 'Safe', yet violent? Women's experiences with obstetric violence during hospital births in rural Northeast India. *Culture, Health & Sexuality, 20*, 815–829.

Das, J. & Hammer, J. (2014). Are institutional births institutionalizing deaths? [Blog post]. *World Bank Blog: Economics to End Poverty*. 20 November. Retrieved from: http://blogs.worldbank.org/futuredevelopment/are-institutional-births-institutionalizing-deaths

Das, J., Hammer, J., & Leonard, K. (2008). The quality of medical advice in low-income countries. *Journal of Economic Perspectives, 22*, 93–114.

Deery, R. (2008). Community midwifery 'performances' and the presentation of self. In B. Hunter & R. Deery (Eds.), *Emotions in midwifery and reproduction* (pp. 73–89). Basingstoke: Palgrave Macmillan.

Di Angelo, R. J. (2010). Why can't we all just be individuals? Countering the discourse of individualism in anti- racist education. *InterActions: UCLA Journal of Education and Information Studies*, *6*(1). Retrieved from: https://escholarship.org/uc/item/5fm4h8wm.

Eide, K. T., Morken, N., & Baeroe, K. (2019). Maternal reasons for requesting planned cesarean section in Norway: A qualitative study. *BMC Pregnancy and Childbirth*, *19*, 102.

Freedman, L. N. (2003). Human rights, constructive accountability, and maternal mortality in the Dominican Republic: A commentary. *International Journal of Gynaecology and Obstetrics*, *82*, 111–114.

Freedman, L. P. (2016). Implementation and aspiration gaps: Whose view counts? *The Lancet*, *388*(10056), 2068–2069.

Government of India (2011). Census of India.

Government of India (2015–16). *National Family Health Survey, India Factsheet.* International Institute for Population Sciences.

Government of India (2015–16). *National Family Health Survey, State Fact sheet Bihar*. International Institute for Population Sciences.

Hall, J. (2013). Developing a culture of compassionate care – The midwives voice? *Midwifery, 29*, 269–271.

Jeffery, P. & Jeffery, R. (2010). Only when the boat has started sinking. A maternal death in rural north India. *Social Science and Medicine*, *71*, 1711–1718. doi: 10.1016/j.socscimed.2010.05.002

Jha, P., Larsson, M., Christensson, K., & Svanberg, A. S. (2017). Satisfaction with childbirth services provided in public health facilities: Results from a cross-sectional survey among postnatal women in Chhattisgarh, India. *Global Health Action*, *10*(1).

Kaur, J. (2012). The role of ensuring women's reproductive rights: An analysis of the Shanti Devi judgment in India. *Reproductive Health Matters*, *20*(39), 21–30.

Kitzinger, S. (2006). Birth as rape: There must be an end to 'just in case' obstetrics. *British Journal of Midwifery*, *14*, 544–545.

Madhiwala, N., Ghoshal, R., Mavani, P., & Roy, N. (2018) Identifying disrespect and abuse in organizational culture: A study of two hospitals in Mumbai, India. *Reproductive Health Matters*, *26*(53), 36–47. doi: 10.1080/09688080.2018.1502021

Manzoor, S. (2011). My wife and baby died in labour. *The Guardian.* 10 September 2011. Retrieved from: www.theguardian.com/lifeandstyle/2011/sep/10/usman-javed-wife-baby-died-hospital

Mayra, K. (2019). Nursing and midwifery regulation in India.

Mayra, K. & Kumar, A. I. K. (2017). Perceptions of antenatal women, husbands and health care providers on husband being birth companion during childbirth: A qualitative study. *Public Health Open Access*, *1*(1).

Mayra, K., Matthews, Z., Padmadas, S., & Sandall, J. (2019). Drivers of disrespect and abuse during childbirth and recommendations for respectful maternity care in India: Nurse midwives' perspectives and experience. Ongoing PhD thesis, University of Southampton.

Matthews, Z., Ramakrishna, A., Mahendra, S., Kilaru, A., & Ganapathy, S. (2005). Birth rights and rituals in rural South India: Care seeking in the intrapartum period. *Journal of Biosocial Science*, *37*, 385–411. doi: 10.1017/S0021932004006911

Merry, L., Small, R., Blonde, B., & Gagnon, A. J. (2013). International migration and caesarean birth: A systematic review and meta-analysis. *BMC Pregnancy and Childbirth*, *13*, 27. Retrieved from: www.biomedcentral.com/1471–2393/13/27

Nayak, A. K. & Nath, A. (2018). There is an urgent need to humanize childbirth in India. *Economic and Political Weekly*, *53*(2).

Olza, I. (2013). PTSD and obstetric violence. *Midwifery Today International Midwife*, *105*, 48–49, 68.

Patel, P., Makadia, K., & Kedia, G. (2015). Study to assess the extent of disrespect and abuse in facility based childbirth among women residing in urban slum area of Ahmedabad. *International Journal of Multidisciplinary Research and Development*, *2*(8), 25–27.

Raj, A., Dey, A., Boyce, S., Seth, A., Bora, S., Chandurkar, D., … Silverman, J. G. (2017). Associations between mistreatment by a provider during childbirth and maternal health complications in Uttar Pradesh, India. *Maternal Child Health Journal*, *21*, 1821–1823. doi: 10.1007/s10995–017–2298–8

Randive, B., Sebastian, M. S., De Costa, A., & Lindholm, L. (2014). Inequalities in institutional delivery uptake and maternal mortality reduction in the context of cash incentive program. Janani Suraksha Yojana: Results from nine states in India. *Social Science and Medicine*, 123. doi: 10.1016/j.socscimed.2014.10.042

Rao, K., Srivastava, S., Warren, N. E., Mayra, K., Gore, A., Das, A., & Ahmed, S. (2019). Where there is no nurse: An observational study of large-scale mentoring of auxiliary nurses to improve quality of care during childbirth at primary health centres in India. *BMJ open*, 9(7), e026845.

Sadler, M., Ruiz-Berdun, D., & Rojas, G. L. (2016). Moving beyond disrespect and abuse: Addressing the structural dimensions of obstetric violence. *Reproductive Health Matters, 24*(47), 47–55. doi.10.1016/j.rhm.2016.04.002.

Sen, G., Reddy, B., & Iyer, A. (2018). Beyond measurement: The drivers of disrespect and abuse in obstetric care. *Reproductive Health Matters*, *26*(53), 6–18.

Slade, P., Balling, K., Sheen, K., & Houghton, G. (2019). Establishing a valid construct of fear of childbirth: Findings from in-depth interviews with women and midwives. *BMC Pregnancy and Childbirth*, *19*, 96.

WHO. (2016). *World health statistics*. Geneva: World Health Organization.

10 Birth choices in Eastern Europe and Russia

Daniela Drandić, Nicholas Rubashkin, Tamara Sadovaya and Svetlana Illarionova

About the authors

I (Daniela) am a pro-choice researcher and advocate at Croatia's largest non-profit organisation representing parents: *RODA – Parents in Action*. I work to improve maternity care in Croatia and in the Central and Eastern European Region. I am passionate about antenatal education, maternal choice and autonomy. I am also a board member of Human Rights in Childbirth and have headed campaigns on improving maternity care in Croatia, including #PrekinimoŠutnju (Break the Silence), a campaign featured in international media reports in 2015. In 2019, I coordinated the development and launch of Expecting, a mobile application for pregnant families. I live in Croatia with my partner and three children.

I (Tamara) have been a practising midwife since 1992 and I am the founder of the Centre of Traditional Midwifery and Family Medicine in Moscow, Russia. I initiated and managed the 'Gentle Birth' project in several maternity hospitals in Moscow. I provide continuous education for midwives. I tell my story in detail below.

I (Svetlana) am a new graduate midwife who completed my Bachelor of Midwifery at Monash University, Melbourne, Australia in 2017. I have three children, all born in Australia. My first child was born by caesarean section. My subsequent babies were born at home. Martina Goerner (featured in Chapter 11) and Ulyana Kora were my midwives for my third birth in 2014. I now live in Ufa, Russia, and support women as a doula while in the process of getting professional registration as a midwife. I translated and supported Tamara to write this section.

Four births in four languages: one woman's international journey to vaginal birth after caesarean section

Daniela Drandić

> Women who refuse to agree to major surgery just because their healthcare systems are refusing to offer them options on vaginal births are turning to alternatives, including unlicensed homebirth and unassisted birth.

> Standing by idly while this happens, without addressing the underlying reasons is not responsible public health management, it is pushing a growing problem under the carpet.
>
> (Daniela Drandić)

A story of four births

The story of my four births is a story of failures – my own, and that of the system that I expected to look out for me. It is also a story of overcoming, of taking calculated risks, and ultimately, of triumph. My maternity care experiences shaped my career and education over the past ten years, especially my work as a professional maternity care advocate. *I own all of what happened, good and bad.*

I was born and raised in Canada and I moved to Croatia three years before becoming pregnant with my first child. My language skills were good, but my preparedness for the overtly patriarchal Croatian healthcare system was poor. From the outside, the Croatian healthcare system reports low perinatal and maternal mortality rates, with a caesarean section rate of around 10–15%. The system is firmly controlled by medicalised care, with four-weekly prenatal appointments involving routine vaginal exams and an ultrasound by an obstetrician. Midwives work within the hospital system, where fragmented care and obstetric control is the norm.

Foreign midwives discretely attend homebirths in Croatia in that grey zone of 'a-legality'. They are licensed in other EU countries but not Croatia, which does not issue licences to independently practising midwives (yet).

My first pregnancy and birth

I was 25 when I first became pregnant. This was an exciting time for my partner and me. Throughout my pregnancy I kept hearing that my baby was breech – I was told that meant she was sitting bum-down instead of head-down. My mum was breech so I didn't think this was a big deal – embarrassingly, I didn't even know that babies were supposed to be head-down. I was very thorough with my prenatal care; in addition to attending regular checks with my ob-gyn, I had extra ultrasounds at a private clinic. Nobody made me think my baby being breech was concerning and, at a time before online information on topics like breech birth was widely available, I had nobody to ask.

I knew women who had water births in hospital. While I thought they were crazy, I still asked my obstetrician about them. She said, 'It's exhibitionism; just because someone in the Netherlands gave birth in a tub now we all should, nonsense, humans don't give birth in water'. That was that.

At 38 weeks, at the first hospital appointment, the doctor on duty told me to come for a planned caesarean section two days later. I was shocked. Nobody had even mentioned caesarean sections before that point. I asked whether baby could change position. He said, 'There is a 12% chance she will change position, basically it's impossible'. I later learnt that he made that up. I looked at my partner in panic, motioned that the doctor was crazy and that we were leaving. I called the private doctor's clinic I attended for ultrasounds to get a second opinion. The doctor confirmed my baby was breech and said,

> Young doctors are very good at caesarean birth. They are not, however, good at vaginal breech birth. Nobody is anymore, and one day when the power goes out and women come to us with breech babies, we won't know what to do. But my advice to you, dear, is let them do a caesarean section. You can always have a vaginal birth next time.

I had my first caesarean. I negotiated my care beforehand – I would be awake (with regional anaesthesia), have my partner with me and get skin-to-skin with baby. In what I learnt later was a standard 'bait and switch', none of that happened. Unbeknown to me, all caesareans were performed under general anaesthetic because the anaesthetists didn't know how to do regionals. My partner wasn't allowed in the building. I saw my baby for the first time hours after she was born. I subsequently learnt that it was standard practice to falsely assure all women that their requests would be met.

I spent the first few weeks and months after her birth confused, thinking it was my fault and that I had done something wrong. I didn't know that I was experiencing trauma-related symptoms caused by the birth. I had trouble bonding with my baby. She had trouble adapting to life outside the womb. I later realised that despite my dates being 39+5 weeks, my baby was actually quite small and looked like she was born early-term. My trust in the system went from a ranking of 100 to almost zero – they had failed me and lied to me at every chance.

Safety and health during caesarean sections

The experiences of women in Eastern Europe reflect mine. In Croatia, as in many of the Eastern European countries, the proportion of women having a repeat caesarean section is growing (Devarajan, Talaulikar, & Arulkumaran, 2018). Caesarean rates have been growing steadily in Croatia over the past 20 years. The latest figures for 2017 show a rate of 24.85% (an increase of 7% from 2016) (Rodin, Draušnik, Cerovečki, & Jezdić, 2018). At country-level, the proportion of women who are giving birth after caesarean section is also rising, and in 2017 it was 9.73%; at the same time the VBAC rate continues to decrease and was 26.18% in 2017 (Đelmiš, Juras, & Rodin, 2018).

Having another go

Two and a half years later, I was pregnant again. By this time, I had joined an advocacy group and began training as a peer-to-peer breastfeeding counsellor. I began to learn about midwives and homebirth.

The bullying during antenatal appointments escalated. At my nine-week appointment, the nurse snapped at me for delaying my first appointment. 'Where have you been?' she sighed. At my 12-week appointment, the doctor berated me for questioning a test – saying that her goal was a healthy baby and clearly mine was not. In tears, I decided never to go back to that doctor again, but I quickly learnt that changing doctors was also a challenge. It was apparently considered 'uncollegial' to take on someone else's pregnant patient. I finally found an obstetrician to take me, who didn't fuss too much when I declined most vaginal exams. That said, the mere mention of VBAC caused eye-rolls. I realised my path to VBAC wouldn't be so easy and started looking for other options.

I found a birth centre in Austria, about a three-hour drive from my home. The few prenatal appointments I had there were heavenly – my midwife Eva Maria looked just like Ina May Gaskin (a famous American midwife), the birth centre had a pool and all kinds of equipment to help women work through labour, and I felt safe. My partner was not entirely on board, but he respected my wishes. As I neared 41 weeks of pregnancy, my Austrian midwives began to get nervous – they could not support births after 41+6 weeks of pregnancy. After trying everything, our final option was a local hospital for induction. I could not afford to pay for a midwife and an Austrian hospital.

I went to a Croatian public hospital instead, to see what my options were. I choose a different hospital, one reputed to be the most mother-friendly hospital in the country. Little did I know what hell would break loose when they saw me – a VBAC at 41 weeks. The doctor immediately announced, 'You do not have the legal capacity to make decisions about your care, pregnant women at term are a special legal category'. She asked my partner how he would feel 'being a single father of two children and how it will feel to have your wife bleed to death in your arms?' I was told I was not qualified to ask questions or get answers and endured lots of 'bait and switch'[1] tactics and outright lies, including that my baby weighed well over 4 kg and that my only option was another caesarean section.

My labour began that evening, 12 hours before my planned caesarean. As soon as a midwife realised I was having contractions, she told me to get on a stretcher and started wheeling me somewhere. I thought I might be going to a labour room, but she wheeled me into the operating theatre. My baby was perfectly average in every single one of his measurements. Before whisking him away, the midwife on duty pushed his scrotum into my face and said, 'You have a little boy, mummy'. I guess I should have been ecstatic to have given birth to a boy, as Croatian culture dictates, but all I wanted was to hold him to my skin and for everyone to leave us alone. All I remember was that he smelled better than anything I had ever smelled before. My partner was not allowed in theatre or recovery, so I was left alone and spent two nights after an uncomplicated caesarean section in intensive care. I saw my baby a few times, lasting for a few minutes each time over those two days. We later found out this was norm at that hospital so, not so mother-friendly after all.

I hated myself and I was furious at my partner. We were deceived, misled, betrayed! I should have been stronger, he should have protected me! The birth experience caused problems in my marriage for my mental health. For the next two years, I had flashbacks of rough vaginal exams, night sweats, nightmares about doctors and midwives doing things to me without consulting me. I later realised that what was happening to me had a name – post-traumatic stress disorder.

At my six-week postpartum appointment, I mustered all the strength I had to tell my doctor, 'I am not doing well – I need help'. He told me I would have to just deal with it, that was par for the course to becoming a mother and having a healthy baby.

The politics around VBAC

The cultural and political climate in which a woman births has a significant effect on her access to VBAC. In Central and Eastern Europe, the rising popularity of far-right conservatism is equally manifest in Croatia, pursuing policies to restrict women's reproductive rights that go far beyond access to abortion (Womenlobby.org, 2016).

In this climate, healthcare providers are encouraged to believe that the foetus has greater rights than the mother. They use aggressive and intrusive interventions, affording women limited informed choice (Kukura, 2010). Financially disadvantaged and minority groups in this region are more vulnerable. Language barriers, lack of access to evidence or information and dismissive care-provider attitudes significantly affect these groups (Kukura, 2010). Data specific for Croatia have shown that women with physical and intellectual disabilities get less information and are more likely to be offered caesarean section (Roda – Parents in Action, 2016).

Pregnant again

Four years later, when I found myself pregnant again, I called a midwife in a neighbouring country and booked in. She is fully licensed in her country, but not recognised in mine. Nonetheless, she was willing to take the risk and attend me. I decided I would refuse check-ups with the obstetrician until 12 weeks of pregnancy and I would lie about my pregnancy dates. A few days before my first appointment with my midwife, I started bleeding. I knew my mental health would collapse if I went into hospital so I found a private doctor who had recently opened a clinic nearby and crossed my fingers that he would be a good choice. He and his nurse were amazing and supported me through a physiological miscarriage. I will never forget the unexpected beauty my family and I found in this process of saying goodbye to our little one.

Third (fourth) time's a charm?

Two years later, there I was, pregnant again. It was such a strange time, I had begun feeling pregnant but thought it was the flu, and little birds were suddenly following me around in the dead of winter (seriously!). This time I was older, wiser and I knew exactly what I wanted and how to get it. By now, healthcare professionals were recognising me from my advocacy work and had stopped questioning me. I was no longer *groping through the fog*, trying to understand the risks and benefits of VBAC or repeat CS (Lundgren, Begley, Gross, & Bondas, 2012).

Homebirth and midwifery care are not a part of the Croatian healthcare system, so while women do VBAC at home, there are no available data as to their success rates or outcomes. Outside Croatia, a planned home VBAC with a midwife was statistically more successful than a planned VBAC at an obstetric unit, over all groups (87.6% vs. 69.1%) with no statistically significant differences between the groups regarding serious adverse maternal or perinatal outcomes (Rowe, Li, Brocklehurst, & Hollowell, 2016). Women in Ontario, Canada who planned a VBAC at home with a midwife had a spontaneous vaginal birth rate of 77% (Darling, 2013).

I met with my midwife, the one I previously engaged, at 12 weeks. I told her the truth about my dates because I knew she would not abandon my care. She was happy to attend me despite her legal status in Croatia being ambiguous at best, criminal at worst. She was, however, licensed in an EU country and had the experience and access (in her own country) to everything I needed – including Rhogam after birth, which I might need because of my negative blood type. At my first appointment with the obstetrician, I lied about my dates. He measured my baby by ultrasound as many times as he needed until the measurements agreed with my fudged dates. I nodded my head obediently and declined all vaginal exams, which my doctor begrudgingly accepted. I avoided answering questions and made (what was to him) strange requests, like asking for Rh sensitivity tests three times during pregnancy and where my placenta was in relation to my caesarean scar. I agreed to come into the hospital at 38 weeks for a caesarean, but I simply didn't show up.

My pregnancy was perfect, my midwife divine. I kept busy, travelled, cared for my children and enjoyed my pregnancy. Appointments with my midwife were filled with laughter and ease. I knew quite a bit about pregnancy and birth by now, and I knew she was being thorough and keeping me safe. Appointments became more frequent as I went over 40 weeks, 41 weeks and finally, over 42 weeks. It was a strange feeling, like being illegal, as I knew I could not just walk into the hospital maternity unit if I needed anything. Thankfully, my midwife was supportive and available for regular checks.

Finally, at 42 weeks and five days, just when I had accepted the fact that I would be pregnant forever, the first nudges began. My midwife crossed three borders to be at my side, where she remained just steps away from me through 35 hours of labour. She came with a car full of equipment and medications in case of complications. In my delirium during transition, I started speaking all the languages I know, and she kept up with me. My exhausted midwife and doula held the space through all the hours and tears and fears. And birth I did – a beautiful baby girl with stars in her eyes joined our family, weighing 3100 g and 50 cm long – perfectly perfect in every way. In the end, I gave birth in a pool, which was key to helping me rest between contractions after 35 hours of hard work bringing my baby earth-side. Within minutes my older children were by my side saying hello to their sister. It was hard work, but perfect.

Perhaps most telling from the experience was my partner, who had been a 'Doubting Thomas' from the start (but thoughtfully kept that to himself). Partners play such an important role in this process (Bonzon, Gross, Karch, & Grylka-Baeschli, 2017). Since our homebirth, he has become a midwifery evangelist. A full four years later, my partner's description of the beauty of the hours after our second daughter was born, with everyone tucked away and sleeping peacefully as the winter sun slowly rose, still brings tears to my eyes. Everything had changed forever, but it was also familiar and ours, without stress or fear. On a recent transatlantic flight, he even spent an hour telling his seatmate about our homebirth!

Was birthing after two caesareans at home with a foreign midwife the safest thing to do in a country where independent midwives have no legal standing or status? Probably not. I should have had the back-up of the hospital system; to be able to tell my doctor the truth and get support; to lean on the system my taxes pay for; and to not fear repercussions at every turn. I should have had my wishes and decisions respected in the maternity system – but my experiences had taught me that those were fools' dreams and I had to do what I had to do to get the care I wanted.

Would I do it again? In a heartbeat.

Opening up the possibility for others

I was my midwife's second client to have a successful VBAC after two previous caesarean sections and as we said goodbye after our fourth postpartum visit, she thanked me for being so strong. But without her, her excellent care and her quiet faith in me and the process, it would have all been for nothing. We would meet again – two years later, I would stroke my friend's hair as the same midwife supported her to push out a beautiful big baby at home after three caesareans.

Conclusion

Women who reject the limited surgical options offered by restrictive and coercive healthcare systems are turning to alternatives, including unlicensed homebirth and unassisted birth. Standing idly by while this happens, without addressing the underlying reasons, is not responsible public health management, it is pushing a growing problem under the carpet and putting women's lives at risk. Research supports women seeking midwifery care and homebirth in order to achieve a successful VBAC, but in order for this to be as safe as possible, maternity systems must be open to collaboration with homebirth midwives and putting mothers and babies above professional turf wars and profit.

We are the canaries in the coal mine, the women who have been lied to, coerced and cast aside by maternity care systems. Scaring us into submission is not an option. We will not stand for it any longer.

In the next section, US-based obstetrician Nicholas Rubashkin discusses his journey from birth to his current interest in Human Rights in Central and Eastern Europe.

An obstetrician's perspective on human rights and childbirth in Central and Eastern Europe

Nicholas Rubashkin

> I realised women are the ones who lose when midwives and obstetricians fight or don't work together.
>
> (Nicholas Rubashkin)

About the author

On meeting me (Nicholas) for the first time, patients, fellow birth activists and researchers commonly ask two questions: (1) how did you become interested in the field of obstetrics and gynaecology, and (2) how did you become so passionate about protecting women's rights in childbirth? My interpretation, from the subtexts in both questions, is that I am being asked how a man can come to approach obstetrics and gynaecology from a resolutely feminist perspective. Also, how would a childless, gay man like me, with seemingly little connection with the health and human rights of pregnant women, dedicate my career to this pursuit?

The involvement of men in obstetrics is far from peculiar – men dominate the profession in many regions of the globe. Men (predominantly educated, upper-class and/or white men) established the obstetric profession in Europe and America (and later settler countries Australia, Canada, New Zealand) and regulated the profession of midwifery virtually to the point of extinction. Men continue to dominate and perpetuate hierarchies of gender, race, class and professional status through the mistreatment and abuse of women in every area of our professional practice – from routine gynaecologic visits and pregnancy and childbirth care, to family planning care and abortion.

That said, the deep political engagement of men with pregnant women's health and human rights is rare. In this personal essay, I share my own 'personal is political' journey, through the stories of my American and Hungarian grandmothers, my own mother and my own birth story. The connections across generations of women in my family charted a path towards my humanistic practice of obstetrics, to becoming a respectful maternity care researcher active in the USA and in Central/Eastern Europe, and to my serving as an expert witness in court cases around the world where pregnant women's human rights have been violated. Because we men are all 'of woman born' (to use the title of Adrienne Rich's foundational examination of feminist motherhood), we need not look very far to find the personal and political ways in which we are connected to childbirth.

My American grandmother had nine children in the North Eastern USA in the era of Twilight Sleep. Twilight Sleep was induced by the administration of morphine (an anaesthetic) and scopoloamine (an amnestic) to labouring women to 'relieve' them of perceived suffering (see also discussions about current use in Chapter 8). Twilight Sleep took off in the USA in the early twentieth century amid eugenic concerns that if white women continued to experience the horrors of childbirth pain they would not 'reproduce the race'. In fact, solving the 'problem' of white women's childbirth pain became connected to efforts to outlaw abortion and regulate midwives out of practice (Rich, 2016). By mid-century, nearly all white women would give birth in an unconscious state, tucked away in dark corners of American hospitals (Sandelowski, 1984). Having spent most of her childhood during The Great Depression in an orphanage, my grandmother wanted to build a large, loving family. She never openly expressed regret about the fact that she was put to sleep for the births of all nine of my aunts and uncles, but I inferred, from the joy she expressed to me about attending my homebirth, her disappointment in her own childbirths.

My mother, herself born in the early 1950s during the peak of Twilight Sleep, didn't like her first hospital experience in the early 1970s in the USA. While labouring with my older sister, my mother entered the hospital fully dilated and pushing. While Twilight Sleep was on its way out as a practice, mechanisms surrounding the practice, such as separating women from their families during labour, remained entrenched. My mother, just 20 years old, was separated from my father and had my sister awake and conscious, but alone. My mother was not college-educated or actively involved in the feminist health movement, but something about her hospital birth just didn't sit right with her. She bought an early copy of *Our Bodies, Ourselves* (MLA. Boston Women's Health Book Collective, 2011), and began making a different plan for her birth – with me.

My parents moved to a remote island 20 miles off the coast of Rockland, Maine, where my father secured his first job as a school teacher. A feature of this island made it an attractive place in my mother's eyes: at that time, all babies were born at home on the island with births managed by the local doctor. My mother learned that the town doctor still commonly sedated the women of the island, even in the home setting. My mother, carrying forward the sense of wanting to birth differently, refused the sedation and gave birth to me in the dining room of our little cottage on a fishing island.

It was a story I grew up with that was just very powerful for my mother in terms of being connected to her pregnancy and birth. My American grandmother was also present. She would always tell me on my birthday every year that she gave me my first bath in the kitchen sink, an intimate act that proved transformative for a woman who was put to sleep for all nine of her births. My Dad, absent from my sister's birth, began every school year by giving his students an assignment about 'new beginnings'. My father often completed his own assignments, so he wrote an essay about the challenges of moving to such a remote place, but also the power of witnessing my birth, which was this huge 'new beginning' in his life. When my parents later moved back to the mainland, they decided to have my brother at home. I remember padding across the kitchen one early morning, at the age of four, to find my parents celebrating the arrival of my younger brother.

I like to think that my American grandmother, my mother, and my own childbirth provided fertile ground for my future interests in human rights in childbirth. My career in this area began when, in college, I came out as a gay man. I started taking women's studies classes where a lot of the gay and lesbian studies classes were hosted. I received a scholarship to conduct in-depth readings on the connections between queer and feminist social movements, and I went on to complete a minor in women's studies prior to entering medical school. While feminism helped me develop a language around rigid gender roles and understand how homophobia can be a weapon of sexism, my explorations in women's studies also connected me more deeply to my mother and her experiences. Not just in childbirth, but as a woman who gave up her dreams to follow my father's career, cleaned houses to make ends meet and who really kind of shouldered a lot for our family. I selected medical schools based on the possibility of completing a Master's degree in a social science, and at Stanford I decided on cultural anthropology, with a focus on gender and sexuality. I wrote my master's thesis on gay men who care for lovers dying of HIV or AIDS, but through a gendered lens, by looking at care work as 'women's work'. There's this big question in the feminist movement about how you get men to do women's work. In the HIV space, gay men were doing women's work of caring and I always thought I was going to care for gay men with HIV and do HIV research.

Then I attended my first birth during my obstetrics and gynaecology rotation. The woman I cared for was a young, Mexican immigrant who had crossed the US border when seven or eight months pregnant, and she was alone. Her husband could not stay with her because he worked nights. My Spanish was rudimentary, but enough to communicate with her. I spent the whole labour with her, through the entire night, and it was a really powerful experience. Honestly, I was tingling the next day and I thought, I could do this for a career.

It's funny because that first birth also had so many elements that I now see are part of the profession's problems, or the power dynamics that we're all talking about. The nurse on shift that day was also a homebirth midwife, and she did this subversive thing of not calling the resident in soon enough to catch the baby, so the woman completed her birth totally unassisted. For me, that birth was a powerful metaphor for the human endurance and survival in my own family. My Hungarian grandmother met my Russian grandfather in a refugee camp after World War II. My father was born abroad, and his mother talked about her hopes for a new life in the USA, having crossed the Atlantic in a boat with my young father in her arms.

Six months later, I ran into the same Mexican woman I supported in labour. She ran up to me and said, 'Do you remember me?' We had a nice interaction but, despite my already deep understanding of the power of birth in my family, it was now dawning on me that compassionate treatment during childbirth *really matters* to women. Here I was, a 'lowly' medical student, but she remembered me and my support for her through the labour and birth. So I was motivated to learn obstetrics sensitively. For example, while learning how to do a pelvic exam in medical school, it really mattered to me to know whether the experience could be empowering or something that would turn a woman away from our care. I think that also relates back to my student experiences in medical school, where I was really stigmatised and experienced homophobia, and as a patient having experienced both empowering and really disempowering care. I think I've always just walked that line between my experiences as a gay man, my family background and then my academic training.

I went on to train as an obstetrician and was lucky that my training was holistic and woman-centred. I was lucky to go to the University of California and San Francisco, a globally renowned centre for termination of pregnancy training, so there's a real emphasis on choice and autonomy. Maternal autonomy was definitely valued in the same way I think it should be when compared to foetal health issues. In our programme, we train collaboratively with nurse midwives and we accept homebirth transfers. When I finished my obstetrics training, I joined a small community hospital. This meant going from a high-tech university environment, which was great training, to a small San Francisco community hospital that served about 50% publicly insured women. It was really a midwife-led practice where the midwives were more front-and-centre of care than even the university practice. They handled all the normal cases, and I saw a lot more unmedicated childbirth. During my five years there, the hospital's status was never secure; it was acquired by another corporation that planned to shut the hospital's inpatient services. While the city of San Francisco worked with the corporation to keep the hospital open, the political uncertainty really affected us and the hospital. When a complication happened on the labour unit, a difficult birth, a difficult outcome for a baby, the midwifery programme would automatically face scrutiny, and we obstetricians would be challenged for being too liberal or for having caesarean section rates that were too low (around 20%) compared to the higher caesarean rate of the private corporation that acquired us.

One day, I was the covering obstetrician when a homebirth transfer arrived. I was likely on duty because it was Mothers' Day and I was the only physician in the practice without children. The woman who planned a homebirth lost her baby under my watch and it had a profound effect on me. She had already consulted with many doctors in the department, had been recommended for induction of labour for several days due to having late decelerations on antepartum testing in the setting of a post-term pregnancy. It took several days to get the induction underway, and then the woman developed a fever and more foetal heart issues, all of which ultimately led to an emergency caesarean and a very compromised baby. The baby had head cooling procedures, seizures and eventually passed away the next day. It was a pivotal experience for me in my young career. Looking back, I could've been more clear about some of the risks that were going on, but I worried about infringing her autonomy. When debriefing with us, she was very honest and insightful, saying that she and her husband had been arrogant about their bodies, that they didn't necessarily believe what we were saying and they felt that it [a bad outcome] couldn't happen to them. They also shared that their homebirth midwife was not aligning with us in the information we provided about induction. The care dynamic was really difficult, and I questioned staying true to my knowledge as a clinician, while also respecting a woman's autonomy and working with homebirth midwives. Midwives are not incorporated into the system, which makes it difficult to work together to improve quality of care, because they [midwives] were marginalised and they don't have easy access to medical consultation. When a complication happens, there's no legally protected way that we can all actually get together and say, 'What could we do to improve our care?'

Homebirth is really seen as just a hot potato that no one wants to handle.

The loss of this baby was a personal and professional crisis for me. If people can't trust the care recommendations of our liberal community hospital with high-quality midwifery care and compassionate obstetric consultation, what is really going on here? I was angry with the midwife for what seemed to be actions undermining our care. For my own part, could pushing the woman harder or communicating my concerns better have perhaps changed the ultimate outcome, while still respecting her autonomy? Perhaps most challenging, on a personal and professional level, was working through my own trauma around the case which was being relived through weekly quality improvement meetings. Due to liability concerns, the hospital administration initially considered ceasing accepting all homebirth transfers – a proposal that staff fended off as a practice even though the administration was placing us under heavy scrutiny.

In summary, one homebirth transfer and neonatal death laid bare the challenges and limitations for both pregnant women seeking supported choices in childbirth and for obstetricians and midwives seeking to collaborate effectively to provide safe, evidence-based care. Ultimately, I focused on a human rights perspective which, in turn, focuses on the laws, policies and systems that create dysfunctional and dangerous care dynamics between doctors, midwives and women. I realised that women lose when midwives and obstetricians fight or don't work well together.

Moving back to my Eastern European roots

Around the same time that this neonatal death occurred, I was discovering my Hungarian roots. Once again, the personal and political would provide a way forward for me. I began to learn the language, and then my father and I visited our Hungarian family for the first time in 2010. My father had not been back since he left at the age of two. On the plane trip home, I thumbed through a copy of *The Economist* and read a short article about an obstetrician who became a homebirth midwife. It was from that point forward that I started following the case of Ágnes Geréb.

Ágnes Geréb

Ágnes Geréb trained as an obstetrician in hospitals but gravitated towards offering homebirth to escape poor-quality care in hospitals, especially regarding respect, dignity and family-centredness for women. Ironically, the Lamaze labour technique, which originated in Soviet Russia, would upend decades of Twilight Sleep and transform childbirth as we now know it in Western Europe and America (Michaels, 2014), but have little or no impact on quality of maternity care in the former communist countries of Central and Eastern Europe. Challenges in the region include outdated equipment and provider training, a scarcity of professionals and pharmaceuticals, and communication barriers between professionals and women (Miteniece et al., 2019). Using a similar measure of shared decision-making, our research group found that, when compared to a Canadian population of women, Hungarian women experienced comparatively less shared decision-making around their birth options and higher rates of mistreatment (Baji, Rubashkin, Szebik, Stoll, & Vedam, 2017). Physicians tightly control birth services and midwives struggle to obtain an independent education and professional practice. It was, in this context, that Ágnes Geréb built a thriving homebirth practice in Budapest – her compassionate and competent care represented an important option for women and families seeking care outside the formal health system.

After experiencing three different complications during three homebirths, Ágnes Geréb came under the scrutiny of the Hungarian authorities (Hill, 2010). At this time in Hungary, as homebirth was not legal, the complications were addressed through the application of criminal prohibitions in Hungary. Whenever a homebirth transfer needed to happen, a police car and an ambulance would show up at the woman's home, not only to transfer but to gather evidence and intelligence required for a criminal investigation and prosecution. Only one of the three families who ultimately endured a loss in their homebirth under Geréb's care moved forwards in partnership with the criminal prosecution. Despite that, all three of the transferred cases worked their way through the criminal courts in a sensational and globally publicised trial. In hospital cases concerning the same set of circumstances, obstetricians – if found responsible – would have been faced either a civil malpractice proceeding or a quality improvement project. But Ágnes Geréb, as a homebirth midwife in Hungary, was put through a criminal process. This was concerning because one of the complications may well have resulted after the transfer to hospital, from a Kristeller manoeuvre (pushing down on the woman's fundus in second stage) that was performed by the hospital staff on one of her patients. That's something I've often wondered about in complicated homebirth transfers, where the midwife is ultimately blamed for the outcome. Countries with highly medicalised and non-evidence-based practice are precisely where it is most important to have options for out-of-hospital midwifery care. Yet, these are also country settings where the midwife is more easily blamed for an injury that might have actually occurred in the hospital.

The public dialogue about Ágnes Geréb's case was (and remains) very polarised. She was either the saviour of women or she was a baby killer. I've come to realise that this is an effective way to deflect attention from the systemic problems. This was the reaction of my hospital administrators who, out of liability concerns, wanted to discourage or outright ban homebirth transfers. It is a recurring problem for homebirth transfers in the Netherlands and the USA, where the accusations start and end with a belief that homebirth midwives are killing babies. Homebirth midwives become easy scapegoats in the polarised debates, in itself an injustice and a distraction that can make it very difficult to discern what actually needs to be improved (see the discussions on those distractions in Chapter 14). It may be that the system needs to change course, not the women. Instead, the whole event just becomes a media circus or witch hunt. While certainly there are significant differences between the quality of maternity care in the USA and Hungary, it seemed to me that Ágnes Geréb and her clients were running up against similar systemic dysfunctions that I encountered in the USA around homebirth transfers.

Ternovszky v. Hungary *(before the European Court of Human Rights)*

In 2010, one of Ágnes Geréb's clients, Anna Ternovszky, with the legal team at the Hungarian Civil Liberties Union (HCLU) challenged the severe legal restrictions imposed on homebirth midwifery practice, which Anna said effectively prevented her from utilising homebirth to safely avoid the poor-quality and abusive care in hospitals. Ternovsky, now pregnant with her second child, argued that her human rights were violated by the Hungarian state's refusal to provide legal and regulated homebirth options. Having exhausted domestic legal remedies with no success, the HCLU took Ternovsky's case to the European Court of Human Rights – and won! The *Ternovszky v. Hungary* decision in 2010 (Ternovsky Decision) was the first European Court of Human

Rights decision to specifically address women's right to privacy as including the right to choose the circumstances of their births (ECHR, 2010). Essentially, the Court held that women have the right to decide where, how and with whom they birth. Hungary violated Anna's right to privacy and family life (Article 8 of the European Convention of Human Rights) by failing to provide any regulation surrounding homebirth. Subsequent to *Ternovszky*, Hungary legalised and regulated the provision of homebirth. There were limitations in the judgement; for instance, the Court gave Hungary a wide latitude on implementing a homebirth framework, including by deciding not to cover homebirth under the national insurance plan. Still, I thought it was interesting that a legal mechanism was being used to shift obstetric practice. Hungary is not the only country to have done this (see Chapters 2, 5, 6, 7 and 11).

Having experienced my own complications during a homebirth transfer and arriving at the conclusion that systemic factors played a role, I began to consider how human rights courts, and legislation and policy informed by human rights principles, could help resolve dysfunctional systems of care that pit obstetricians and midwives against each other. I started to see how human rights can be addressed at that big policy level and be a set of values that inform policies and inform clinical interactions.

I thought I was the only person outside Hungary who was following this court case in Hungary. I started to think about a research project that would compare women's experiences of care in home and hospital births in Hungary. Then a call came to attend a human rights and childbirth conference in The Hague, Netherlands. The main objective of the event was to dissect the *Ternovszky* decision and its significance. In 2012, I rearranged my busy clinical schedule to attend. The conference just blew my mind, seeing this whole community of people thinking about the very same that I was contending with in private. At the conference, I met several Hungarian collaborators who spoke on the panel about *Ternovszky*, and this led to my placement at the Semmelweis Medical School in Budapest to conduct my research, funded by a Fullbright research grant.

Gratuity payments to obstetricians for better care

While in Hungary, I adapted English-language maternity care surveys with a group of Hungarian experts (Rubashkin et al., 2017). We surveyed Hungarian women across place of birth about their experiences of evidence-based and respectful care. One of the most challenging aspects of adapting existing surveys to the Hungarian context was the issue of cash 'tips' that women were paying obstetricians for their births. Due to underfunding of the health system, including low provider wages, patients in all healthcare sectors experience higher out-of-pocket payments. However, in maternity care, there is a specific 'gratitude payment', a culturally ingrained practice whereby women make informal payments to secure a continuity relationship with a known provider. For providers, these informal payments now make up a significant portion of their salary. As you can imagine, this can be prone to abuse, and women share stories on social media of being mistreated if they don't 'tip'. The practice of pursuing informal payments is so culturally embedded, it operates like an 'open secret'; not sanctioned by government and not openly discussed between providers and women. Women have lively discussions, over social media, about which providers accept payment, how much they require and whether a provider might directly ask for a payment which is considered more offensive or even illegal. No research group ever asked what the women actually get in return for tipping their obstetricians.

Without official records of informal payments, one of the best ways to study the practice was to ask women. We created survey predictors to track the flow of money through informal cash payments. We found that the culturally appropriate term used by women was 'chosen': a woman will say that she is getting prenatal care with a 'chosen' doctor. 'Chosen' indicates an intention, through encoded language and informal arrangements, to forward an unlawful cash gratuity payment to a doctor. The unlawful component is perhaps why it is considered taboo for providers to ask directly for a payment. Using the same encoded language, we found that, in our nationally representative sample of internet-using women, 60% of Hungarian women tipped their obstetrician with cash following childbirth. We found that the main driver of the probability of payment was whether the doctor showed up, physically, to the delivery. Once there, even doctors who mistreat women would get paid. It didn't matter whether the women had a caesarean or vaginal delivery. The type of delivery didn't affect the probability of receiving payment. If anything, the women who tipped across the board endured more procedures, such as caesarean sections, episiotomies and inductions, but they also reported greater shared decision-making and fewer experiences with mistreatment.

We concluded that while the gratitude payment system in Hungary works as a 'shadow' cash payment system within the national (public) health insurance scheme, it in fact functions more like a (private) fee for service. Women are essentially paying for continuity of care with a 'chosen' obstetrician and, in substance, associating the continuity relationship with safety and evidence. Additionally, we found that women used cash payments to make informal arrangements to receive an epidural, as the rate in Hungary is very low. Women who paid informally had an epidural rate of 13% when they delivered vaginally. The group who paid informally also had a higher rate of inductions (32%), so we are concerned about the undertreatment of women's pain while they are being exposed to more painful obstetric interventions (Baji et al., 2017).

Where women are mistreated, a strong conflict develops over whether they should tip after childbirth. Paying a tip is such a strong practice in Hungary that it creates a dilemma for women who feel they received low-quality care. While working on this survey, Human Rights in Childbirth received an inquiry from a Hungarian woman who planned to tip her obstetrician. The obstetrician scheduled and rushed the induction; she received a caesarean section just six hours into hospitalisation. She then developed a wound seroma which her provider misdiagnosed, after denying that the woman was even having a problem. Despite having a likely unnecessary caesarean and her surgical symptoms denied, she paid a tip. For her second delivery, the woman returned to the same obstetrician who had a good reputation despite her previous experience. She wanted a VBAC, but the obstetrician refused to meet or discuss it with her. He scheduled a caesarean instead. When she developed a bad cold and cough, she requested he delay the surgery, but her doctor refused. After the surgery (through which she coughed uncontrollably), she asked for an ultrasound examination of the incision prior to leaving the hospital, as with her first caesarean, but he refused. With all her coughing, the woman ultimately experienced a wound evisceration: soon after returning home, she found that her intestines had come out of her incision. Wound evisceration is a life-threatening surgical emergency which this woman was lucky to survive. While many details of this case will never be known (the woman requested her records and none of the details of the wound evisceration were documented), it is possible that the physician's desire to schedule the delivery, which relates to receiving a cash gratuity and his rejection of her concerns, contributed to this woman's life-threatening complications.

Many women in Central and Eastern Europe are experiencing medicalised and extremely traumatising care. The status of women and attitudes to women in Hungary is shockingly different to the rest of Europe (RODA, 2015). Right now, there's a big push for Hungarian women to have more children, and that's related in part to (eugenic) beliefs about population decline and anti-immigrant sentiments. There's a different emphasis in Hungary on women's traditional roles in the domestic sphere as being to have children and to reproduce the nation.

In my research, advocacy and through serving as an expert court witness, I hear shocking stories of physical and verbal abuse in hospital care in Central and Eastern Europe. This was really surprising to me, even as someone who had been following the Gereb and Ternovszky cases. Actually living and researching in the region helped me put the *Ternovsky* Decision into perspective. In Central and Eastern Europe, homebirth is a safety valve for a woman to obtain respectful and evidence-based care, but in a very different way to the USA.

For Roma women (Gypsies), for instance, homebirth could be an important option because they experience significant racism in the Central and Eastern Europe healthcare systems. Roma women are forcibly sterilised, relegated to segregated maternity wards where they are neglected or receive inferior care and verbally abused while in labour (Janevic, Sripad, Bradley, & Dimitrievska, 2011). On the other hand, Roma women live in segregated settlements that lack electricity and clean running water, potentially compromising safe homebirth care. Further complicating the situation, if a Roma woman has a fast labour and births at home, the child welfare authorities can threaten to take their children away.

In Eastern Europe, majority white Hungarian and Roma women face significant challenges accessing quality out-of-hospital birth options that don't put their families at risk. Birthing outside the guidelines or the system creates its own set of problems. When women are driven out of the medical system because of fear and mistrust, it becomes even harder for the midwives to transfer when needed. Women lose in these situations because the system is strict, oppressive, traumatising, racist and the midwives fearful. I have noticed, however, no matter where you look, in Brazil, Hungary, Australia and the USA, where medical and surgical intervention in childbirth are just out of control, there's still this embodied knowledge that women have and protect when it comes to childbirth. I think of my mother and that birth concept she had that birth happens through a vagina and women take that as a given (Dweik, Girasek, Toreki, Meszaros, & Pal, 2014).

In the last few years, I began testifying in court cases where women's rights in childbirth have been violated. I have submitted written testimony to cases in Central and Eastern Europe, Latin America and the USA. I have appeared in person, as an expert witness, in court cases in the USA, including in the states of Alabama, Washington and Louisiana. In Louisiana, I testified on the behalf of a midwife who had come up for review before the medical board. I thought it was shocking that a doctor had to be the expert on her behalf. This was because she reported to the medical board and not a midwifery board. I had to learn a little more about the standards relating to homebirth care so I could be an adequate expert for her. This is inappropriate. She requires a homebirth midwifery expert, and that expert opinion should be valued in its own right by a court of law. Midwifery regulations should always provide for autonomous and self-governing practice. Doctors do not know or understand midwifery standards of care for homebirth. Human Rights in Childbirth recently funded my travel to the Philippines to provide expert testimony on behalf of a couple who experienced a stillbirth due to the unsafe and inappropriate use of oxytocin to stimulate labour.

Right now, the USA is experiencing a maternal health crisis which is delineated by race (and racial discrimination). I think that part of the way forward is to support a revival of midwives of colour who serve and support women of colour where they live, whether in black neighbourhoods or on Native lands. Midwives of colour are undermined by the same stereotypes that are used to attack their communities of origin; for instance, Black 'grand' midwives in the Southern USA were denigrated as dirty and disease-ridden, like the Black families they served (Fraser, 1998). Diversity has been purposefully stamped out and we have a one-size-fits-all model that has taken over most of the world. There is a growing realisation that we need to meet women where they're at; a core principle of midwifery with the potential to deliver health equity and transform lives, because midwives of colour are on the front lines dealing with the tapestry of issues, whether challenges of gentrification and loss of housing for black women or establishing birth centres on Native American land. There is also a changing narrative around doulas happening in some organisations, where administrators are calling it more than just birth work. It says a lot about community resilience and empowerment, and being a part of the solution to racial disparities through compassionate, continuous care (McLemore & Warner Hand, 2017).

On risk and choice

Risk is an essential topic to discuss, but we need to ask: at what point does a discussion on risk turn into a tool of power? There are circumstances where it is clearly being deployed as a tool of power: when risks are distorted or exaggerated, when women are told that they have to comply for the baby and the risks inflated to coerce a decision.

There's also a middle ground, where obstetricians (and some midwives) counsel women by engaging in a risk–benefit conversation, where it is not immediately obvious but is also an act of power asserted over women. Right now, care-providers have the power to decide which risks to present and how to frame them so a woman feels like she cannot refuse. The risk–benefit conversation may be accurate but, by being incomplete, is in effect coercive. As obstetricians, we have been trained to think that engaging in a risk–benefit conversation is all that is needed, but this conversation is really just one element of person-centred care. Women want supported options and they want to talk about their fears and their hopes. They also need to have a rights-based conversation. This does not happen in a risk–benefit discussion. My view is that the focus on risk–benefit discussions is another act of power – where other aspects of person-centred care are deliberately suppressed or excluded (Rubashkin, Warnock, & Diamond-Smith, 2018). The more robust discussions of risk happen where it really involves a woman's preferences, future pregnancy plans and her culture. That just doesn't really happen, and that's the direction where care should go.

The past struggles between midwifery and obstetrics were around the belief that pregnancy is an inherently pathological condition doctors need to control, the science of which midwives couldn't possibly understand. Risk is today the new terrain of the interprofessional power struggles. It is obstetricians who get to decide what high-risk is (Kukla et al., 2009) and how it is defined. It seems like just about every woman today has some kind of risk factor that justifies our involvement. Once involved, we get to determine the content of conversations discussing risk, and whether that risk justifies intervention. For example, if you have a BMI of 30 and a 15% risk of gestational diabetes, we decide whether you need an induction of labour. Weight, age and race are becoming categories used to either limit women's birth options or blame them for poor outcomes (McLemore, 2018). Risk is a slippery concept that can morph from appearing as an evidence-based tool for discussion to a tool of power very easily and without anyone realising.

Although my personal and professional journey and my work as a researcher and an expert witness have all afforded me insight into the struggles of midwives, I still love to manage medical and surgical complications of pregnancy. My background has given me a clear perspective about how and when the tools of medicine and surgery should be applied. My training and practice in collaboration with midwives and the time I spent in Hungary under the mentorship of midwifery researchers have all helped me to think a bit more like a midwife. This is unique in my profession. Midwives understand obstetricians better than we understand midwives because midwives are forced to understand us and navigate their work around us. In my view, a lot of the polarisation between our professions has to do more with obstetrician's lack of exposure to autonomous midwives. The synthesis and the tension that we experience between our different philosophies is actually productive. To work effectively, we need to see it as a productive tension, as opposed to right/wrong polarisation, because bringing the different perspectives and philosophies together is representative of the reality of childbirth. Neither of us is wholly right nor wholly wrong. The scientific training process and policy processes need to be more integrated in order to develop a complete picture and provide holistic care. We need our autonomous spheres, but we also need more opportunities where we can all come together.

In the next section, Tamara Sadovaya supported by Svetlana Illarionova give us a brief look into what is happening in Russia when it comes to women's choices and birthing choices.

A postcard on birth from Russia

Tamara Sadovaya, translated and supported by Svetlana Illarionova

The birth of a new paradigm in Russia

In 1979, on the sunny coast of Crimea, under the morning rays of the sun, one of the first babies was born in sea water. This baby initiated a new era in which women made public their desire to give birth without violence and birth outside the system. The founder of the water birth experience in Russia was engineer Igor Charkovsky who, with his supporters, organised a club called 'Healthy Family'. His followers pursued a healthy lifestyle, including the practice of water birth at home. This Russian movement is now 40 years old. Over time, the experience changed. Women who gave birth independently at home, usually with their husbands and without the presence of professional midwives, told stories about birth that were both wonderful and without pain and violence. Many of them found their vocation and later became professional midwives. So, homebirth midwifery practice in Russia was based on rejection of the public maternity care practices. This rejection was sometimes excessive and very painful because women often encountered violence and cruelty during their first facility birth. The system presented as a soulless conveyor belt to many people. The formation of maternity care service, led by midwives, in defiance of the public medicalised obstetric system, inevitably led to conflict.

Tamara's experience of running away from the system

In the late 1980s, a young woman named Tamara Sadovaya gave birth to her first child in an ordinary Soviet maternity hospital. According to the obstetric standards of that time, all went well. Tamara had a seven-hour labour, during which she was subjected to the following: (a) a single intramuscular injection of drotaverine (pain relief); (b) amniotomy without indication in the first stage; (c) classically managed pushing on her back in the second stage; (d) Kristeller manoeuvre (fundal pressure to push the baby out); (e) episiotomy; and (f) the feeling of being a soulless object that was manipulated as she gave birth. The result was a healthy boy of 4 kg, which was not put on Tamara's chest even for a minute. While she was left lying in the hallway with an icy water bottle on her abdomen, her baby was left alone and screaming on a changing table. She was allowed her baby the next day, every four hours for a feed. For her next pregnancy, Tamara chose to birth at home. This birth was not a conscious choice; rather, it was an escape from the system, a response to the fear of entrusting herself and her baby to people in white coats. The birth took place at home with just Tamara and her husband. This experience was so joyful it inspired both Tamara's future choice to give birth to her third child at home and her desire to become a midwife.

After her first pregnancy, Tamara understood very well that she would never return to this organisation called a maternity hospital. But never say never! Twenty years later, she returned in a professional capacity to change the system and create the opportunity for women to have a joyful childbirth.

Implementation difficulties in post-Soviet Russia – inspiration, naivety, risks

In the 1990s, post-Soviet maternity hospitals continued to follow the old paradigms of care which disrespected women. Obstetricians denied the simplest requests by women, such as a request to move in labour or adopt alternative birth positions.

The first homebirth midwives did not have a medical education. Enthusiasm, inspiration and an unwavering faith in the power of women's bodies was expressed by those fearless midwives. This faith was the driving force behind the growing popularity of homebirth. According to unofficial statistics, the planned homebirth rate in Moscow was 4% at that time. Today, the homebirth rate is lower because midwifery models of care like the one Tamara runs have expanded to give women humanised options in hospital.

Most homebirth midwives entered medical colleges in Russia in the 1990s. After completing their midwifery courses, however, they could not imagine working in the public obstetric system and continued to practice illegally as the official maternity healthcare system categorically rejected homebirth. Women who transferred from home to a hospital seeking specialised medical care were subjected to psychological pressure and humiliation.

Tamara finished a medical college degree and created a family club for parents. The family club was one of the first non-commercial gatherings of like-minded parents who pursued homebirths and a healthy lifestyle. Tamara conducted birth preparation classes and supported new homebirth clients through this club. She enjoyed years of midwifery practice helping women to give birth at home. She is inspired by the happy expressions of women holding their babies in the minutes after birth. She received satisfaction from the fact that the women were happy with motherhood and that many of them decided to have more children.

Assimilation into the system

In 2002, Tamara founded the Centre of Traditional Midwifery and Family Medicine. Midwives and doctors tried to implement the safest possible homebirth with the participation of two midwives, or a midwife and a family doctor, and the support of an ambulance service. This was a difficult five years which involved battling systemic resistance, multiple inspections and investigations by public supervisory bodies, the Department of Health and interprofessional conflicts with hospital administration.

At the same time, the work of Tamara's Centre showed good outcomes. None of the women or babies had complications in birth or with their health as a result of having a homebirth. Despite this, the Centre endured multiple investigations from the Department of Health between 2002 and 2006. At the end of 2006, Tamara reached an agreement with the Head of Moscow obstetrics. They agreed to develop the first birth space in Moscow where a woman could birth in a home-like environment with the support of a Centre midwife. The practice of the Centre changed. In hospital, women were offered a wait-and-see philosophy of care, limited routine interventions, free movement in labour, the ability to use a bath and have a water birth, routine skin-to-skin for mother and baby for at least one hour after birth, delayed cord cutting and supported to breast-feed on demand. This same project, 'Gentle Birth', is now offered in 12 different maternity hospitals in Moscow and in some other cities in Russia. Since 2007, Tamara's Centre has had more than 7000 births with a caesarean section rate below 12% and significantly lower use of syntocinon and epidural anaesthesia compared with Moscow city maternity hospitals. Most importantly, the Centre's outcomes include healthy babies and high maternal satisfaction with the birth experience.

Today, the midwifery models of care in Russia are still not common. Obstetricians are the main specialists who are responsible for birth outcomes. Maternity care is fragmented, many protocols are outdated and medicalisation of birth is high. Few obstetricians accept the wait-and-see philosophy of non-interference in labour. Midwives operate as assistants to obstetricians. They cannot independently provide full antenatal or postnatal care, or support the birth on their own. Homebirth is essentially illegal, although prosecution does not follow unless there is a significant adverse event. Some women choose to give birth at home on their own or with an attendant who may or may not have a medical education. Homebirth is not discussed much for the protection of the midwives and women. Recently, a midwife in Russia faced extensive investigations over a homebirth case. These investigations have had a significant flow on impact on other midwifery practices, which has resulted in an underground, fearful environment when it comes to homebirth.

A way forward

Daniela

- Women need genuine alternatives and options, or they will turn to unlicensed providers or freebirth
- Safe care will require maternity care providers to collaborate and put mothers and babies above professional turf wars and profit
- Coercion will not work and using fear and misinformation to make women do what the system prefers only leads to distrust and disengagement
- Recognise women have the right to determine what happens to their bodies and respect this, no matter how difficult

Nick

- We need to set research priorities that integrate the perspectives and experiences of women, midwives and doctors
- We need upstream conversations that help us more thoughtfully determine which risks we present to women and how we do that
- Stop using risk as a tool of power and have rights-based conversations with women too
- We need to meet women where they're at and have more midwives of colour and other ethnic diversities there to support women with their cultural needs as well as their physical needs

Tamara and Svetlana

- We still have a lot to do to bring the midwifery profession to life! We need contemporary standards of practice and better education for midwives
- We need to develop a strong professional body so midwives can advocate at government level
- We want to be available to serve every woman anywhere in our big country
- It's time for us to unite with midwives and other professionals who are looking for another way to practise that focuses on the interests of women and babies and makes us develop, learn new things, grow and improve, be able to make decisions and be responsible and accountable for the results of our work

Note

1 Bait-and-switch is a common but unlawful business practice of advertising or making representations that are fraudulent to entice consumers to purchase a good or service. It is especially prevalent in industries where consumers are not able to assess the quality of the good or service they are acquiring prior to consumption, such as the provision of maternity healthcare services. The 'bait' is the promise or representation that a particular service (such as skin-to-skin or waterbirth) will be offered. The 'switch' occurs when the woman arrives in hospital only to discover that the advertised services are either not offered or not available, and she is pressured to consider unwanted or unacceptable alternatives.

References

Baji, P., Rubashkin, N., Szebik, I., Stoll, K., & Vedam, S. (2017). Informal cash payments for birth in Hungary: Are women paying to secure a known provider, respect, or quality of care? *Social Science and Medicine, 189*, 86–95.

Bonzon, M., Gross, M. M., Karch, A., & Grylka-Baeschlin, S. (2017). Deciding on the mode of birth after a previous caesarean section – An online survey investigating women's preferences in Western Switzerland. *Midwifery, 50*, 219–227. doi: 10.1016/j.midw.2017.04.005.

Darling, E. P. (2013) Vaginal birth after cesarean section: Outcomes of women receiving midwifery care in Ontario. *Canadian Journal of Midwifery Research and Practice – Revue Canadienne de la Recherche et de la Pratique Sage-femme, 10*(1), 9–19. Retrieved from: http://ojs.library.ubc.ca/index.php/cjmrp/article/view/184065.

Đelmiš, J., Juras, J., & Rodin, U. (2018). Perinatalni Mortalitet u Republici Hrvatskoj u 2017. godini [Perinatal deaths in Croatia in 2017]. *Ginecologia et perinatologia, 17*, 1–33.

Devarajan, S., Talaulikar, V. S., & Arulkumaran, S. (2018). Vaginal birth after caesarean. *Obstetrics, Gynaecology and Reproductive Medicine, 28*, 110–115.

Dweik, D., Girasek, E., Toreki, A., Meszaros, G. & Pal, A. (2014). Women's antenatal preferences for delivery route in a setting with high cesarean section rates and a medically dominated maternity system. *Acta Obstetrica et Gynecologica Scandinavica, 93*, 408–415.

ECHR. (2010). *Ternovszky v. Hungary*. 67545/09. Strasbourg: ECHR.

Fraser, G. J. (1998). *African American midwifery in the South: Dialogues of birth, race, and memory*. Cambridge, MA: Harvard University Press.

Hill, A. (2010). Hungary: Midwife Agnes Gereb taken to court for championing home births. Gynaecologist faces five years in Hungarian prison, prompting protests over authorities' hardline childbirth policy. *The Guardian*.

Janevic, T., Sripad, P., Bradley, E., & Dimitrievska, V. (2011). 'There's no kind of respect here'. A qualitative study of racism and access to maternal health care among Romani women in the Balkans. *International Journal for Equity in Health, 10*, 53.

Kukla, R., Kuppermann, M., Little, M., Lyerly, A. D., Mitchell, L. M., Armstrong, E. M., & Harris, L. (2009). Finding autonomy in birth. *Bioethics, 23*, 1–8.

Kukura, E. (2010). Choice in birth: Preserving access to VBAC. *Penn State Law Review, 114*, 955–1001.

Lundgren, I., Begley, C., Gross, M. M., & Bondas, T. (2012). 'Groping through the fog': a metasynthesis of women's experiences on VBAC. *BMC Pregnancy and Childbirth, 12*, 85.

Mclemore, M. R. (2018). What blame-the-mother stories get wrong about birth outcomes among black moms. *Children's Health Matters.* Online: Center for Health Journalism.

Mclemore, M. & Warner Hand, Z. (2017). Making the case for innovative reentry employment programs: previously incarcerated women as birth doulas – A case study. *International Journal of Prisoner Health, 13*, 219–227.

Michaels, P. (2014). *Lamaze: An international history*, Oxford: Oxford University Press.

Miteniece, E., Pavlova, M., Rechel, B., Rezeberga, D., Murauskiene, L., & Groot, W. (2019). Barriers to accessing adequate maternal care in Latvia: A mixed-method study among women, providers and decision-makers. *Health Policy, 123*, 87–95.

MLA. Boston Women's Health Book Collective. (2011). *Our bodies, ourselves.* New York, NY: Simon & Schuster.

Rich, M. (2016). The curse of the civilised woman: Race, gender and the pain of childbirth in nineteenth-century American medicine. *Gender & History, 28*, 57–76.

Roda. (2015). Human Rights in Childbirth Eastern Europe Conference. In: Ateva, E. (Ed.), *Human Rights in Childbirth Eastern Europe Conference*. April 2015, Zagreb, Croatia.

Roda – Parents in Action. (2016). Majčinstvo i žene s invaliditetom [Motherhood experiences of women with disabilities]. [Online.] Zagreb: Roda – Parents in Action. Retrieved from: www.roda.hr/media/attachments/udruga/projekti/ppzird/Majc%CC%8Cinstvo_i_z%CC%8Cene_s_invaliditetom.pdf [accessed 6 April 2019].

Rodin, U., Draušnik, Ž., Cerovečki, I., & Jezdić, D. (2018). Porodi u zdravstvenim ustanovama u Hrvatskoj 2017. godine [Childbirths in healthcare institutions in Croatia in 2017]. Retrieved from: www.hzjz.hr/wp-content/uploads/2018/07/Porodi_2017.pdf.

Rowe, R., Li, Y., Brocklehurst, P., & Hollowell, J. (2016). Maternal and perinatal outcomes in women planning vaginal birth after caesarean (VBAC) at home in England: Secondary analysis of the Birthplace national prospective cohort study. *British Journal of Obstetrics and Gynaecology, 123*, 1123–1132.

Rubashkin, N., Szebik, I., Baji, P., Szanto, Z., Susanszky, E., & Vedam, S. (2017). Assessing quality of maternity care in Hungary: Expert validation and testing of the mother-centered prenatal care (MCPC) survey instrument. *Reproductive Health, 14*, 152.

Rubashkin, N., Warnock, R., & Diamond-Smith, N. (2018). A systematic review of person-centered care interventions to improve quality of facility-based delivery. *Reproductive Health, 15*, 169.

Sandelowski, M. (1984). *Pain, pleasure, and American childbirth: From the twilight sleep to the Read method, 1914–1960.* Wesport, CT: Greenwood Press.

Womenlobby.org. (2016). Croatia: Women's rights under threat. [Online.] Retrieved from: www.womenlobby.org/Women-s-rights-in-Croatia-under-the-threat-after-parliamentary-elections-in [accessed 27 June 2019].

11 The modern-day witch hunt

Hannah Dahlen and Jo Hunter

> By day I am a highly respected professor. By night I assume the shadowy form of the 'other', of the dark revolutionary. I have become a modern day witch. My pyre is not made of wood and flame but of shame and blame which blisters the soul just the same.
>
> (Hannah Dahlen, 2019)

About the authors

My (Jo Hunter) journey to becoming a midwife began as a consumer who was considered by the medical model to have risk factors. My informed choice to give birth at home was supported by my midwife, and I went on to have three beautiful, straightforward homebirths. My interest in the topic of midwife persecution started in 1998 after the homebirth of my second child. My midwife, Maggie Lecky-Thompson, had been reported to the regulatory body and subjected to a lengthy and very public investigation which ultimately led to her deregistration as a midwife. As the past Convenor of Homebirth Australia, I heard from many midwives across Australia seeking support after being reported to the regulatory body. Soon after becoming a midwife, I supported several midwifery colleagues through investigations, some which seemed absurd at best and vexatious at worst. In my fourth year of private practice, I myself was reported to the Australian Health Practitioner Regulation Agency (AHPRA) by personnel at the hospital to which I transferred my client. I had restrictions placed, with immediate effect, on my registration while a long, drawn out investigation was conducted. After almost a year of investigations, the conditions were removed and AHPRA advised that it was satisfied that I was a competent midwife. During this investigation, ambulance officers made false allegations about my resuscitation practice in relation to a baby born at home. When it was later realised that my practice and their interactions with me had been recorded, the ambulance service apologised for their false statements.

I (Hannah Dahlen) told my story earlier in this book. I was Jo's principle supervisor for her Honours thesis, which explored the experiences of private midwives who are being reported to AHPRA in Australia. I also work as a private midwife in Sydney supporting women who mostly give birth at home. So, by day I am the highly respected Professor Dahlen, but by night, I have discovered just how darkly my activities are viewed by the system.

Introduction

There is a rise in the reporting of private midwives who attend homebirths around the world. Their stories appear in newspaper articles and now also in peer-reviewed research. While laws in most countries protect women's rights to give birth where they choose and to have the provider of their choice, the harsh reality is that there is much that gets in the way of women's rights to self-determination. While authorities may not be able to compel women to avoid a homebirth, in most cases they can easily target their midwives, and by doing this, cut off a lifeline to the women, which has the same effect as dissuading them from their choices. We call this out for what it is: a modern-day witch hunt.

The history of witch hunts from the Middle Ages to today

In the 1400s, witch hunters Kramer and Sprenger wrote that no one does more harm to the Catholic Church than midwives (Ehrenreich & English, 2010). While historians continue to debate the extent to which the witch hunts of the Middle Ages targeted midwives (Purkiss, 1996), there is no doubt that midwives were caught up in the hysteria of that time. Midwives were deeply trusted and embedded in the community as the holder of secrets, facilitator of abortions and contraception, and discreet manager of adoption services for babies born out of wedlock. The midwife posed a significant threat to the puritanical and patriarchal control that the church wanted to assert, through the lens of morality, over women's bodies. Ehrenreich and English (2010) also argue that the witch presented a triple threat to the church: (a) she was a woman and unashamedly so; (b) she was part of an organised underground of peasant women; and (c) she was a healer whose practice was based in empirical study. In the face of the repressive fatalism of the church, she held out hope of change and progress in the world.

We see echoes of this perceived 'triple threat' today, in the way that midwives who attend homebirths are targeted. Most if not all of these midwives are women who loudly and unashamedly declare themselves feminists. The organised underground of peasant women has been replaced with the political activism and social media/social groups midwives engage in. The care that midwives provide at homebirths is being increasingly shown by research to be optimal in contrast to the highly medicalised mainstream options. Midwives often represent hope to women who struggle in the face of the repressive fatalism of the medicalised model which tells them that their bodies are flawed or dangerous to their babies. For these women, having a midwife means that they are capable of birthing their babies and birth trauma need not be their reality.

Recently, Federici (2018) argued that the witch hunts of the Middle Ages were about more than the persecution of midwives. They represented the birth of the medical profession, the development of the mechanical view of the word and the triumph of the patriarchal state structure, but they also stood at the crossroads of a cluster of social processes that paved the way for the rise of the modern capitalist world (Federici, 2018). Federici said that women stood in the way of a developing capitalist system that needed a massive workforce. To achieve this, women needed to be confined to reproduction and unpaid domestic labour. To achieve this, the patriarchal systems of the day subordinated women to men and punished those who refused to comply. As Federici (2018) points out, violence against women became normalised in the subsequent years with increased incarceration of women in mental hospitals, and through forced sterilisation and lobotomy practices. Federici (2018) argues that the witch hunts are far from over but are today disguised in other forms, such as through an escalation of violence against women (femicide), which has seen an unprecedented increased in recent years and is becoming more public and brutal, many taking on forms often witnessed in war time. The witch camps in the north of Ghana and killing of the women in Tanzania for allegedly being 'possessed' if they have red eyes (a hazard that comes with cooking over open fires), along with dowry murders, rapes and the jailing of women activists are all a feature of a woman's life today, not some far distant past (Federici, 2018). It is most likely that a witch was never anything more than a feature of fairy tales, yet this image of the pointy-hat-wearing witch, and that of women roped to, and burnt at, stakes, can prevent us from seeing the perpetuating witch hunt against women who stand up, stand out and actively reject the patriarchy. The midwife who supports women to give birth at home and who often earns a private income from this is one such person. She stands up, she stands out and she challenges deeply held beliefs that women are inherently flawed when it comes to pregnancy, birth and mothering, promoted by institutions and individuals with significant monetary investment. Federici (2018) goes on to describe how witch hunts target women by exaggerating alleged crimes to mythical proportions, terrorising society with highly publicised punishments, isolating victims, discouraging resistance and making masses of people afraid to engage in practices that until then were considered normal. The witch was both the 'socialist' and terrorist of her time. The witch was and is the midwife, yesterday, today and most likely tomorrow too.

So what form does this modern-day witch hunt take and what effect does it have on the women who are targeted?

The trials of Hanna Porn in the 1800s

Eugene Declerq (1994) wrote about the trials of midwife Hanna Porn in the 1800s in Massachusetts, USA. Porn served a primarily Finnish-Swedish clientele – wives of labourers – and she had excellent outcomes. Her neonatal mortality rate was less than half that of local physicians and she repeatedly defied court orders to stop practising. Her case was part of a wider agenda to abolish midwifery in the USA which, in reality, has been fairly successful until recent times. After her tenth trial in four years, the judge sentenced the 48-year-old midwife to three months in the house of corrections. Her crime was simply that she continued to practise when the court had ruled that midwifery was illegal in Massachusetts (Declercq, 1994). As you will have read in Chapter 1, this is still the case in several US states. The judge referred to Porn as an 'irregular practitioner'. This, ironically, is fitting and something many midwives would consider a compliment today; however, Declercq (1994) writes that Massachusetts became the centre of the campaign to eliminate midwifery as a profession. Many factors came together to enable this eradication of one of the oldest professions on earth. These factors included: (a) the increasing legitimacy of the medical profession, which involved self-promotion; (b) the deprecation of midwives as dirty and dangerous and the redefining of birth as dangerous; and (c) the availability of Twilight Sleep offering a panacea to the pain of labour and birth (Donnison, 1988; Declercq, 1994; Ehrenreich & English, 2010). Many midwives were prosecuted and fined, but it was Porn alone who persisted in her practice.

Many other cases (court or regulatory) against lay midwives in the USA and registered midwives in countries such as Australia and the UK continue today, and we shall explore some of these shortly. Many are instigated by doctors or hospital care-providers, such as administrators (and even other midwives), but very rarely are they instigated by the women cared for by these practitioners. For example, in a study we undertook in Australia interviewing in-depth eight privately practising midwives (PPMs) who attended birth at home, none had been reported by the women they cared for (Hunter, 2018).

Porn fought the charges repeatedly, signed her own name to birth certificates as a midwife and remained a popular, busy practitioner. When she was finally jailed, the four doctors who gave evidence against her increased their patient intake (in number of births) by 86% in the following two years. Porn was tried before an all-male jury and convicted for her 'persistent determination to carry on the work'. She continued practice, even after being released from jail, but underground and in a much diminished way, no longer posing a threat to doctor's incomes. Within four years of release, she died. There are sad parallels to the 2019 case of Irish midwife Philomena Canning, which is discussed later in this chapter. To add to the tragedy and poignancy of the story, it appears that Porn died attending a birth, doing what she loved (Declercq, 1994) and in some ways remained unwilling to be beaten by the system that hunted her down. The public example made of Porn likely hastened her own death, but also had the required effect of making midwives fearful and helping to hasten the demise of the profession. The rest, as they say, is history (or herstory), as midwives in the USA continue to fight, to this day, for their right to practice in many states (see Chapter 1).

The modern-day witch hunt

In this next section, we share the stories of four midwives from four countries, to illustrate the witch hunt is alive and well. Although today it may not involve burning upon a pyre, there are other painful and traumatic ways that careers are destroyed and lives deeply affected. In 1995, Marsden Wagner wrote an article on the global witch hunt (Wagner, 1995). He talked about the investigation of health professionals in many countries accusing them of dangerous maternity practices to maintain control over maternity services. The key issues, he said, underlying each case were money, power, gender and choice. Of the 20 cases Wagner was involved in, 70% concerned midwives, 85% were women and the unifying feature of all the cases was that at least some of their practice was considered not mainstream ('irregular'). Wagner insists that the evaluation of professional behaviour must be based on deviations from practice based on scientific evidence rather than on deviations from peer or medical controlled opinions of what constitutes good practice (Wagner, 1995), especially when these peers are not always evidence-based in their practice.

One would have thought, over the past 25 years, we would see a resolution of this issue, but sadly, what I step you through next will show the opposite. I (Hannah) have written previously about homebirth being 'fear's Petri dish' (Dahlen, 2011). Homebirth is loved because it supports women's agency and physiology, midwifery autonomy, trust in birth, and the absence of the obstetric gaze; the very elements that some of our obstetric colleagues find incredibly threatening. We show below just how effectively that fear can be used to undermine midwives.

Norway

Cathrine Trulsvik was recently banned *for life* from attending homebirths; her punishment for deviating from policies restricting women's choices in childbirth. In her cosy little house on a cold December day in 2018, over a plate of freshly baked cinnamon rolls made by her daughter Ingrid, this strong, humble Norwegian mother and midwife told me (Hannah) her story. Below is an adaption of a Facebook post about Trulsvik.

Trulsvik's professional licence was restricted by a 'limited authorisation', which means she can no longer attend homebirths as a midwife. The limitation on her licence and scope of practice was imposed when she supported women who chose to remain at home as against the Norwegian national guidelines for transfer to hospital. The guidelines are not based on evidence, but on prevailing medical opinion. They also violate a woman's human right to bodily autonomy; that is, the right to decide whether to transfer to hospital or receive medical treatment. Two births were reported to health authorities – not by the women or their families, but by personnel at the receiving hospital. The Norwegian Board of Authorization decided to limit Tulsvik's authorisation to practice, a decision later upheld by the Norwegian Health Authority, which claimed that 'the midwife should have *persuaded the patient* to transfer to hospital'. The two cases are described below.

Case 1

In this case, despite a great outcome, the hospital reported Trulsvik for breaching Norwegian guidelines, which assert that women must be transferred to hospital if labour isn't progressing according to Friedman's curve (four-hour action line partogram). The woman, in her first pregnancy, was having a prolonged early labour lasting three days with irregular contractions and intermittent long breaks (a few hours at a time), during which time she slept, ate and recuperated. The woman was happy with the pace of, and the breaks during, her labour. The baby moved well with a normal heart beat detected and documented according to protocol. On the third day of labour, her membranes broke with clear liquor noted and she was dilated to 9 cm. An hour later, although she was fully dilated, the head was not yet on the pelvic floor and she did not have the urge to push. Baby was fine with movements and a good heartbeat. Her labour paused again, so she ate a little and slept for a few hours. When she awoke and still didn't have an urge to push, she agreed to transfer to the hospital (which was just 450 m away) that same evening. An oxytocin drip was initiated and, after 45 min, the woman gave birth to a girl with Apgars of 9 and 10. She had no postpartum bleeding or perineal tears. The parents are happy with the birth. Trulsvik was nevertheless reported.

Case 2

In this case, despite a great outcome, the hospital reported Trulsvik for supporting a woman beyond the guidelines, which say that 11 days over the due date is the limit. The woman the subject of the complaint was 12 days past her due date. At 40+5 weeks, the woman and baby were checked at the hospital on Trulsvik's request. The woman reported being poorly treated at this visit, saying the treating doctor tried to scare her by saying 'she was not fit to give birth at home because her first child (11 years ago) was delivered by vacuum extraction'. When the woman attended at 12 days past her due date for a check-up, she was told that she was 'not allowed' to go home. As the ultrasound on the same day showed all was well, the woman objected. Nevertheless, hospital staff reportedly continued to threaten her with statements about how dangerous her actions were for her baby. She reluctantly conceded, under pressure, to the insertion of a Foley's catheter to induce labour and was only then 'allowed' to go home. After an hour, her contractions started and she asked Trulsvik to attend her. Trulsvik arrived immediately with another colleague and, an hour later, her baby was born in perfect condition in water. In her joy at meeting her baby, the mother inadvertently pulled the cord too hard so it broke off before the placenta was born.

When the placenta did not come within a few minutes, Trulsvik called an ambulance, although there was no bleeding or urgency. Norwegian guidelines say health providers can wait for up to an hour for the placenta to come before needing transfer. The woman was given a syntocinon injection as per protocol, and she uneventfully birthed her placenta on arrival at the hospital 30 minutes later. There was no extra bleeding (maybe 500 ml all together). The parents reported a hostile mood in the room as they discussed their choice of homebirth and Trulsvik's role in supporting them. The parents were happy with their choice and disappointed in hospital staff behaviour. The hospital nevertheless reported her.

Trulsvik was one of the handful of Norwegian midwives that support approximately 200 babies born at home in Norway each year. She has engaged a law firm to assess the Norwegian guidelines, to determine the possibility of auditing the guidelines with greater focus on human rights in childbirth and professional autonomy when it comes to supporting women.

The United States of America

Elizabeth Catlin, New York, was arrested and charged in November 2018 for practising midwifery without a licence while serving the reclusive Mennonite community of greater New York. The State of New York requires midwives to be Certified Nurse Midwives (CNM) or Certified Midwives (CM) and Catlin is a Certified Professional Midwife (CPM) (see discussion in Chapter 1). This makes it difficult for women to have homebirths, with just three non-hospital birthing centres and few licenced midwives practising in New York City. Catlin can practise in some other US States where CPMs are permitted, but not in the state of New York. Catlin's arrest and prosecution animated the normally quiet Mennonite community to attend the court hearing and raise money to support her defence. A Mennonite elder called the prosecution a 'humanitarian crisis' (Gastaldo, 2019).

Catlin's story, which was covered by the *New York Times* in March 2019 (Pager, 2019), bears an eerie resemblance to the story of Hanna Porn 200 years ago. If convicted, she faces up to seven years imprisonment. In her defence, Catlin asserted that her service was only restricted by the fact that New York did not recognise her midwifery certification. She pleaded not guilty to all the charges.

The *New York Times* report also interviewed over a dozen of the women that Catlin had cared for over two decades and none had complaints about her. 'The care that she gave was like a mother. She knew exactly how you felt', said Kaylene Hoover cited in (Pager, 2019). Catlin was devastated by the prosecution. 'My life has ground to a halt', she said 'My passion has been taken away' (cited in Pager, 2019).

Ireland

I (Hannah) have never met Irish midwife Philomena Canning who, at one time, worked as a private midwife in Australia. In early 2019, I viewed a heartbreaking video that she made from her hospital bed as she lay dying with ovarian cancer. In that video, Canning pleaded with the National Office of Nursing and Midwifery of the Health Services Executive (HSE) to cease an unsubstantiated investigation, cover her legal fees and clear her name so she could die in peace. Canning died shortly after that video.

Canning's case is an example of how the state can unduly extend midwifery investigations, without substance, in order to place unnecessary financial and emotional pressure on a practitioner that is considered 'irregular'. Canning's only crime, through a five-year investigation, appeared to be her plans to open a birth centre in Ireland. In 2014, the HSE suspended Canning from practising as an independent midwife, revoked her indemnity insurance and ordered her to hand over all her records. At the time, Canning had 29 women on her books, some just weeks away from giving birth. Jo Murphy-Lawless writes:

> This was no mistake as we first thought, but turned out to be a sophisticated and ruthless hunting down of a midwife with an impeccable record of care by a group of midwife administrators in the state's HSE, the operational arm of the public health services. It was initiated, we have always believed, in fear and panic on their part that Philomena's long-hoped for plans for an independent birthing centre with fully independent insurance were nearing fruition.
>
> (Murphy-Lawless, 2019)

There are limited options for midwifery-led care in Ireland, where only a handful of private midwives attend homebirths. The State covers insurance for independent midwives provided they agree to a set of protocols which severely restrict the women they can take for homebirth. Canning was prosecuted following two normal births at home with minor complications. Neither of the women complained. Canning, the women in her care and midwives supported her, but she lost her case even though an expert hired by the HSE said that Canning's care was without reproach. In 2015, without warning, all charges were dropped and Canning's appeal costs paid in full by the HSE. Shortly after, however, the HSE commenced a 'systems analysis' of the two cases that were previously investigated. Canning was informed that, until the investigation was concluded, her name could not be cleared and she could not return to practice. Canning sold her home to pay her legal fees in what developed into a long and torturous process for almost five years

(Murphy-Lawless, 2019). As she lay dying, Canning made a public plea: she asked for her lawyers to be paid, the 'systems analysis' dropped and her good name restored so she could die in peace. After the video was published, Canning reached a settlement with the HSE. On 3 March 2019 she issued a statement on Facebook, which ended with a message for pregnant women:

> Finally, I want to say to every pregnant woman out there, and every woman who wishes to be: you have within you the great gift of creation. Therein lies enormous power and potential. Aeons of time and tides have pushed against your centre of power – sometimes gently, sometimes not. Only woman can have dominion over birth, yet she is made to battle continuously to guard her territory, or to gain access to it. Every woman has the right to be supported by her healthcare providers in the birth of her choosing – just as she has the best interests of her baby at heart. Your inner compass will show you the way. Look to it. Listen to your intuition. Sit in the centre of your courage: fear may be part of the journey but courage will overcome it every time. And please listen to my words. You were born to do this. You were born to do this.
>
> (Philomena Canning, 2019)

Twenty days after publishing this statement, Canning's battle with the authorities and ovarian cancer was over (Gleeson & Holland, 2019).

For the women of Ireland and their midwives, the battle over their bodies goes on.

Australia

In October 2018, a picture circulated in social media of a proud mother sitting in her bath at home holding her surprise twins in her arms. The post on Facebook had 15,000 likes and 1700 comments. According to the mother, Brooke King, she had declined ultrasounds so neither she nor her midwife knew she was expecting twins (Lever, 2018). In addition, as King was still breastfeeding when she became pregnant (and so was not regularly menstruating), neither she nor her midwife were able to estimate her date of conception. With her belly growing a good size, neither she nor her midwife thought that there was anything out of the ordinary. The twins were born early, at 35 weeks, and transferred to hospital, after one began experiencing respiratory difficulties (not unusual for twin babies).

King's happiness was short-lived. Her midwife, Martina Görner, was reported to AHPRA and immediately suspended from practice. Investigators attended her practice in Melbourne, without notice, to remove files, computers and mobile phones. After three months of delay, during which time Görner was the subject of significant online attacks and biased newspaper reporting, she was notified that AHPRA was reopening nine previously closed notifications against her, no doubt to conduct a 'systems analysis' not unlike what Canning faced in Ireland. None of these notifications were initiated by her clients and one was obviously personally motivated. In frustration, Görner handed in her registration shortly after.

In the aftermath, Brooke King had a lot to say about the treatment of her midwives, which we have summarised below (King, 2019):

> My darling surprise twins came into this world in such a hurry, with just 1 hour of active labour and birthed gracefully into our bath at home. We expected a placenta and instead were blessed with a twin. Both midwives were suspended, controversy was ignited and their story circulated all over the world, with over 1.5 million views, comments and likes.
>
> So why was their birth such a big deal? Because it shocked people. Because it highlighted the underlying birthing culture we have all unknowingly become a part of. A culture that has led us to believe that a natural and instinctual approach to birth is not safe, desirable or achievable. A culture that has unknowingly taken a stronghold over our beliefs and ingrained in us a subconscious fear around our ability to carry and birth our babies. Now we simply enter 'the system'. Get pregnant, get your schedule, get told where to be, at what time, who is going to touch you, poke you, scan you, and tell you if your baby is 'normal'. And we don't question it because we are led to believe that it is all very necessary … rather than being told the truth, which is that it is all optional, and each mother should evaluate and individually select the right care options for her and her baby. The system has taken away the single most important question that every expecting mother should be asking herself … 'how do I want to carry and birth my baby?' What specific tests, scans and advisors will make ME personally feel safe and empowered and using each of her choices accordingly.
>
> We may be excelling in the technology department but we are failing in our humanness. There is no greater time in a mother's or baby's life that they need personalised, connected, loving human care than at birth. At a time when they have never felt so vulnerable, raw and instinctual mothers need to feel heard, they need to feel safe and they need to feel in control of their birthing space. Mothers have the right to accept and decline care according to their individual circumstances and they should be encouraged to use their instincts for what their body and baby needs.
>
> The twins' birth was controversial because it was a clear reminder of what pregnancy and birthing can be when we go back to basics. It was proof that not all pregnancies and births need the one-size-fits-all approach that we are offered. For some women being within a hospital environment makes them feel safe, and they are able to relax and achieve the birth they deserve and desire, and for that we are all grateful … but what about the women that need a different type of care to achieve the birth that they deserve and desire?

These are the women that we find seeking alternative birthing options such as birthing houses, home births and free birth. These mothers have very different needs in order to have a successful birth and to feel safe in their birthing space. These mothers need to feel heard; they need to feel in control, and they need to do things in a way that feels right for them. Unfortunately, though these mothers birthing options are slowly being removed, the AHPRA policies are becoming too tight and too regimented for private midwives to truly fulfil these mothers birthing rights. Take for example my midwife Martina, she did nothing but accept mine and my husband's informed pregnancy and birthing choices, which is our right, but for that she has lost everything. She had to close her business, lay off her staff, move from her home and spend over $40,000 on legal advice. Yet 6 months later, has not been proven guilty of anything and is still unable to work. And 6 months later AHPRA has still not spoken to my husband and I for our account on the events. This is not right and sadly her situation is not unique.

We should be empowering and equipping private midwives to successfully help mother's birth at home but instead the private system is being cracked down on and carers are being reprimanded for doing nothing but supporting birthing women rights. There can't be a one-size-fits-all policy for midwives when their patient's needs, and birthing rights, are so vast. And it is completely unethical to take their licence away for supporting a women's birth rights. If we don't get this right, we will see an increase in fearful midwives refusing birthing women care, and in turn these mothers will have no one to care for them and will choose to freebirth. This does not sound like a desirable outcome.

So where does this leave future birthing mothers?

(King, 2019)

The experiences of privately practising midwives who have been reported to the regulator in Australia

Moving into private practice can be confronting, as I (Hannah) experienced a shift from being celebrated as a midwife and academic (even recently receiving an Australian Medal from the Queen), to being viewed with suspicion and hostility. I saw it in the eyes of former colleagues and in the attitudes of staff when I transferred women to hospital or had to consult with them.

In Australia, the majority of homebirths are attended by PPMs, with the remaining supported at one of the 14 publicly funded homebirth programmes (Catling-Paull, Coddington, Foureur, & Homer, 2013). Hannah and Jo are among this small number of PPMs (around 250 dotted around the country) who attend women at home in a private capacity. Jo has been reported to AHPRA, and Hannah continues to practise with the Sword of Damocles' hanging over her head.

The small number of PPMs that are registered for practice is not commensurate with the level of regulation and practice scrutiny to which they as a profession are, and have been, subjected over the past decade. It is fundamental to the philosophy of private midwifery practice to support individual women who take responsibility for their pregnancy and birth. On occasions, this means supporting the informed choices of clients who choose care that falls outside professional guidelines. This puts PPMs in a vulnerable professional position, and may be contributing to the significant number of PPMs reported to AHPRA. We estimate, from conversations and social media reports, that over half the PPMs in Australia have been reported to AHPRA and some reported numerous times.

Homebirth midwives are 'doubly tainted'

PPMs endure a stigmatisation that other maternity care professionals do not experience. In the sentinel work on stigma, Goffman defines it as 'an attribute that is deeply discrediting with a particular social interaction' (Goffman, 1963, p. 3). Work which is both physically disgusting and/or contrary to our moral perceptions will be viewed as stigmatised (Hughes, 1971). Monteblanco (2017) describes this as out of hospital midwives being 'doubly tainted': they work in close proximity to women's genitals and their work is seen as morally questionable as they are perceived to be putting mothers and babies in jeopardy by providing care outside of the hospital. Hospitals (despite evidence to the contrary) are framed in modern discourse as clean places where care providers can distance themselves from contamination and the genitals of women by using sterile instruments and equipment. Mainstream maternity care providers are perceived as not coming in direct contact with women's body parts or operating in conditions considered physically unclean settings (the home). In comparison, the homebirth midwife is seen as undertaking 'dirty', dangerous work (Monteblanco, 2017) by supporting what many, despite the evidence, believe puts the baby's life in danger. Ironically, a paper has been published recently showing babies born at home have a healthier microbiome than those born in hospital (Combellick et al., 2018).

In addition, there is a moral attitude that rightly pervades in society that children should be preserved as most precious. In the 1980s, the president of the American College of Obstetricians and Gynecologists (ACOG) described homebirth as a form of child abuse (De Vries, 1996), thus perpetrating the historically disparaging view that the midwives attending homebirths are child abusers.

The history of midwives, as we briefly discussed above, is one of being constantly challenged and threatened with extinction. Legal processes have, and still are, been used to try to control the practice of midwives, especially those who dare to challenge mainstream care and assumptions of safety. In the following section we briefly demonstrate this through Jo's study into the reporting of PPMs in Australia.

The reporting of PPMs in Australia

In recent years in Australia, PPMs have been increasingly reported to AHPRA, mostly by other health professionals, as the stories above illustrate. The aim of my (Jo's) research for my Honours was to explore the experiences of PPMs in Australia who have been reported to the AHPRA. In-depth interviews with eight Australian PPMs were undertaken and analysed using thematic analysis. This was the first study to explore this issue in depth in Australia. We found that the reports to AHPRA occurred when midwives supported women who chose care that was considered outside the recommended Australian College of Midwives Consultation and Referral Guidelines (2014). As other chapters have discussed the evidence for the safety of homebirth, we will not revisit this here.

PPMs who attend homebirths are a marginalised, minority group in the dominant medicalised culture of birth in Australia (Wagner, 1995; Edwards, 2008; Edwards et al., 2011). PPMs still do not have access to insurance for homebirth, nor is homebirth funded or rebated as are other aspects of maternity care. Many PPMs lack access to public hospitals and find it impossible to obtain visiting rights, despite health policy directives for this provision (NSW Government, 2015).

In Australia, the views of the medical establishment impact the regulation of PPMs. In 2009, the Australian Medical Association advocated very strongly for written collaborative agreements with a medical practitioner to be mandated as part of the Government's reforms (Commonwealth of Australia, 2009), while PPMs are required to collaborate with doctors (Nursing and Midwifery Board of Australia, 2017). It is not mandatory for doctors to reciprocate. In fact, doctors do not have to collaborate at all if they do not wish to. This places midwives in a position of being subordinate to, and dependent on, obstetricians to be able to practice.

PPMs are mostly judged by nurses, midwives and consumers who have never worked or given birth within the private midwifery model of care and therefore do not understand the intricacies of private midwifery practice. They also will have never attended a birth at home. The regulators expect PPMs to practise in the same way that midwives within the system do, but without the immediate support, equipment, facilities and assistance available to midwives who work in the system. PPMs are expected to adhere to the standards of a system that does not employ them and that largely shuns their work.

It is in this environment that PPMs, the vast majority of whom are women, practice.

'Caught between women and the system'

An overarching theme that emerged from my (Jo's) study was 'caught between women and the system', and it described the participants' feelings of working as a PPM in Australia. The data analysis revealed six themes and several subthemes: (a) the suppression of midwifery; (b) a flawed system; (c) lack of support; (d) devastation on so many levels; (e) making changes in the aftermath; and (f) walking a tightrope forever.

Some of the findings of the study are briefly outlined below.

The suppression of midwifery

Many of the PPMs we interviewed felt that private midwifery practice only existed with permission of the medical establishment, with medicine dominating and holding power over maternity care and midwifery. One PPM commented that she overheard the doctor who reported her say words to the effect of, 'You get rid of the midwives and then the women have to come to the hospital' (M3). Another PPM, who transferred a woman from home to hospital and was supporting her client's right to decline treatment said, 'The doctor reported me for being "obstructionist" and interfering with what they wanted to do'. Several of the PPMs felt that mainstream care providers believed PPMs practise dangerously, with one midwife stating, 'They think we're all cowboys'.

Many PPMs in this study described their experience of being reported and investigated as 'a witch hunt':

> It just feels like such an injustice. Because that's how it feels, like I'm just being burnt from the bottom up for doing everything that I believe in and everything that means anything to me.

Participants shared how it felt to go through an investigation and assumed guilty until proven innocent:

> You're caught up in the whole system and off you go with, you know, hours and hours of your life, writing reports and photocopying your notes and sending them in and for someone to then go, oh, there's nothing to answer to, like Captain fucken obvious. Really? There's nothing to answer to?

A flawed system

All the PPMs described the system as flawed, with some describing the investigation process as impersonal, 'I had no face to face contact. Didn't speak to anyone on the phone. Didn't attend anything'. Other PPMs said the process took a really long time:

> I know one of them took four years, after the four years, that's when I got the conditions put on my registration … I felt like I was just left to worry. I just don't understand why investigations need to take so long.

There was a lack of communication from AHPRA representatives and the process was intimidating: 'AHPRA turned up on my doorstep … the letter in their hand, hand delivering it, with the taxi out the front, running'. Several PPMs said, as Brooke King did (above), that investigators did not involve the women whose care was at the centre of the complaints.

> Do they ever talk to the women? … If they talk to any of my clients or read my notes, they'd see … she made me read this and made me sign that … that's what we do. Give them all the risks and all the options.

When eventually cleared of charges or complaint, PPMs said that they did not receive an apology or feedback: 'All I got was a letter, they didn't even say sorry for the last two years'.

Midwives also talked about the fact that complaints were anonymous and how unjust this is given the lack of accountability:

> I suspect who it is, but no. It was anonymous. It was a big brave person who didn't sign their name to it … I was just so angry that they should even be addressing an anonymous report.
>
> Investigate the people who are making the report in the first place … it just seems ridiculous to me that any Joe Blow could make a report about somebody and take somebody's life through such hell and trauma and not even be accountable to put their name to it.

Lack of support

Seven of eight of the participants said they felt unsupported through the process of investigation, whether professionally, practically or emotionally. The majority found 'most of the support in colleagues and others who've been there', but also felt a distinct lack of support from professional organisations.

PPMs described the enormous amount of paperwork involved in an investigation and the short time frame given to respond:

> I had to get together everything from university transcripts to all the professional development I'd done since [I'd become a midwife]. It was a large volume of work … the actual process I had issues with, they wanted a lot of information in a very short period of time.

PPMs suggested that legislation should include a duty of care whereby midwives have a moral and legal obligation to ensure the safety and well-being of the women and babies in their care. Therefore, if the woman declines recommended guidelines, the midwife must continue to support that woman and her family without the risk of being reported and losing her registration for doing so:

> They could do something that puts in place that we have a duty of care to the women so this shit doesn't happen to start with. That if this woman wants to have her baby at home then that's okay, and that we can come in and do an appropriate transfer and we're not strung up for it.

Seven of the PPMs suggested the need for 'an in-between' point for PPMs, saying the smallest of incidents are being investigated at a high level. They point out that, if hospital employees were involved, many of the reported incidents would be addressed in person and not immediately escalated to AHPRA. None of the PPMs suggested that they were against regulation or an incident being investigated; however, most thought the level at which the investigations occurred was excessive:

> If they had somebody that could actually go through these reports before they get to the HCCC or AHPRA, there's got to be something in the middle.

Devastation on so many levels

Every PPM talked at length about how distressing the process of being reported to AHPRA was and how 'it was devastating on so many levels'. This devastation included feelings of fear of 'being reported all the time' and 'what it would mean for the future'. The devastation also included feeling 'really, really paranoid' and that being reported was 'very personal and insulting'. Finally, devastation was couple with feelings of shame: 'is it my fault? Should I have done things differently?'

Every PPM said that being reported and investigated had affected their mental health and well-being, reporting guilt, shame, fear, loss of confidence, anxiety, depression and PTSD. Five PPMs referred to losing confidence after being reported and how difficult this was for them.

> The one thing I've had in my 25 years as a midwife is feeling really confident with what I know and what I don't know and I find that really challenging since the reporting.

Many experienced anxiety over what would happen to them and their ability to cope during and after the investigation:

> I'm finding it's affecting me to the point that I don't know that I can go on, because I can't you know, when you're in that sort of anxious state then you can't pay attention to anything.
>
> I walked out of that hospital with PTSD from the hospital. Because the next day when I went back, I had a panic attack walking in the hospital because there was a security guard that stood outside and I thought they were waiting for me.

Seven of the PPMs discussed the negative impact that being reported had on their family and their relationships. Partners would ask 'Why do you keep doing this to yourself?'

Another stated:

> My husband doesn't want me to do births anymore, definitely not. Because he gets angry. He just gets really, really angry. He gets what it's like to be a family member and have the experience. He gets how much my women appreciate me, but he doesn't get me. He feels like I'm sacrificing myself, which I'm not at all.

Making changes in the aftermath

After being reported, PPMs made changes to their practice and, in some cases, their careers. Midwives either fight on or give up after being reported.

> I just gave up because I'm not going to win … I just said I was guilty of everything … they were petty little things and I went, you know what, just, I'm guilty, I don't care because at the end of the day you're going to find me guilty anyway. It's going to cost me a shit load of money to fight this and I can't do this anymore.
>
> I don't care anymore Jo to be honest. I'm just, I know I'm going to get reported. You know, I'm damned if I do and I'm damned if I don't. So, I just think, I don't necessarily book a woman whether she's a VBAC or not. I book a woman because she's a woman and she wants the care I can provide.

Four PPMs said that being reported made them 'practise more defensively'.

> I try not to let it affect my clinical decisions because I think I'm quite solid clinically. But I do definitely look more into, how would this stand up in court? Rather than just the evidence or the woman's choice … I think about whether if I had to stand up in front of a professional counselling situation, would woman's choice wash.

PPMs said they felt they needed a career back-up plan in case a future report affected their livelihood. Due to 'being self-employed and the only wage earner' they thought it necessary 'to have a back-up plan'. The PPMs felt that the current political climate around private practice is such that, once they'd been reported, it remained a cloud over them forever:

> It's the climate. I think the way the climate is at the moment, I think there's a lot of complaints happening. And I do feel like we're walking a tightrope all the time.

Participating PPMs said they believed that, once a complaint was made against them, they would never end:

> It's now on my record that I've had two complaints. So if I ever get a third, it's very different to investigating someone who's never had a complaint before.

All PPMs recognised that the current political climate is limiting choice for women and the result is a rising freebirth rate in Australia:

> The women are between a rock and a hard place. Now the problem is I think a lot more women are freebirthing because the midwife won't support them, because they're scared.
>
> Basically, the women told me that they were going to freebirth if I didn't go. And the reason they weren't going to go into the system was because they were so traumatised, by the system.

Conclusion

In this chapter, we have shown that the global witch hunt is not a thing of the past. The attacks on midwives are ongoing and the effects on midwives attending homebirths are intense emotional and psychological distress. Understanding the effects of the process of investigation is important to improving the quality of professional and personal support available to PPMs reported to regulatory authorities. It would better to streamline processes. It is becoming increasingly difficult for PPMs to support the wishes and needs of individual women and also meet the requirements of both the regulators and an increasingly risk-averse health service.

A way forward

- Legislation is needed to make clear that midwives have a duty of care to attend women, even when they decline recommendations, and midwives must be protected when they fulfil this duty of care
- Midwives being reported to regulatory authorities need strong professional support and more streamlined and efficient investigatory processes that reduce unnecessary escalation. Professional bodies can play a role in this
- Supporting homebirth as a mainstream option will make it seem less obscure and hence less likely to be unreasonably targeted by facility personnel
- Investigations need to be quick and clear with regular communication maintained during the process
- Women who have received the care that is the subject of the reporting should be interviewed for their input

- Bringing PPMs into mainstream care by offering visiting rights and access to ongoing education and debriefing will help them not feel as unsupported and alienated from mainstream care

References

Australian College of Midwives. (2014). National Midwifery Guidelines for Consultation and Referral – 3rd Edition Issue 2. Retrieved from: www.midwives.org.au/resources/national-midwifery-guidelines-consultation-and-referral-3rd-edition-issue-2-2014 [accessed 10 May 2019].

Catling-Paull, C., Coddington, R. L., Foureur, M. J., & Homer, C. S. E. (2013). Publicly funded homebirth in Australia: A review of maternal and neonatal outcomes over 6 years. *Medical Journal of Australia, 198*, 616–620.

Combellick, J., Shin, H., Shin, D., Cai, Y., Hagan, H., Lacher, C., ... Dominguez-Bello, M. (2018). Differences in the fecal microbiota of neonates born at home or in the hospital. *Scientific Reports, 8*.

Commonwealth of Australia. (2009). *Improving maternity services in Australia, The Report of the Maternity Services Review, 2009*. Canberra: Commonwealth of Australia.

Dahlen, H. (2011). Perspectives on risk or risk in perspective? *Essentially MIDIRS, 2*, 17–21.

De Vries, R. G. (1996). *Making midwives legal: Childbirth, medicine, and the law*. Columbus, OH: The Ohio State University Press.

Declercq, E. (1994). The trials of Hanna Porn: The campaign to abolish midwifery in Massachusetts. *American Journal of Public Health, 84*, 1022–1028.

Donnison, J. (1988). *Midwives and medical men*. London: Historical Publications.

Edwards, N. P. (2008). Safety in birth: The contextual conundrums faced by women in a 'risk society', driven by neoliberal policies. *MIDIRS Midwifery Digest,* 18(4), 463–470.

Edwards, N., Murphy-Lawless, J., Kirkham, M., & Davies, S. (2011). Attacks on midwives, attacks on women's choices. *AIMS Journal,* 23(3), 3–7.

Ehrenreich, B. & English, D. (2010). *Witches, midwives and nurses: A history of women healers* New York, NY: The Feminist Press.

Federici, S. (2018). *Witches, witch-hunting and women*. Oakland, CA: PM Press.

Gastaldo, E. (2019). Midwife arrested for delivering babies: Mennonites are making a rare public stand in her defense. *Newser*, 7 March.

Gleeson, C. & Holland, K. (2019). Pioneering midwife Philomena Canning dies. *The Irish Times*, 23 March.

Goffman, E. (1963). *Stigma: Notes on a spoiled identity*. Englewood Cliffs, NJ: Prentice-Hall, Inc.

Hughes, E. C. (1971). *The sociological eye: On work, self, & the study of society*, Vol. 2. New York, NY: Aldine-Atherton.

Hunter, J. (2018). The experiences of privately practising midwives in Australia who have been reported to the Australian Health Practitioner Regulation Agency: A qualitative study. Honours thesis, Western Sydney University.

King, B. (2019). My surprise twin homebirth. Brooke King's website. Retrieved from: www.surprisetwinhomebirth.com/ [accessed 11 December 2019].

Lever, C. (2018). After successfully delivering twins, midwife Martina was suspended. Now mums are fuming. *Mamamia*, 15 November.

Monteblanco, A. D. (2017). Midwives on the margins: Stigma management among out-of-hospital midwives. *Deviant Behavior*, *39*(12). https://doi.org/10.1080/01639625.2018.1438061.

Murphy-Lawless, J. (2019). Philomena Canning: A midwife vindicated. *Birth Practice and Politics Forum*, 6 March.

NSW Government. (2015). Provision of Private Midwifery Services by Eligible Midwives in NSW Public Hospitals. Retrieved from: www1.health.nsw.gov.au/pds/ActivePDSDocuments/GL2015_014.pdf

Nursing and Midwifery Board of Australia. (2017). Safety and Quality Guidelines for Privately Practicing Midwives. Retrieved from: www.nursingmidwiferyboard.gov.au/Codes-Guidelines-Statements/Codes-Guidelines.aspx [accessed 15 December 2017].

Pager, T. (2019). She helped deliver hundreds of babies. Then she was arrested. *The New York Times*, 5 March.

Purkiss, D. (1996). *The witch in history and society: Early modern and twentieth century representations*. London: Routledge.

Wagner, M. (1995). A global witch-hunt. *The Lancet, 346*, 1020–1022.

12 Birth trauma

The noxious by-product of a failing system

Maddy Simpson and Agy Cater

> I literally felt my soul shut down in order to get through it – similar to when a rape victim needs to shut down their connection to their body.
>
> (Agy Cater)

About the authors

Maddy is a midwife and PhD candidate. Her thesis is focused on gaining a better understanding of psychological birth trauma and the development of post-traumatic stress disorder following childbirth. Maddy became interested in this area while completing her Master's degree. She attended a workshop on traumatic birth experiences and was disturbed to learn from the workshop facilitator that when undertaking a study on traumatic birth, she received requests to participate from women in their 60s and 70s. These women were so negatively affected by their birth experiences that, years after the event, they were reliving the experience and needing to share their stories. As her final project for her Master's degree, Maddy completed and published a literature review on psychological birth trauma and has continued this work as part of her PhD study.

Agy is a consumer who gave birth to her baby and suffered birth trauma. Her story appears throughout the chapter to illustrate the points Maddy makes.

Introduction

The birth of a baby is often associated with elation, love and joy. It is the start of a new adventure, a time of change, transition and growth. Women become mothers, couples become families and a new generation begins. However, for more and more women and their families, birth is not a positive, life-affirming moment and can leave deep emotional and psychological scars. Their negative birth experiences live with them forever and have the potential to adversely impact on many areas of their lives. This is referred to as birth trauma. As you will have already read in previous chapters, birth trauma is a major motivator for women who birth outside the system in future pregnancies. We see birth trauma as the poisonous gas that is escaping from the coal mine (mainstream care) and slowly killing the canary.

What is birth trauma?

Birth trauma is a subjective experience, described as being in the eye of the beholder (Beck, 2004a), which reportedly occurs in 20–48% of women (Ford & Ayers, 2011; Harris & Ayers, 2012) following childbirth. Sorensen and Tschetter (2010) describe birth perception as a subjective judgement of a woman's global birth experience, indicating personal satisfaction with the birth process and outcome. The more serious side of birth trauma is PTSD. According to Simpson, Schmied, Dickson and Dahlen (2018), 'PTSD is defined as the development of a certain cluster of symptoms, such as persistent, involuntary and intrusive memories, avoidance of stimuli, recurrent distressing dreams, dissociative reactions, altered mood state and intense or prolonged psychological distress following exposure to a traumatic event that represents an actual or perceived threat to the life of an individual'. A review of the literature shows that, around the world, about 30% of women are experiencing symptoms of PTSD following birth (Simpson & Catling, 2016). Of those, between 1.7% and 9% of birthing women meet the full diagnostic criteria for PTSD following childbirth (Beck, Gable, Sakala, & Declercq, 2011; Denis, Parant, & Callahan, 2011; Ford & Ayers, 2011). PTSD following childbirth and experiencing symptoms of PTSD have been shown to have a negative impact on mental health outcomes and breastfeeding and is linked to disruptions in mother–infant bonding (McDonald, Slade, Spiby, & Iles, 2011; Ionio & Di Blasio, 2014).

In a second literature review, we assessed the risk factors for developing PTSD. We found significant risk factors associated with symptoms of PTSD including a prior traumatic event, pre-existing emotional issues and/or mental health disorders, complex pregnancy or pre-existing medical conditions impacting pregnancy, antenatally reported fears about labour and/or birth, financial factors (low socio-economic status/no access to medical insurance), demographic factors, operative birth (caesarean section, particularly emergency caesarean section, or instrumental birth), neonatal complications, preterm birth, fear for the safety of the neonate, traumatic obstetric event/birth experience or maternal complications during labour, low level of support during labour, sense of loss of control during labour, perception of pain during labour and birth, low social support during the postnatal period, increased postnatal physical pain, trauma and maternal morbidity, symptoms of depression after birth, not exclusively breastfeeding or breastfeeding as long as planned, and postnatal consultation with a mental health professional (Simpson et al., 2018).

Birth trauma is a global phenomenon, with dedicated research originating from the United Kingdom, Australia, Canada, the USA, Europe and the

Middle East (Sorenson & Tschetter, 2010; Beck et al., 2011; Denis et al., 2011; Ford & Ayers, 2011; McDonald et al., 2011; Stramrood et al., 2011; Harris & Ayers, 2012; Verreault et al., 2012; Boorman, Devilly, Gamble, Creedy, & Fenwick, 2014; Taghizadeh, Irajpour, Nedjat, Arbabi, & Lopez, 2014; Ionio & Di Blasio, 2014; McKenzie-McHarg, Crockett, Olander, & Ayers, 2014; O'Donovan et al., 2014). The impact of a psychological and emotional birth trauma can continue long after birth. For some, the consequences can last a lifetime (Taghizadeh et al., 2014). When describing their traumatic birth experiences, women used terminology such as 'birth rape' and 'obstetric violence' (Kitzinger, 2006; Elmir, Schmied, Wilkes, & Jackson, 2010; Fernández, 2013).

To illustrate what can potentially turn birth into a traumatic event for women and families, Agy contributed aspects of her birth story below.

Agy's story

Agy's story is, sadly, not uncommon. Agy describes leaving hospital physically healthy a few days postbirth. However, aspects of her labour and birth negatively impacted on life for herself and her family in the days that followed, something she attributes to her care during labour and birth. She describes it as 'a very sensitive topic for our family' that has been 'an ongoing emotional hurdle for me for the past 13 months'.

Below are extracts from Agy's correspondence to the hospital at which she birthed, describing her experience in labour and birth.

> From the time I was admitted into my own birthing suite right up until I birthed my baby (12 hours in hospital) I felt harassed, questioned, coerced, undermined and bullied in every aspect of my labour. My doula and husband – who attended the birth and were my advocates – were also undermined, harassed and bullied throughout this time, not to mention threatened, while I was made to feel like I was not entitled to receive basic human rights including declining the type of care I wished to have.
>
> The constant haranguing from your staff, bullying, questioning and coercion created such a stressful environment for everyone in my birthing space, but most obviously – me. I was very upset emotionally during my labour as I felt completely unsupported by hospital staff and lacked trust in staff that were looking after me. I was continuously bullied and questioned in regards to every decision I made and then finally coerced into things I did not want to go ahead with simply because staff gave me no other choice. I felt completely unsafe, frightened, and like things were just happening to me without giving any thought to how I felt and whether I was willingly consenting. Your team went against my direct and clear wishes in regards to many points that we voiced at the time and wrote in our birthing plan, in addition to the constant bullying and coercion, which resulted in me feeling completely unsafe, alone and

> terrified – as I had lost all faith in the team that was looking after me and my baby – not to mention our best interests.
>
> Once in my birthing suite care was taken over by [Midwife 1]. [Midwife 1] created a very unpleasant environment as soon as we entered the room. I made it clear in my birth plan that communication was to be between the midwives/doctors and my husband/doula throughout my labour in regards to my care. [Midwife 1] did not honour this from the start. She was discussing performing a vaginal exam on me in order to check how dilated I was, not to mention advising me of all the different pain relief that I could receive – again, all things I had clearly noted in the birth plan that I did not want to discuss unless I so advised. All these things were basic decisions my husband and I made beforehand in order for me to be able to be stress-free in my labour, knowing that I had my husband and doula making the right decisions for me.
>
> I wanted my birth to be a sacred space with no fear, open heart and doing what's best for baby and I without interventions. Within half an hour of being in the birthing suite [Midwife 1] did a great job of making me feel like I was doing something wrong, when she even requested to see a bottle of massage oil my doula was using to rub my back and neck for me and started listing all the ingredients. Again, only half an hour later after I was moved to my birthing suite and half an hour after we had already declined a vaginal exam, [Midwife 1] again pressured for a vaginal exam to see the progress of my labour – which we declined again – alongside declining her advice of foetal heart monitoring. [Midwife 1's] persistence regarding foetal heart monitoring did not cease, and to be left in peace we agreed to it through abdominal palpation.

Agy goes on to describe unnecessary conflict with staff, constant obstruction of her choices for simple things, like use of water immersion during her labour, and a 'bait and switch' attempt:

> Between 4:30 p.m. and 8 p.m. my husband and doula were requesting that I be able to use the bath for pain relief. At this point the midwives kept pressuring the vaginal exam and advising that they would not allow me to get into the bath unless I had the exam. They were also creating lots of pressure around the situation, stating that if I did not consent to a vaginal exam they would have to send me home as they need to be able to see what stage of labour I am at to confirm that I am definitely in labour. I am not a midwife but I am educated enough to know that the timing, length and strength of my contractions was more than enough to see that I was very much in labour. After already more than 14 hours of labour (including home labour) I was getting very upset that I was being withheld from using the bath as pain relief – as that was my intended pain relief. Regardless of the amount of discussions we had with the midwives between the three of us, none of them were accepting our reasoning and

> I was coerced into providing consent. The midwives were being very disrespectful to our wishes, where they knew my husband, doula and I were a team, and regardless of this, would wait until my husband and doula were out of the room before they would question me more and try to coerce me into making decisions I didn't want to make, nor even wanted to discuss in such a vulnerable state. It felt like I was being taken advantage of simply because I didn't have my support people with me in the room. The midwives made it very obvious that they thought I was being 'tricked' into doing things I didn't want to do by my husband and doula, when the reality was the midwives themselves were trying to trick me into providing consent for things I didn't feel comfortable doing, and quite frankly was not in a position to be making those decisions in the middle of intense labour. I eventually gave in and had a vaginal examination against my wishes. The midwives found I was 9 cm dilated.
>
> With the vaginal examination over I was still using the shower only as pain relief and getting frustrated with my husband as to why the midwives STILL were not allowing me to use the tub, even after I agreed to provide them with a vaginal exam just so I could use it. My husband then confided in me again stating that the midwives were now arguing that I was not allowed in the tub because I had a history of heart palpitations. In now hearing this news I was absolutely enraged and felt betrayed by carers we were supposed to be able to trust. I was coerced into a VE so I could get into the tub. I provided consent for a VE on coercion, and now they were using another thing against me getting into the tub.

Agy's private cardiologist and the hospital's obstetricians had cleared her for a vaginal delivery. Agy expressed frustration and fear caused by interpersonal conflict with hospital staff:

> Again, I felt like I had been taken advantage of and was feeling scared about my safety and care with the way the midwives were manipulating us.

Agy was further and constantly pressured by clinicians to accept interventions without medical indication and contrary to her express preferences, such as continuous electronic foetal monitoring, augmentation of labour, insertion of a urinary catheter, forceful vaginal examinations and instrumental delivery in the operating theatre. Notably, these are common factors associated with traumatic birth experiences, in addition to the low-quality relationships she had with her care providers. She felt frustration and anger at not being supported and feared for herself and her baby. She felt that she was being put in an unnecessarily stressful and traumatic situation:

> At this point the energy in the room was very negative and the midwives were being very disrespectful to my husband, doula and myself. The language and tones being used, as well as the constant pressure and speaking

> down to us was not only belittling, but frightening, complete and utter bullying and disgusting from people who are supposed to have your best care at heart. How was I supposed to feel as a woman in strong labour, being faced with constant bullying pressure and coercion into making decisions for myself and my baby that I did not want to make, not to mention bullied into believing that the choices I was making with my husband were the wrong choices. I am a human being with human rights. It is a basic right of every human being to be able to say yes or no to anything that happens to their body – regardless of what staff at the hospital want or believe. I was never given this basic right and made to feel threatened by hospital staff who were in the room.

At this point, Agy was presented with yet another clinician who made her feel distressed and unsafe:

> [Obstetrician] was anything but pleasant to us from the moment she stepped into my birthing space, making us all feel overpowered, ordered around and treating us like we had no idea what we were doing let alone the right to make safe decisions for ourselves. She was negative, bossy, forceful, rude, arrogant and a downright bully, insisting (unrealistically) that I birth my baby on her clock.
>
> The environment was very uncomfortable once [Obstetrician] got involved in my labour. She was ordering midwives around and not allowing them to do their job. Myself and my support team kept asking our midwife for advice and her sincere opinion so that we could make better informed decisions without [Obstetrician's] biased views, and [Obstetrician] kept answering questions for them not allowing any midwives to give us advice and ensuring that the power was in her favour for the situation to unfold her way. We all saw our midwives hesitate to answer any questions while glancing at [Obstetrician] nervously and hesitate to disagree with [Obstetrician] at times where I needed their support and voice the most.

Agy describes the pressure and harassment to pass urine if she wanted to avoid having a urinary catheter inserted:

> The obstetrician ordered me into the toilet to try and empty my bladder. Being in the midst of intense labour and at this point emotional and fearful as I felt like everything depended on me passing urine, each time I sat on the toilet, the pressure of the baby would initiate a contraction. With my husband beside me, I was trying to pass urine when a contraction hit me and [Obstetrician] stormed into the toilet turning the light on, yelling that if I had not yet passed urine then I wasn't going to, and ordering me to get off the toilet and onto the bed so that she could insert a catheter. With that I got so upset and my husband very enraged that

> [Obstetrician] was not only being so rude, but that she was being completely careless not even giving me a chance to pass urine as I was hit with a contraction. My husband got up from beside me and turned the light off, yelling at [Obstetrician] that she had not even yet given me a chance, nor was it polite for her to be walking in on someone on the toilet and turning a bright light on, on a labouring woman. He slammed the door on her to give me some privacy so I had some sort of a chance to try and pass urine. With the environment becoming so stressful and being unsuccessful at passing urine on the toilet, I wanted a good chance, and thought maybe I could try passing urine in the shower if I could relax. Again with no success, I sadly was ordered out by [Obstetrician] to have a catheter inserted …
>
> The amount of stress and bullying [Obstetrician] was placing on us, I had no choice but to give in to the insertion of a catheter and another vaginal examination. Over the time that I was labouring the support team and I were tirelessly asking for midwives and [Obstetrician] to give us privacy to discuss our options and make decisions together – all of these but a few completely ignored, unheard and dismissed. Midwives and [Obstetrician] were becoming rude, impatient, pushy and had no desire to give us any privacy or time to discuss as they kept ignoring our needs. They all simply kept standing on top of me, trying to coerce me or change my mind, and any moment my support team would leave my side, they would barrage me with a tone of questions and information to try and persuade me to do what they wanted.

Agy then goes on to describe the loss of control over her birth experience, when the obstetrician 'took over the room', insisting she had been labour too long with no progress, despite now being fully dilated:

> She told me that she was ready to take me down to theatre to try and get the baby out with forceps. I had not even had a chance to give birth to my baby. Everyone in the room was barking orders at me since I entered the birth suite, I was under high stress from midwives and [Obstetrician] continuously barraging me with information and decisions to make – completely disregarding my requests and my choices – and I was not given the privacy I so desperately wanted and my husband kept asking midwives to give us. Trying to cling on to some sort of control over the type of birth that I wanted, my husband, doula and I kept requesting for more time to allow me to relax and try to bring the baby down to pushing stage. The obstetrician was completely against this and kept arguing that I am in danger, my baby was in danger (neither one of us were in danger at the time as heart rates were stable and I was coping well), I was too tired (even though I had not once complained about being tired) and even though I had absolutely no urge to push, kept advising that I needed to start pushing the baby out. With enough stress on my shoulders this was

another breaking point for me when I was well informed about the way a woman's body works and the dangers I would be under if I were to push a baby out without my body being ready.

After an hour of passive decent had passed, my disappointment lay heavy as I was forced by [Obstetrician] to start active guided pushing – against my own body's will to do so. [Midwife 2] was kind enough to direct me with pushing whilst I was on the birth stool. With this position being unsuccessful, I was directed back to laying semi-reclined on the bed to continue directive pushing with vaginal pressure to guide me. As non-invasive as [Midwife 2] had been through my whole labour, it was at this point of her directive pushing that she threw her fingers inside my vagina to show me how to push – with such force that I screamed out in pain with how traumatic this was for me. Not only did I feel like a piece of meat, but as much as I lacked trust in the care I was receiving up to this point, this was something that completely broke me and has caused many PTSD moments for me since my child's birth. My husband still recollects this scream of pain and terror from me and breaks into tears every time, my mother also – therefore you can only imagine how it has affected me. For people who I am supposed to trust with my care, [Midwife 2] let me down at this point the way I was butchered inside with no care of the effect on me …

During this time, Agy experienced more negative interactions with the obstetrician as well:

… [Obstetrician] was in and out of the room, constantly barraging me with bullying comments that if I don't give birth soon she will be wheeling me down to theatre for a forceps delivery and if that didn't work a caesarean. Each time I tried to get privacy to discuss the risks and benefits of each thing that was proposed to me with my support team, the midwives and [Obstetrician] ignored our requests and continued pressuring or telling us that they've given us enough time, even though they did not provide privacy to discuss at all. With again, no other choice but to adhere to [Obstetrician's] demands I again was bullied into providing consent for the syntocinon regardless of what I wanted.

I was put in the lithotomy position – again, against my will of wanting to be on my knees or all fours in the second stage. In this position I had at least three people bending my legs towards my head and pushing into me so hard every time I had a contraction and pushed (I cannot recall who these three were, but I remember at least one midwife). I had [Obstetrician] and [Midwife 2] both taking turns in hammering their fingers into my vagina with each contraction to 'guide' my pushing, even though I lay there completely helpless and held down by a team of people supposedly looking out for my safety and felt like a complete piece of meat with every thrash and tear into my vagina.

> I literally felt my soul shut down in order to get through it – similar to when a rape victim needs to shut down their connection to their body. I could feel [Obstetrician] ripping and stretching me fiercely inside the vagina between each contraction and I was doing everything I possibly could to try and push my baby out to get out of this environment and into safety, to the point where my eyes were weeping …

At the time that Agy gave birth to her daughter, she does recall a positive interaction with a midwife who came on duty:

> … this new midwife was a breath of fresh air for me. I did not come to know her name until I was lying in my recovery room hours later, however [Midwife 3] was an amazing light for me when everyone in the room was treating me like an animal. I remember seeing her behind [Obstetrician], quietly mouthing positive reinforcements and smiling and acknowledging me and the hard work that I was doing as a labouring woman in such an environment. She was giving me thumbs up, showing me how far the baby was away and honestly I believe that if it wasn't for her being in the background and allowing me to cancel all the people out in front of me with their viciousness and unkindness, I don't know if I would have had the natural birth I wanted in the end. She gave me the strength to get through it through her smiles and quiet encouragement, and for that I will always be truly grateful, however it is disgusting that I didn't get to have that kindness and care throughout …

However, at the same time, Agy continued to feel bullied into procedures and interventions that she did not want:

> [Obstetrician] was now starting to bully me, stating that my perineum had suffered major tearing already, including inside my vagina and pressuring me for an episiotomy – again another thing I was against. She kept advising that if I didn't do this my injuries could be even worse, and they are already very bad – I have to mention here that I do believe all the fierce fingers thrashing and ripping me inside during every contraction felt like they did a lot of damage, not to mention being forced to push a baby out before my body was ready. [Obstetrician] led me to these injuries herself, and now she was coercing me to have an episiotomy. With again no strength to fight and with obvious injuries, I had no choice but to give consent for this as well, and before the syntocinon could kick in I had delivered my baby …

Agy describes her birth experience as follows:

> Throughout the whole labour I felt frightened and out of control, and without appropriate support or care. I felt cheated and manipulated by

> my health carers and had absolutely no faith in them. The clinicians went against my direct and clear wishes regarding many different points in my birth plan and just generally during labour, which resulted in my fear increasing as I believe the things that were happening to me should have only occurred if things were getting very serious. The emotional impact of this birth experience on myself has been enormous, and has had repercussions for my whole family. I experience flashbacks daily of many aspects of the birth and regularly feel severe anxiety, with trauma flashbacks each time my baby cries intensely. I have struggled to bond with my baby and found day-to-day tasks sometimes insurmountable, as a result of the high levels of anxiety.

What makes birth traumatic?

A factor frequently reported as contributing to traumatic birth experiences, as demonstrated in Agy's story, is the interactions between woman and health care providers during labour and birth. Agy's clearly describes how she felt unsupported, ignored, undermined and fearful. Sorenson and Tschetter (2010) have analysed how Quality of the Provider Interactions (QPI) can influence the birth experience. They found that healthcare provider behaviours that are perceived as negative or unsupportive, and interpersonal interactions of low quality, correlated with women's experiences of perinatal trauma symptoms and depression. If women felt that they had low QPI with their care providers it affected their long-term memories of negative and traumatic birth experiences (Sorenson & Tschetter, 2010).

Harris and Ayers (2012) also report on interpersonal interactions with healthcare providers during labour and birth, and the impact of these interactions on the woman's experience. In their study, the authors examined and identified 'hot spots' in the reports women gave when describing birth experiences as negative or traumatic. The most frequently reported hot spots concerned interpersonal conflict with care providers. The women most frequently reported feeling ignored, unsupported or abandoned by care providers (Harris & Ayers, 2012).

Agy describes her traumatic birth experience as negatively impacting on not only herself but her family. She calls it as a very 'sensitive subject' within her family. Elmir et al. (2010) found that traumatic birth experiences had extreme consequences for women and their partners. They reported that women described feeling overwhelmed, angry, disappointed and had a sense of loss. The experience of a traumatic birth caused women to disconnect from their partners and infants, and experience symptoms of depression, including suicidal ideation. Again, the overwhelming cause of the birth trauma was the poor or unsupportive care from midwives, nurses and doctors. In other studies women described the care they received as 'dehumanizing, disrespectful and uncaring' (Elmir et al., 2010).

Another constantly repeated theme in Agy's story is the lack of autonomy, control and choice afforded to her. Women's perception of a lack of autonomy through external locus of control, non-involvement in decision-making, lack of choice, being restrained and not having expectations met also contributed to birth becoming a traumatic event for women (Nicholls & Ayers, 2007).

What is life like after a traumatic birth experience?

Not surprisingly, traumatic birth experiences are associated with fear of childbirth, also known as secondary tokophobia, which can result in either avoiding pregnancy or labour (e.g. requests for elective caesarean section) (Borg Cunen, McNeill, & Murray, 2014). Women who develop these fears may choose not to have any more children, or they seek stringent birth planning for future pregnancies so as to avoid another traumatic experience. Traumatised women who again become pregnant live in constant fear and anxiety through that subsequent pregnancy (Beck, 2004b; Ayers, Eagle, & Waring, 2006). Women also report experiencing sexual dysfunction, linked to the fear of becoming pregnant and having to birth again (Nicholls & Ayers, 2007). While some request a caesarean section to avoid another traumatic labour, others choose to freebirth or attempt a homebirth regardless of risk factors.

PTSD: the extreme end of the birth trauma continuum

PTSD following childbirth is shown to cause difficulty for women when relating to, or bonding with, their infants. PTSD symptoms in the postnatal period are associated with difficulties initiating positive interactions between mothers and infants (Ionio & Di Blasio, 2014). McDonald and colleagues (2011) found that women with PTSD symptoms were more likely to perceive their child as difficult and experience higher levels of parenting stress. Maternal PTSD symptoms have also been found to cause anxiety in the infant (Cigoli, Gilli, & Saita, 2006). Women who experience postnatal PTSD self-report difficulties interacting and bonding with their infants; for example, they report a negative perception of their infant as well as negative bonding styles ranging from avoidant, or rejecting, to overprotective and anxious (Beck, 2004b; Ayers et al., 2006; Nicholls & Ayers, 2007).

Women with postnatal mental health disorders, such as PTSD, show impaired ability to interpret infant emotions, causing them to be less sensitive to the needs of the infant (Webb & Ayers, 2015). Women who experienced higher rates of PTSD symptoms at two months after birth displayed more intrusive behaviours towards their infants during play phases in an attempt to build a relationship through physical contact with their child (Ionio & Di Blaso, 2014). In response, their infants showed less interest in nearby objects and more avoidance behaviours, such as physically distancing themselves from the adult.

Birth trauma, particularly when associated with symptoms of PTSD, not only interferes with mother–baby bonding, it can significantly impact women's quality of life and interpersonal relationships. Women frequently report that their birth experiences and subsequent PTSD injuries damaged or impaired the important relationships in their lives. Relationships with partners or spouses became fraught when women felt they were not getting adequate support or their experiences were not understood (Ayers et al., 2006). Women also reported relationship strain caused by lack of intimacy, loss of self-esteem following birth, disagreements, poor communication and blaming partners for events during the birth (Ayers et al., 2006; Nicholls & Ayers, 2007).

Birth trauma and PTSD symptoms following birth also create friction in women's relationships with their wider social network. Women describe losing social connections due to lack of trust, lack of desire to socialise and feeling trapped in their 'own little world' (Ayers et al., 2006). Women will sometimes, as a coping mechanism, isolate themselves from mothers who have not experienced traumatic birth (Beck, 2004b).

Not only does birth trauma negatively impact on women's relationships and support networks, it also has the potential to affect their ability to function as they did before their traumatic birth experience. Some attempt to strictly control their environment, confine themselves to the home to cope with heightened levels of fear, create regimented daily routines and impose high standards upon themselves to achieve perfection (Ayers et al., 2006). In this context, subsequent attempts to both avoid hospital as the source of their trauma, and choose homebirth, make sense. If midwives were part of creating that trauma (as in Agy's case), then freebirthing (without the support of a midwife) is also a logical extension of this trauma.

On a physical level, women with postnatal PTSD symptoms described feeling mutilated, doubtful about their bodies, extremely drained from physical pain and depressed (Ayers et al., 2006), as well as reporting more physical ailments after birth (Ayers, Radoš, & Balouch, 2015). Agy describes her feeling in graphic detail, using terms like 'rape' and 'being ripped apart'.

Emotionally, women described feeling helpless, humiliated, shocked, violated dehumanised, inadequate, angry, numb, detached, depressed and even suicidal following a traumatic birth (Beck, 2004b; Ayers et al., 2006; Nicholls & Ayers, 2007). They describe just going through the motions of daily life and feeling isolated, anxious and depressed after their traumatic birth experiences (Beck, 2004b).

Potential healing and protective factors against birth trauma

While Agy's story demonstrates the many elements that cause birth to become a traumatic event for women, there is also research that points to factors that contribute to positive and empowering birth experiences for women and their families. While still in its infancy, the research offers some food for thought around factors such as interpersonal relationships and birth environment. In addition, there are indications that a subsequent positive birth experiences facilitates recovery and encourages a woman to feel empowered, strong and confident again (Beck, 2004b). This is supported by Thomson and Downe's (2010) research on the redemptive quality of a positive birth experience.

Support for women during labour is an important factor in influencing the birth experience (Ayers et al., 2015). It correlates with studies relating low QPI during labour and birth to the development of a traumatic birth experience and PTSD after childbirth. This factor can be facilitated by increasing awareness and educating clinicians on the importance of high-quality interpersonal skills and collaborative support when providing intrapartum care. Lack of social support and poor-quality care in labour is continually recorded as a risk factor for PTSD development in current literature. Midwifery continuity of care has been identified as a potential protective factor. Further research into midwifery-led continuity of care models could potentially help to reduce the current rates of childbirth-related PTSD symptoms experienced among women (Simpson et al., 2018).

Finally, the birth environment can also reduce the likelihood of a traumatic birth experience. Homebirth or birth in a home-like setting is identified as a potential protective factor against PTSD development (Simpson et al., 2018). Furuta, Sandall, Cooper and Bick (2016) identified homebirth as a protective factor against developing postnatal PTSD symptoms and Haagen, Moerbeek, Olde, Van Der Hart, and Kleber (2015) noted that women who birthed at home were the least likely cohort to report traumatic childbirth experiences. Stramrood et al. (2011) stated that, initially, their study comparing birth in a home-like and hospital environment showed that birthing in a home-like setting was protective against women developing PTSD symptoms. However, they noted that when controlling for the less-complex nature of homebirth, the protective factor is nullified. However, we would argue that as homebirth is associated with less intervention it is potentially protective against birth trauma. You will have read in Chapter 6 about the much lower rates of birth trauma and PTSD noted in women who had a homebirth compared to hospital birth experiences in the national Australian Homebirth Survey. When women choose to birth outside the system following a traumatic birth they may well be trying to protect themselves from repeating the trauma in subsequent births.

The way forward

- We need to increase awareness of risk and protective factors for PTSD following childbirth by clinicians
- Governments must support the development and testing of predictive models for PTSD symptoms following childbirth

- Further research into the benefits of midwifery-led continuity of care or birthing at home or in a home-like environment at reducing rates of PTSD symptoms is needed
- Promoting breastfeeding and/or immediate skin-to-skin contact and mother and infant bonding may help to mitigate PTSD symptoms
- Ensuring throughout pregnancy, birth and the postnatal period that women have appropriate social support and compassionate care-provider support

References

Ayers, S., Eagle, A., & Waring, H. (2006). The effects of childbirth-related post-traumatic stress disorder on women and their relationships: A qualitative study. *Psychology, Health & Medicine, 11*, 389–398.

Ayers, S., Radoš, S. N. & Balouch, S. (2015). Narratives of traumatic birth: Quality and changes over time. *Psychological Trauma: Theory, Research, Practice, and Policy, 7*, 234–242.

Beck, C. T. (2004a). Birth trauma: In the eye of the beholder. *Nursing Research, 53*, 28–35.

Beck, C. T. (2004b). Post-traumatic stress disorder due to childbirth: The aftermath. *Nursing Research, 53*, 216–224.

Beck, C. T., Gable, R. K., Sakala, C., & Declercq, E. R. (2011). Posttraumatic stress disorder in new mothers: Results from a two-stage U.S. national survey. *Birth: Issues in Perinatal Care, 38*, 216–227.

Boorman, R. J., Devilly, G. J., Gamble, J., Creedy, D. K., & Fenwick, J. (2014). Childbirth and criteria for traumatic events. *Midwifery, 30*, 255–261.

Borg Cunen, N., McNeill, J., & Murray, K. (2014). A systematic review of midwife-led interventions to address post partum post-traumatic stress. *Midwifery, 30*, 170–184.

Cigoli, V., Gilli, G., & Saita, E. (2006). Relational factors in psychopathological responses to childbirth. *Journal of Psychosomatic Obstetrics and Gynecology, 27*, 91–97.

Denis, A., Parant, O., & Callahan, S. (2011). Post-traumatic stress disorder related to birth: A prospective longitudinal study in a French population. *Journal of Reproductive & Infant Psychology, 29*, 125–135.

Elmir, R., Schmied, V., Wilkes, L., & Jackson, D. (2010). Women's perceptions and experiences of a traumatic birth: A meta-ethnography. *Journal of Advanced Nursing, 66*, 2142–2153.

Fernández, I. O. (2013). PTSD and obstetric violence. *Midwifery Today*. Eugene: Midwifery Today, Inc.

Ford, E. & Ayers, S. (2011). Support during birth interacts with prior trauma and birth intervention to predict postnatal post-traumatic stress symptoms. *Psychology & Health, 26*, 1553–1570.

Furuta, M., Sandall, J., Cooper, D., & Bick, D. (2016). Predictors of birth-related post-traumatic stress symptoms: Secondary analysis of a cohort study. *Archives of Women's Mental Health, 19*, 987–999.

Haagen, J. F. G., Moerbeek, M., Olde, E., Van Der Hart, O. & Kleber, R. J. (2015). PTSD after childbirth: A predictive ethological model for symptom development. *Journal of Affective Disorders, 185*, 135–143.

Harris, R. & Ayers, S. (2012). What makes labour and birth traumatic? A survey of intrapartum 'hotspots'. *Psychology & Health, 27*, 1166–1177.

Ionio, C. & Di Blasio, P. (2014). Post-traumatic stress symptoms after childbirth and early mother–child interactions: An exploratory study. *Journal of Reproductive & Infant Psychology, 32*, 163–181.

Kitzinger, S. (2006). Birth as rape: There must be an end to 'just in case' obstetrics. *British Journal of Midwifery, 14*, 544–545.

McDonald, S., Slade, P., Spiby, H., & Iles, J. (2011). Post-traumatic stress symptoms, parenting stress and mother–child relationships following childbirth and at 2 years postpartum. *Journal of Psychosomatic Obstetrics & Gynecology, 32*, 141–146.

McKenzie-McHarg, K., Crockett, M., Olander, E. K. & Ayers, S. (2014). Think pink! A sticker alert system for psychological distress or vulnerability during pregnancy. *British Journal of Midwifery, 22*, 590–595.

Nicholls, K. & Ayers, S. (2007). Childbirth-related post-traumatic stress disorder in couples: A qualitative study. *British Journal of Health Psychology, 12*, 491–509.

O'Donovan, A., Alcorn, K. L., Patrick, J. C., Creedy, D. K., Dawe, S., & Devilly, G. J. (2014). Predicting posttraumatic stress disorder after childbirth. *Midwifery, 30*, 935–941.

Simpson, M. & Catling, C. (2016). Understanding psychological traumatic birth experiences: A literature review. *Women and Birth, 29*, 203–207.

Simpson, M., Schmied, V., Dickson, C., & Dahlen, H. G. (2018). Postnatal post-traumatic stress: An integrative review. *Women and Birth, 31*, 367–379.

Sorenson, D. S. & Tschetter, L. (2010). Prevalence of negative birth perception, disaffirmation, perinatal trauma symptoms, and depression among postpartum women. *Perspectives in Psychiatric Care, 46*, 14–25.

Stramrood, C. A. I., Paarlberg, K. M., Huis In 'T Veld, E. M. J., Berger, L. W. A. R., Vingerhoets, A. J. J. M., Weijmar Schultz, W. C. M., & Van Pampus, M. G. (2011). Posttraumatic stress following childbirth in homelike- and hospital settings. *Journal of Psychosomatic Obstetrics & Gynecology, 32*, 88–97.

Taghizadeh, Z., Irajpour, A., Nedjat, S., Arbabi, M., & Lopez, V. (2014). Iranian mothers' perception of the psychological birth trauma: A qualitative study. *Iranian Journal of Psychiatry, 9*, 31–36.

Thomson, G. M. & Downe, S. (2010). Changing the future to change the past: Women's experiences of a positive birth following a traumatic birth experience. *Journal of Reproductive and Infant Psychology, 28*, 102–112.

Verreault, N., Da Costa, D., Marchand, A., Ireland, K., Banack, H., Dritsa, M., & Khalifé, S. (2012). PTSD following childbirth: A prospective study of incidence and risk factors in Canadian women. *Journal of Psychosomatic Research, 73*, 257–263.

Webb, R. & Ayers, S. (2015). Cognitive biases in processing infant emotion by women with depression, anxiety and post-traumatic stress disorder in pregnancy or after birth: A systematic review. *Cognition and Emotion, 29*, 1278–1294.

Part 2

Working towards a solution

13 What are women's legal rights when it comes to choice in pregnancy and childbirth?

Farah Diaz-Tello and Bashi Kumar-Hazard

> Each time a woman stands up for herself, without knowing it possibly, without claiming it, she stands up for all women.
>
> (Maya Angelou)

About the authors

Bashi is an Australian consumer and human rights lawyer and the Chair of Human Rights in Childbirth, and she has told her story in the Introduction and in Chapter 9.

Farah Diaz-Tello, JD, is a US-based human rights lawyer whose career has been dedicated to the pursuit of reproductive justice, and in particular on pregnancy and its many outcomes. She believes that the struggles over bodily autonomy and basic dignity unite all pregnant people, regardless of whether they choose to continue a pregnancy or how to give birth. She was catalysed to devote her feminist activism to rights in childbirth after her own experiences of mistreatment in birth, and having an abortion (which she recounted to the US Supreme Court in an amicus brief in *Whole Woman's Health v. Hellerstedt* in 2016). The scars from her birth have long since healed, and as Farah has since had two subsequent affirming and empowering experiences of birthing, she hopes to contribute to healing the system as well. The following is an edited extract of Farah's birth story as chronicled in the Winter 2017 edition of *Narrative Inquiry in Bioethics* (Diaz-Tello, 2017):

> Every birth story is about transformation, and mine is about a transformation from being a reproductive health activist and associating ob/gyn care with agency and autonomy, to recognizing the coercive power of our institutions, providers and the state over those giving birth. I went to law school out of a notion that rules and systems work, fed by a belief instilled by my immigrant parents that good things come to those who follow instructions and persevere. The series of closed doors I faced in pregnancy, in spite of the favorable law, was a harsh awakening.

I was in my first semester of law school when I got pregnant. It was 2006. In my naivety, I figured prenatal care and birth would be just like the rest of the reproductive health care I received from a combination of university health services and feminist reproductive health centers. I'd visit conscientious professionals who would explain things to me; I'd do my own research, ask questions, and make decisions that would be respected.

My options were circumscribed from the beginning. I live in an area with exceptional access to health care providers, but the only place that took Medicaid through my managed care organization was nearly an hour away by bus. Appointments were done by cattle-call, so a 9:00AM meant showing up at 8:30AM to be seen for five minutes at 11:00AM. I often felt dismissed and scolded; my questions were unwelcome. I hated that everyone called me mami. Finally, after being yelled at for not submitting to a test that had never been scheduled or even offered to me, I vowed I wouldn't let anyone treat me that way again, even if it meant catching my own baby alone. I found a homebirth midwife who agreed to accept me as a client late in the second trimester. After months of nonsensical insurance bureaucracy, I got insurance approval for a homebirth. Despite the fact that my midwife was a certified nurse-midwife and already an approved Medicaid provider, case managers and utilization review officers were shockingly uninformed about what a homebirth entailed, questioning my emergency plans, my midwife's credentials and my reasons for choosing a homebirth.

My battle had only just begun. After laboring for days without progress and finally running out of energy, I decided to transfer to hospital. My midwife warned me on arrival that we were now on their turf and their terms. The hospital was renowned for being midwife-friendly, but I could hear them murmuring about a homebirth transfer. My midwife had admitting privileges and continued to oversee my care, but I was shocked by the subtle and unsubtle ways she had to yield her power to the institution. After I was given an epidural, we were mostly left alone and I slept through the night. But with the dawn came the shift change. My epidural was wearing off and I was in shocking, agonizing pain. Someone, somewhere – the anesthesiologist, I think – decided that it was time to move to a cesarean. I wasn't given a choice; I wasn't even given a reason. To this day, it remains a mystery to me why I was subjected to a major surgery without any indication of danger or distress to my baby. My memory is an unreliable narrator, but I do remember some things. I remember everyone but my husband and midwife leaving the room, and her hurriedly trying to help stretch my cervix the remaining half-centimeter to avoid a cesarean. I remember the flurry of activity as they prepared me for surgery, and the way nobody even acknowledged when my husband asked if there was any other way. I remember the way my midwife grabbed the obstetrician by the sleeve of his white coat when he walked in, introduced himself as the person who would be doing my c-section, and turned to walk out. 'I think she might have questions,' she said. Frozen and in shock, I remained speechless. The final preparations in the operating room were a further exercise in invisibility: everyone in the room was there because of me, but no one saw me. But I wasn't the only one who was invisible at this point. There was the nurse who finally understood that the reason I was writhing in pain was not because of contractions but because the IV had infiltrated in my arm. She was disregarded. There was my midwife, the formidable woman with decades of experience catching babies, reduced to pleading with the young male anesthesiologist not to replace the IV in my elbow because I wanted to breastfeed. He did it anyway. A fog had descended over me. Everything felt like a movie or a nightmare that I futilely hoped I could wake from. My baby – despite being unnecessarily taken to NICU and then being transferred to the nursery for hours without anybody telling me what was going on – was perfectly healthy. I was physically healthy. Two other women got the 'shift-change cesarean' at the same time I did. As I lay stunned and trembling from cold and morphine in the recovery room, I overheard nurses helping a man excitedly getting outfitted to accompany his wife in surgery. Minutes later, I heard them explaining to him in hushed voices that she had experienced a seizure on the table as he watched.

I went into pregnancy believing that knowledge is power, that women have a fundamental right to mastery of their own fates and bodies, and that health care providers are there to help us exercise this agency. I came out of it with the realization that not all health care providers feel this way. The experience forged a connection in my mind as I returned to my studies weeks later: birth, like other aspects of our reproductive lives, is about a balance of power. And in our society, the balance of power is determined, among other factors, by race, class, and gender. I was called to the law to equalize that balance of power for women, and yet had just been through an experience in which being disempowered seemed not only commonplace, but a component of the protocol. I was galvanized to do something about it.

Introduction

In 2019, at the time of writing, Marshae Jones, a young, African-American woman residing in the USA, was shot in the abdomen during an altercation. She lost her pregnancy. While she mourned her loss, in a twist that made global headlines, Jones was charged with manslaughter. The shooter went free after an attempt to indict her proved unsuccessful. According to Lieutenant Danny Reid:

> The only true victim in this was the *unborn baby*. It was the mother of *the child* who initiated and continued the fight which resulted in the *death of her own unborn baby*.

> Lt Reid added that the child 'had no choice in being brought unnecessarily into a fight where she was relying on her mother for protection'.
>
> (BBC News, 2019, emphasis added)

The struggle at the heart of Ms Jones's case is the struggle for recognition as a person under the law, a fundamental human right acknowledged by Article 6 of the Universal Declaration of Human Rights and numerous authoritative recognitions of human rights. For some, unborn foetuses should be endowed with that recognition under the law – a *juridical personhood* – from the earliest stages of pregnancy, even before the cell formed by the union of egg and sperm have implanted in a woman's uterus. In the USA, proponents of foetal rights state that their intent is to prohibit abortion. In Australia, the pursuit of foetal rights are often shrouded in claims about the purported safety of the unborn foetus.

In either case, the practical effect of juridicial personhood goes far beyond prohibiting abortion: women are stripped of their human rights and deprived of their own personhood under the law. By the time pregnant women are ready to give birth, there seems to be a prevailing assumption that they have surrendered their right to decide what happens to their bodies to a medical stranger.

How did we get to this? How, in the twenty-first century, in two Western, wealthy democracies with laws underpinned by the philosophies of liberalism, equality and individual freedoms, can legal systems and principles lead to a woman being prosecuted as the perpetrator of an act of violence against her own body? For present purposes, what are the implications of such prosecutions for all women?

When the state can interfere in a pregnant woman's decision-making capacity in the name of the pregnancy she carries within her own body, the state is given a virtually unlimited power to dictate the terms of pregnancy, including decisions as fundamental, and as personal, as how women choose to give birth.

Extending state jurisdiction into the womb

Pregnancy and childbirth, and all of the decisions they entail, are as old as humanity itself, predating any law. The idea that the law should address a pregnancy at all, much less in a way that controls or punishes women on the basis of pregnancy, is a relatively modern contrivance.

Throughout most of the history of places governed by English common law (including the USA and Australia), women were excluded from the public sphere under a system of *coverture*, in which a woman's personhood under the law was entirely subsumed by that of the men in her life. At its simplest, this meant that women had no independent civil or property rights, protections or privileges. It also meant, by reason of our exclusion from the public sphere, that the law had little to say about 'women's matters', such as pregnancy, miscarriage, abortion and birth. Foetuses, like the women who carried them, were essentially treated as the property of the man with whom a woman was identified: either as a vector for the patrilineal transfer of wealth in the case of a wife, or as actual property in the case of enslaved women (Ojanuga, 1993).

How then, did the law come to address human life *in utero* and, with it, the control of a woman's body? The answer lies in the attempts by medical practitioners to professionalise the scope and practice of medicine.

Throughout history, reproductive healthcare – including relief for menstrual complaints, prevention and termination of pregnancy, and care during childbirth and postpartum – was generally provided by midwives. In both the USA and Australia, midwives were historically viewed with suspicion and faced persecution because of their destabilising role in a patriarchal society (see Chapter 11).

In the USA, these midwives were the women who were ostracised and executed as witches in the early colonial days, the Grand Midwives who brought their African midwifery traditions with them in the trans-Atlantic slave trade and attended births for black and white women alike, the immigrant women attending births of the poor and working class in overcrowded slums during the Industrial Revolution, and the indigenous midwives who carried on their traditions even as they were forcibly removed from their homelands and subjected to systematic genocide (Oparah & Bonaparte, 2016).

In Australia, midwives were painted as illiterate, incompetent working-class women working in secrecy without training, and blamed as the cause of maternal and infant mortality (Bogossian, 1998).

By the mid-1800s, physicians in both countries had begun to define their practice in order to consolidate professional power. Pregnancy, which had previously been viewed as 'women's concerns', presented the medical profession with an opportunity to territorially control a continually refreshing professional (and economic) territory. The nascent medical profession claimed this territory by advocating for legal systems that recognised them as experts and their rivals as criminals (Federici, 2018). In the UK and Australia, early attempts by women to do the same for midwifery – by establishing a regulatory and educational base for midwifery practice – were actively resisted until the latter half of the nineteenth century (Bogossian, 1998).

Prior to the law-building efforts of the medical profession, it was generally not considered a crime for someone to end a pregnancy prior to quickening (the onset of perceptible foetal movement) (Means, 1971). Some early common law statements identified post-quickening abortion as a misdemeanour, but generally an infant had to be born alive for criminal liability to follow. In fact, it was commonplace to see advertisements in newspapers offering contraceptives and abortifacients for 'feminine complaints'. Soon after, however, the American Medical Association mounted its first anti-abortion campaign in the USA, claiming superior knowledge of the foetus to seek criminal penalties for midwives, herbalists and other healthcare providers (known as *irregulars*) who performed abortion (Siegel, 1992). In the United Kingdom (and Australia), the medical profession was influential in the development of the law on abortion from the early 1800s, which it used to both establish professional status and further their own professional interests (Keown, 1998).

In many states, this meant that midwives who had served their communities for decades became criminals overnight. Catching babies became the province of the medical profession, and ending pregnancies became the crime of abortion.

These prohibitions set the stage for the interprofessional and territorial disputes over reproductive practice and women's bodily autonomy in the 1960s and 1970s. Feminists pushed for access to contraception and decriminalisation of abortion as a means of ensuring women's autonomy and ending unnecessary deaths and injuries from clandestine abortions. Women begin to seek out the services of midwives, such as Ina May Gaskin (Gaskin, 2002), in a bid to resist medicalised childbirth options.

Foetal protection and pregnancy prosecution

As pregnancy and birth became the exclusive province of the medical profession, the laws to maintain the scope and control that the medical profession has had over women's bodies, continues to be tested and expanded. For better or for worse, bringing these matters into the legal forum has forced courts to contend with whether and when the law may exert jurisdiction over a foetus, and at what point it can extinguish the rights of a pregnant person.

The criminalisation of pregnancy and birth is used as a means to control certain communities, including people of colour and people living in poverty. It provides a cost-effective means for socially controlling the marginalised in order to maintain certain (perceived) social standards. Even today, pregnant women of colour living in poverty are the most likely to experience criminal penalties for their pregnancies, in particular people who use drugs to cope with social difficulties.

In the USA since the mid-1800s, laws concerning access to abortion have been primarily concerned with control over procedures and providers (If/When/How: Lawyering for Reproductive Justice, 2017). In *Roe v. Wade* 410 U.S. 113 (1973), the first US case to frame the constitutional right to end a pregnancy which, in turn, led to the decriminalisation of abortion, the US Supreme Court observed that the states did not pervasively hold the view that a foetus is an entity with legal rights warranting protections. From this observation, the Court reasoned that a foetus is not a 'person' entitled to rights under the Constitution, but that the state has an interest in the protection of *potential* life. This interest becomes stronger as a pregnancy progresses, such that at the point of foetal viability, the state could prohibit abortion provided that women are still permitted to end a pregnancy if their life or health is in danger if the pregnancy continues.

In response, opponents of abortion set into motion a long-term plan, across the globe, to establish the notion of legal status for foetuses in as many places in the law as possible, including the criminal law, medical malpractice, inheritance and even public benefits. This plan began with seeking the passage of feticide, or 'unborn victims of violence', laws that treat harm to the foetus as tantamount to harm committed upon a born person. The aim was to develop a vastly changed legal landscape. That way, if the superior courts were to revisit the issue of whether foetuses were considered constitutional persons, they could rule differently, permitting the criminalisation of abortion not as an unlawful medical practice, but as a homicide. Currently, there are 37 US states with laws that criminalise harm to foetuses by conferring a legal status on the foetus. These laws are passed in the name of protecting pregnant individuals from violence, but in virtually every state where they exist, they have been used to justify criminalising women on the basis of pregnancy outcomes (Paltrow & Flavin, 2013).

In Australia, a similar pattern of criminally pursuing foeticide was initiated which, in the absence of express High Court guidance on the issue, remained the province of respective state legislatures and courts, with limited consideration given to the impact on the civil and constitutional rights of women. In cases involving vehicle accidents occasioning injury to pregnant women, courts have noted the absence of any clear or consistent rules in relation to the legal status of the foetus (*R v. King* (2003) 59 NSWLR 472). In the resulting legal lacuna, judges have assigned a legal status on the foetus which, in these cases, were each described as the 'unborn victims of violence' (*R v. Iby* (2005) 63 NSWLR 278). These legal precedents have since been used to inappropriately extend the jurisdiction of coroners to enable the investigation of stillbirths that take place in the home with consequent police-led investigations (*Barrett v. Coroner's Court of South Australia* [2010] 108 SASR 568). Its use has since been extended, with some states using the concept to restrict access to abortion, introduce mandatory prenatal reporting of pregnant women by health professionals, and the development of criminal laws for 'unborn victims of violence', including from harms purportedly committed by the pregnant woman herself (Crimes Amendment (Zoe's Law) Bill 2017 (NSW)).

Convicted for refusing a caesarean section

In 2004, Melissa Rowland was charged in Utah for the murder of one of her twin babies. Prosecutors claimed that, because Rowland refused a timely caesarean section, one of her twin babies was stillborn. They filed murder charges under a statute establishing a foetus as a person for the purposes of criminal prosecution. Following a public outcry, Rowland was offered a plea bargain. She pled guilty to lesser child endangerment charges and faced up to five years of incarceration (Minkoff & Paltrow, 2004).

Prosecutors said Rowland's behaviour showed a depraved indifference to the value of human life. In particular, it was claimed she refused the surgery when it was recommended because she was vain and didn't want to scar. They could not explain why, 11 days later, she consented to the same surgery.

Rowland said hospital staff were cruel and hostile to her, and she was terrified of 'being gutted from breast bone to pubic bone', which is why she left that hospital and went elsewhere. Even before the prosecution, Rowland was vulnerable. She was abandoned by her birth parents. At 12 years of age, she was dumped in a mental hospital by her foster parents. She had her first delivery – also twins – at just 14 years of age. Through no fault of her own, she struggled with mental illness, a history of poverty, homelessness and drug abuse and she had previously birthed – and lost – her children when she was just herself a child. Society had failed her as a child and was now punishing and incarcerating her as an adult.

The public outcry that followed this and a spate of similar cases prompted the American Congress of Obstetricians and Gynecologists (ACOG) Ethics Committee to warn that: 'In the absence of extraordinary circumstances, circumstances that, in fact, the Committee on Ethics cannot currently imagine, judicial authority should not be used to implement treatment regimens aimed at protecting the fetus' (ACOG, 2005).

It is not clear, however, if these statements are actually influencing change among the medical profession. In 2007, in a study involving a convenience sample of ACOG obstetricians (n = 229) and health lawyers (n = 126), over 51% of respondents favoured use of judicial authority to coerce pregnant women into enduring medical treatment (Samuels, Minkoff, Feldman, Awonuga, & Wilson, 2007). In that study, respondents read a vignette about a pregnant woman who was refusing a caesarean section despite being told that her foetus would die without surgery. Several different scenarios were then presented, changing the circumstances surrounding either the woman or her reasons for the refusal (such as, say, religious reasons). Respondents were invited to indicate the likelihood that they would seek a court order if the woman refused in each of the presented scenarios and to provide a description of themselves. Researchers found that the respondents who described themselves as religious, Republican-voting, or 'pro-life' were significantly more likely to use court orders in several scenarios. In an ordinary regression model, being 'pro-life' was the only variable consistently associated with obtaining a court order for the healthy mother–healthy child scenario. The same respondents were significantly less likely to use a court order if (a) the woman was described as a lawyer, (b) the foetus had Down syndrome, (c) *the husband supported her decision*, (d) the mother refused on religious grounds, or (e) the operation was associated with a tenfold increased risk to the mother's life.

Criminally prosecuted for induction of labour

Anne Bynum was charged with concealing a birth and abuse of a corpse for inducing a labour that ended in a stillbirth (*Bynum v. State*, 546 S.W.3d 533 (Ark. Ct. App. 2018)). Bynum was a single parent living in her mother's home and working a minimum-wage job when she became pregnant. After Bynum's mother indicated that she would be kicked out if she were pregnant, Bynum decided to place the child for adoption with a friend, and even hired a lawyer to complete the adoption process. When she became too big to hide the fact that she was pregnant, and concerned that she would become too attached to place the baby for adoption, she obtained and took medications to induce labour. The baby was stillborn at approximately 33 weeks' gestation. Unsure how to proceed, she contacted her lawyer, who told her she should seek medical help. Bynum packaged the remains in a plastic bag and, knowing that she could not drive because she was lightheaded from the delivery, fell asleep. When she awoke, she saw her son off to school and went to the hospital to be examined, taking the foetal remains with her.

Several days later, she was arrested for concealment of a birth, a crime that had only been used twice in the previous hundred years, as well as abuse of a corpse for having placed the foetal remains in a bag. At trial, the prosecutor attempted to portray her as having ill intent towards the pregnancy. The fact that Bynum had previously terminated a pregnancy was used against her; according to the prosecutor, this showed her intent to have an abortion and conceal the delivery. After four minutes of deliberation, she was sentenced to the maximum sentence, six years in prison. Bynum appealed the conviction, and the appellate court ultimately ruled in her favour on the basis that her abortion history unjustifiably prejudiced the jury against her, and that whether she took abortion-causing medications was irrelevant to whether she had or had not concealed a birth. However, the court stopped short of finding that the facts did not amount to a crime: hiding the birth from her mother, for any amount of time, even when she called her lawyer and reported the stillbirth as soon as possible without engaging emergency services, could be potentially prosecuted. Although the conviction was overturned, she must submit to court-mandated supervision whenever she wants to be with her son.

Criminally prosecuted for an unassisted birth

Allissa Pugh was charged with manslaughter after a breech delivery during which the baby did not survive. When Pugh went into labour well before term, she thought that she was having a miscarriage. It was not until she went to the toilet and felt a foot emerging from her body that she became concerned. She knew from birthing classes that breech babies could experience complications. She quickly pulled her baby out while pushing, and then attempted to resuscitate the baby after it emerged. Pugh did not summon assistance because the baby never cried or moved. She was prosecuted on a theory that she acted recklessly by not seeking medical assistance when she discovered she was having a breech delivery, by pulling on the baby and by not summoning aid after the delivery. She was sentenced to two and a half years of incarceration, followed by probation.

Pugh's conviction was overturned three years later, with the court recognising that it would be difficult to define 'reasonable' conduct in labour, and to impose a duty to seek aid on behalf of a foetus would have ramifications for the fundamental, constitutionally protected right to refuse unwanted medical care, including during birth. This favourable outcome for Pugh and strong repudiation of the notion that a pregnant woman can be required to submit to medical intervention on behalf of a foetus was a rare acknowledgement that some people opt to deliver without any assistance (*Commonwealth v. Allissa Pugh*, 969 N.E.2d (Mass. 2012)).

Of note, however, is the fact that the court specifically emphasised that it was not presented with a case in which a woman proceeded with a homebirth despite being warned, meaning that people who opted to deliver at home despite contraindications might find themselves charged with manslaughter in the event of a poor outcome. Thus, while the case ended in a favourable outcome for Pugh, there is a risk that the court sees the fundamental rights of pregnant individuals as potentially circumscribed by foetal interests, such that there might be some circumstances in which a homebirth might be a prosecutable offence.

Conviction for concealing a birth

In 2010, Keli Lane was convicted for murdering her two-day-old infant, Tegan, in a jury trial where no body was found, no cause of death established, no forensic evidence presented of the manner or time of death, no reasonable motive given for committing the crime and no witnesses alleging a history of violence on the part of the defendant. The prosecution introduced evidence of her previously concealed pregnancies to formulate a theory that led to the conviction. The theory was that when Lane fell pregnant five times over the course of seven years in the 1990s, she had sought 'a permanent solution' to all the pregnancies: by terminating the first two pregnancies, adopting out the babies from the subsequent pregnancies and, as a natural corollary to those behaviours, purportedly murdering Tegan two days after she gave birth to her in a hospital. The prosecution claimed that Lane did this to conceal her pregnancies in order to pursue her privileged lifestyle and her ambitions to become an Olympic sportswoman. Lane maintains her innocence, claiming that she gave Tegan to the baby's biological father. The trial judge, who clearly disagreed with the jury's verdict, noted that two of the pregnancies occurred when Lane was a teenager, and that she had elected to abort the pregnancies to avoid disappointing her parents who had very high expectations of her. Her pain, isolation and trauma in those early pregnancies and abortions, which appeared to inform her later decisions to not only conceal the pregnancies but to attempt to have the baby she could not have, were acknowledged as a form of 'repetition compulsion' by the prosecution's psychiatrist (*R v. Lane* [2011] NSWSC 289: para 29). Concealing a pregnancy does not, however, actually establish the elements required to convict her of murder. Despite the lack of evidence, after a four-month trial, and media speculation, the prosecution won the day. Lane is still serving an 18-year sentence in Sydney, Australia for murder and for lying under oath.

Birthing rights without remedies?

As lawyers working to protect the reproductive rights of women, a question we are frequently asked is: what are people's rights in birth?

This is a trick question. There are many statements of the rights of birthing people created by advocacy organisations (such as the Respectful Maternity Care Charter), and adopted by states (such as laws in Latin America prohibiting obstetric violence). The truth, however, is that the most important right possessed by a person giving birth is the right to be afforded all the same rights with which every other human being is endowed.

The notion that every person has the right to the resources they need for a safe and healthy pregnancy and birth, as well as the freedom to make decisions about their pregnancy and birth free from discrimination, coercion or violence, should be a given, as it is for anyone seeking medical treatment. It would be unthinkable for a physician to call a man a bad father, or even threaten to report him to child protection authorities, for refusing a recommended course of care without which his children may be rendered fatherless. It would likely never occur to a man that his physician might seek permission from the state to have him forcibly sedated and operated upon, or might perform a genital or rectal examination without first seeking consent. It is also highly unlikely that a man's capacity to parent is called into question because he has refused medical treatment. And yet these degradations are routinely reported by people giving birth, in particular, women of colour, women of lower socio-economic circumstances and women with disabilities.

The rights that pregnant women enjoy include autonomy-based rights to make decisions about one's own body without coercion, manipulation or deception, freedom from unwanted restraint or touching – even when that means declining potentially lifesaving medical intervention – and freedom from unwarranted state intrusion into private family life. They also include entitlements to support, such as the right to the highest attainable standard of health, and to protection for pregnancy, childbirth and the postpartum period as moments in the life course that are both vulnerable and pivotal.

It is helpful to consider the context in which people experience violations during childbirth, including coercion, demeaning comments, abuse, unconsented examinations or procedures, misleading information and discrimination, especially when compared with the healthcare non-pregnant people might seek. Based on how pervasive mistreatment and abuse in labour and birth are, it would be an easy mistake to make to believe that people lose their rights upon becoming pregnant, or at some point during pregnancy. That is not the case. Rather, what they lose on account of pregnancy is the sympathies of the legal systems they would resort to for protection and redress: constitutional courts and civil courts.

Civil rights

In the USA, most people's concept of what they think of as their 'rights' derives from the protections of the Constitution, and more specifically, the amendments that describe the freedom of religion, freedom of peaceable assembly, the right to vote, the guarantee of equal protection under the law, and so forth. But the US Constitution, written in the eighteenth century, making it the oldest 'living' constitution, is a product of the time it was written, and reflects the political anxieties of those times. Some of these concerns persist today – such as overreach by tyrannical government, arbitrary seizures of property and persons and suppression of political dissent – but the differences in the society for which it was written and in which it is currently being interpreted are substantial. For one thing, the community of 'we the people' was much smaller than it currently is: for much of American history, only white men were considered legal persons. Enslaved Africans were considered property until the 1860s with the passage of the 13th, 14th and 15th Amendments to the Constitution. Native Americans were not considered persons under the law until the Indian Citizenship Act was passed in 1924, and women were essentially considered an extension of the men in their lives, gaining suffrage when the 19th Amendment was ratified in 1920.

Australians, for the most part, depend on the ratification of international human rights instruments and creation of federal legislation to derive the individual 'rights' and protections purportedly enjoyed at law. The Australian Constitution was written in 1901 by white men, in circumstances that bore little relevance to the indigenous inhabitants of the country. It was primarily concerned with protecting both the British occupants from new intruders and the territorial sovereignty of established state governments. A first order of the newly created Federal Parliament was to implement a unified white Australia policy that endured for over 50 years and continues to inform institutional policy today (Kendall, 2008). While white women were simultaneously given federal suffrage, indigenous people were not considered persons at law until a referendum was passed in 1967! This early division between white women and women of colour proved to be a defining element in maintaining institutions of government underscored by exclusion on the basis of race. Buoyed by a belief in the theory of eugenics, the white Australian women's movement formed alliances with educators, scientists, doctors and politicians to strongly advocate for segregation, sterilisation of the 'unfit' and immigration restrictions (but not universal birth control). White women continued to support the preservation of government institutions and education and health policies that maintained the racial divide, even where to do so was to effectively undermine the rights of all women. This included surveys to identify the 'feeble-minded', forced sterilisations, redirecting education funding to the 'more worthy' and, of course, the forced, mass removal of indigenous children – Australia's Stolen Generation (Carey, 2009a, 2009b, 2012).

As a result, in both countries, two primary gaps leave women vulnerable to mistreatment in birth: lack of specific gender-based protections for pregnant women, and abdication of responsibility for the prevention of harm by non-state actors.

The US jurisprudence on sex equality is relatively new, beginning with cases in the early 1970s. These cases established that, in order for the state to discriminate on the basis of sex, it must provide an 'exceedingly persuasive' reason for making the distinction. This upended more than a hundred years of cases justifying excluding women from public life (such as jury service, learned professions and well-paying work) on the basis that they were inherently ill-suited to powerful roles. Indeed, women's presumed capacity to become pregnant was frequently cited as a reason to deprive them of rights to participate in public spheres. Women's proper role was the propagation of the human race, so this discrimination was deemed natural, as well as beneficial to women and society (see, e.g., *Bradwell v. Illinois*, 83 U.S. 130 (1872) (Bradley, J., *concurring*) (ruling that a married woman could be denied a licence to practise law based, in part, because '[t]he natural and proper timidity and delicacy which belongs to the female sex evidently unfits it for many of the occupations of civil life').

While later case law suggests that imposing a burden or punishment on the basis of pregnancy may be considered impermissible sex discrimination, the lack of clear law or settled jurisprudence has meant that courts have failed to recognise attempts to force women to undergo unconsented medical interventions or to punish them for adverse pregnancy outcomes as inherently discriminatory and diminishing of women's personhood under the law. There is at least one reported case in which a woman sued a hospital and a number of state officials, alleging that they had conspired to violate her constitutional rights by forcing her to undergo an unconsented caesarean section under court order. Her claim was denied; the court reasoned that the state can prohibit abortion under some circumstances after viability, and '[b]earing an unwanted child is surely a greater intrusion on the mother's constitutional interests than undergoing a caesarean section to deliver a child that the mother affirmatively desires to deliver' (*Pemberton v. Tallahassee Memorial Regional Center*, 66 F. Supp. 2d 1247 (N.D. Fla. 1999)).

In Australia, in the absence of a constitutional charter of human rights, courts have relied instead on the application of common law 'rights' in interpersonal relationships, whether expressed in the law of tort or contract or in respect of property rights. To the extent that these 'common law rights' were connected to property and economic interests, they remained inaccessible to the majority of women and were interpreted without consideration of the consequent impact on women. Freedoms (such as the freedom of movement, freedom from discrimination, freedom of assembly and freedom of association) could not be enforced, save to the extent that their infringement may constitute an actionable wrong such as an interference with property rights or a tort.

In the 1970s and 1980s (and in the face of substantial resistance), the Australian Government adopted legislation aimed at prohibiting discrimination on the grounds of sex and race in strictly confined public spheres of operation. A body responsible for overseeing and implementing these laws was also created but which has since endured significant administrative and funding constraints over time, thereby limiting its overall effectiveness as a much-needed institution for procuring systemic or cultural change. For the most part, the legislation provided the means for individuals to bring actions against both state and non-state actors seeking accountability for harms caused by discrimination. The narrative of reducing racism and sex discrimination to the behaviours of a few errant individuals, purportedly easily managed through private accountability mechanisms, has proved an easy distraction from understanding and addressing systemic discrimination in Australia. In one reported case, a mother alleging discrimination and a breach of human rights by a tertiary hospital's refusal to accommodate her in its homebirthing service by reason of her age and number of previous births was dismissed on the grounds that the medical advice was sound. The mother, who was not comfortable with receiving medicalised treatment, was forced to birth without skilled assistance.

This leads us to the second gap in constitutional protections for both countries, that is, the lack of accountability for harms caused by non-state actors. The gap is particularly vexing given that interactions with healthcare providers, where tensions over decisions regarding birth are most likely to manifest, are generally considered private transactions. Both Constitutions generally protect individuals *from the government*; therefore, except under limited circumstances, harms caused by private individuals or institutions – even ones that implicate rights otherwise protected by the Constitution – are not constitutional violations. For instance, in the US Constitution, even though the right to be free from unwanted bodily intrusions is considered a fundamental right protected by the 14th Amendment, a person cannot sue a physician or hospital for violation of the Constitution. In such a situation, they must file suit in civil courts.

Tort and breach of contract

Without a robust system of human rights accountability for gender-based discrimination in pregnancy and childbirth, women are left to navigate the civil justice system. In this system, people seek accountability directly from the individual who has wronged them through a lawsuit for monetary damages either by alleging a tort (such as battery, medical malpractice, or failure to provide informed consent) or a breach of contract.

Ordinarily, any unconsented touching – even if that touching is life-saving medical care – can enliven the tort of battery. Physically restraining a person in a limited space against their will or preventing them from leaving can constitute false imprisonment. Ceasing care for a patient at the very moment they are most in need of care can constitute patient abandonment, a form of malpractice. But access to justice through the civil courts has proven challenging for women who have experienced such mistreatment and coercion (Abrams, 2013).

Initiating a case within the civil justice system has often proven inaccessible because the system is devised around value structures created for non-birthing people. For example, the types of harm people are most likely to face as a result of coercion in birth, including psychological trauma, sexual dysfunction, nerve damage or inability to carry future pregnancies to term (whether from physical harm or phobia) may not be considered compensable harm. Moreover, the expertise of obstetrician-gynaecologists is privileged – even in the arena of physiological birth, where midwives are the providers with the most specialised training and experience. That is, if an obstetrician-gynaecologist opines that a foetus was in danger based on their observation during the birth or a review of the medical record, this opinion creates a presumption that is difficult for the plaintiff to overcome. As a result, it can be extremely difficult for women to find lawyers willing to bear the costs of litigating cases for harms caused to the woman by early or unnecessary interventions in childbirth.

Most medical negligence suits are brought on a 'contingency fee' basis. This means that the lawyer is paid a percentage of the client's monetary award if they win, and does not get paid if they do not. The contingency fee system is intended to facilitate access to justice for people who cannot afford to pay an attorney an hourly rate, allowing them to recoup litigation costs from the person who harmed them. However, the practical result is that lawyers will not take cases that are unlikely to result in a significant award of damages, especially if they include expenses like expert witnesses. In Australia, this deterrence is exacerbated by the adoption, by state legislatures, of statutory defences and procedural requirements which again elevate the opinions of obstetrician-gynaecologists. If, for example, an obstetrician can assert, as a defence, that a treatment option occasioning harm to women is a treatment option readily deployed by the profession, the plaintiff will be forced to assume the costs, incurred by both sides, of pursuing the litigation. These procedural constraints can, over time, create a disincentive among medical practitioners to explore innovative practice and to speak up about colleagues who are practising unethically.

Even so, women have been taking on the mistreatment they experienced in birth, and finding varying levels of success in US Courts.

Forced caesarean section occasioning assault and battery

By the time she was pregnant in 2011, Rinat Dray had had two previous cesarean sections. She wanted to have a vaginal birth after cesarean (VBAC). Her religious community values large families, and she wanted to avoid the risks to her health and future fertility of another surgical delivery. She availed herself of New York's laws requiring reporting of hospital-level caesarean and VBAC rates to find the hospital with the lowest caesarean section rate and highest rate of VBAC success. She chose Staten Island University Hospital because of its favourable rates, despite the hospital's considerable distance from her home in Brooklyn.

She engaged a provider willing to support her VBAC, but he was not present on the day she came to the hospital in labour. From the moment she arrived at the hospital, she encountered pressure to have a caesarean section. After several hours of labour, the physician presented an ultimatum: consent to surgery immediately or be reported to child welfare authorities and subjected to court-ordered surgery. However, the hospital did not seek a court order. Instead, an unconsented surgery was pursued under to an undisclosed hospital policy that applied to pregnant patients. The ob/gyn noted in Dray's file:

> I find the woman has decisional capacity ... I have decided to override her decision not to have a cesarean section, her physician ... and hospital attorney ... are in agreement.

Despite her pleas, Dray was wheeled into surgery, operated upon and suffered a bladder laceration as a result.

Deprived of due process of law, Dray sought justice by suing for malpractice. The private hospital argued that the forced surgery was justifiable because the state has an interest in the protection of potential life. It failed to account for the fact that it did not seek authorisation from the state to vindicate that interest. After more than five years of litigation (at the time of this writing), Rinat Dray has still not been afforded justice (*Dray v. Staten Is. Univ. Hosp.*, 160 A.D.3d 614 (N.Y. App. Div. 2018)).

Forced episiotomy occasioning assault and battery

In 2013, when Kimberley Turbin engaged her care provider at Providence Tarzana Medical Center in Tarzana, California, she explained that as a survivor of sexual assault, she did not want any personnel to touch her without prior permission. While she was restrained in stirrups, on her back and in the final stages of pushing, however, her doctor positioned himself on a stool between Turbin's legs, took out a long pair of scissors and announced that he was going to perform an episiotomy. A video of the exchange between Turbin and her doctor was captured on video by Turbin's mother (who could also be heard encouraging the doctor to ignore Turbin's objections). Turbin posted the video on YouTube in frustration when the hospital denied her claim for assault and battery (Complaint for Assault and Battery: *Turbin v. Abassi*, BC580006 (Cal. Super. Ct., filed Apr. 27, 2015)). The video went viral on social media.

In the video, Turbin can be heard begging the doctor not to cut her and firmly saying 'no' several times. When he does not respond, she pleads with him: '[B]ut why?' she says, 'Why can't we just try?' The doctor positions the scissors in front of her vagina and makes a downward slashing motion with his hand while asserting that, without a cut, Turbin would tear down to her 'butthole'. There is no evidence to support his claim. Turbin is physically restrained so cannot even close her legs to protect herself. As Turbin again calls out 'No!', he raises his voice, and says 'What do you mean "Why"? I am the expert here!' The doctor proceeds to slash Turbin's perineum 12 times, after which he reaches into her vagina and pulls out the baby. He did not ask or receive consent for any of those procedures. It was only after the video went viral that the hospital and the doctor in question responded appropriately to Turbin's complaint.

Other forms of commonly reported forced interventions during childbirth include unconsented vaginal examinations, labour induction, membrane stripping or breaking, vacuum-assisted or forceps-assisted delivery, or manual removal of the placenta. Most of these treatments are not even discussed before the women were subjected to them.

Forcing treatment by threatening child removal

Michelle Mitchell of the Commonwealth of Virginia filed a battery lawsuit after experiencing coercion and threats during her birth in June 2010. With a family history of delivering large babies without incident, Mitchell was happy preparing for birth through childbirth education and the assistance of a doula. Her obstetrician, however, pushed her to have an induction before full term or consent to a caesarean for a macrosomic baby.

Mitchell left her ob/gyn practice and presented to the emergency department of a neighbouring hospital when in labour. All went well, until her medical records were transferred. The treating physician insisted that she consent to a caesarean. Mitchell declined, but signed a form saying she had been warned. The physician was not satisfied. He continued the pressure, resorting to shouting and swearing at her. He eventually threatened to seek a court order to force surgery and to report her to child protection services. Terrified, Mitchell revoked her refusal and submitted to unwanted surgery. The hospital nevertheless reported her an unfit parent, denied access to her newborn and triggered months of humiliating and intrusive interrogations and home inspections by social workers. The investigation was eventually dismissed as baseless.

Mitchell commenced proceedings, arguing that the consent form she signed for surgery was invalid because it had been signed under duress (the threat of court order and child apprehension (*Mitchell v. Brooks*, No. CL13001773–00 (Va. Cir. Ct. Augusta County))). It took years of litigation for her case to even reach a courtroom, and only 20 minutes for a jury to return a verdict favouring the physician. According to one witness to the proceedings, the doctor 'made the best choice for [Mitchell] and her baby'.

As we noted above, in spite of ACOG statements rejecting coercion in obstetric care, studies indicate that doctors who identify as religious, conservative or 'pro-life' were the most likely to seek judicial control over women. This tends to suggest that while obstetricians assert a superior knowledge to trump individual decision-making, they are in fact either consciously or unconsciously pursuing a notion of *moral superiority* – the ideological pursuit of religious, conservative or 'pro-life' beliefs.

As one ob/gyn stated in an official deposition in a lawsuit for a caesarean performed under threat of court order that resulted in psychological trauma for the patient:

> I respect patient's opinion … [But] I have two patients. I don't have just one patient … that is why I disagree with the statement of your, of the American, whatever, ACOG, that the desire of the mother has to supersede the desire of the foetus. I disagree with that … I have an obligation now toward the baby. I've gotta speak for the baby because that is my second patient.

False advertising and non-consented care occasioning assault and battery

There has been at least one case in which a woman in the USA prevailed in a civil lawsuit against a healthcare provider. Caroline Malatesta sued Brookwood Medical Center, an Alabama hospital, for medical negligence, reckless fraud (false advertising) and her husband's loss of consortium (deprivation of the benefit of a family or marital relationship) after she sustained a catastrophic injury during her 2012 delivery (*Malatesta v. Brookwood Med. Ctr.*, 2014-cv-900939 (Al. 10th J.C. 2016)).

Brookwood advertised itself as being amenable to personalised birth plans and equipment to facilitate a physiological labour, including birthing tubs, wireless monitoring and squat bars. On arrival at hospital, however, Malatesta was told her movements would be restrained by continuous foetal monitoring and that she had to deliver on her back. Hospital staff became increasingly hostile toward her, and when she began pushing on her hands and knees, a nurse grabbed her wrists and flipped her onto her back. As the baby was crowning, a nurse pushed the baby's head back into Malatesta's vagina for six minutes so the physician could 'catch' the baby. This caused a tear so severe that it caused permanent, debilitating nerve damage.

Malatesta received a $16 million verdict for her injuries, the first major verdict in a case of obstetric violence. While her case is an outlier, it has sparked a public conversation about deceptive practises and coercion in birth, and may encourage other women to come forward (and encourage hospitals to consider the potential consequences of misleading and abusing prospective patients).

Human rights: privacy and dignity in childbirth

It is now incontestable, in human rights law and principles, that every human being is born free and equal in dignity and in rights. The right to privacy is a form of dignity. It operates as a freedom, built into our social structures, to enable personal choice, association and expression – all without discrimination, and by protecting civil and socio-economic freedoms and equality before the law. In that way, it protects the right to lead a dignified life, to participate as an equal citizen in a democracy, without hindrance.

Anna Ternovsky, a young pregnant mother living in Hungary, asked the European Court of Human Rights to affirm her freedom to choose to give birth at home under Article 8 of the European Convention of Human Rights (ECHR), which protects the right to respect for a private and family life. The Court confirmed that the circumstances of giving birth incontestably formed part of a person's private life for the purposes of Article 8 (*Ternovszky v. Hungary* No:67545/09 (2010) ECHR). The Court found that Ternovsky was in effect not free to choose to give birth at home because of the permanent threat of (criminal) prosecution faced by health professionals who sought to assist her, in this case, a midwife who specialises in providing homebirth services (see Chapter 10). The Court noted the absence of specific and comprehensive legislation on the issue of homebirth in Hungary as contributing to this threat.

At the time, Ternovsky's case was considered landmark for affirming the freedom to choose the circumstances of childbirth as a woman's right to privacy and family life under Article 8 of the ECHR. It also paved the way for a human and legal rights discourse around the state's obligations in relation to regulating childbirth. This was especially relevant to the state of Hungary and the Eastern European nations, where women have long reported systemic and direct abuse and disrespect in facilities during childbirth, while midwives were being criminally prosecuted for supporting them at homebirths.

That said, the limits imposed on the scope of Article 8 in the Ternovsky decision has resulted in that decision becoming a standalone on the rights of women to choose the circumstances of their births in Europe. The Court noted that, in keeping with Article 8's scope as a negative right, national authorities have considerable room for manoeuvre in cases involving complex matters of healthcare policy and the allocation of resources. This 'wide margin of appreciation' has since been used to deny violations, in factual circumstances that were substantially similar to the Ternovsky case, in Russia, Croatia and the Czech Republic.

Looking forward

Given the difficulties that women have faced in asserting their rights in courtrooms and delivery rooms, and the increasing politicisation of pregnancy and birth, it would be easy to fall under the misbegotten impression that pregnant people have fewer rights than others, or that the status quo is a permanent state of affairs. But rather than letting the deprivation of women's rights mire us in despair, we should heed the call to action that they represent. Women cannot afford to stop defending our rights – for ourselves and for each other.

Ongoing attacks on reproductive rights in Australia and the USA, by both state and non-state actors, have precipitated a groundswell of support for reform of laws that criminalise reproductive outcomes and protest against prosecutorial abuses, as well as the election of an unprecedented number of female elected officials. Stark racial disparities in maternal and infant outcomes caused, in part, by disregard for the needs and experiences of women of colour have captured public attention from the international to the local level, thanks to the work of activists and researchers. Artists, journalists, and documentarians have created platforms for women to share their own stories, lifting the veil of silence around mistreatment of women during childbirth. It is working – it has captured the attention of the United Nations Human Rights Committee.

Although there is still a long way to go until we have achieved true equality for all women, a renewed movement for equality and a movement for reproductive rights that includes the full range of possible outcomes of a pregnancy is close at hand. Women are speaking out, and we will not be silenced until we have achieved full enjoyment of our human rights in all aspects of our lives, including in pregnancy and childbirth.

The way forward

- Women must continue to speak up for our reproductive rights – not just for ourselves, but for each other. Remember, in our silence, we are complicit
- Doctors, governments, health professionals and women need to stop making excuses for the way women are abused and mistreated in pregnancy and childbirth: this form of gender-based violence against women can never be justified, minimised or deflected
- Before you judge, condemn or punish another pregnant woman for her choices, ask yourself – knowing the circumstances she is in, would you treat your daughter that way?
- Remember that your rights are interconnected with those of women who may make decisions you would not make for yourself, whether that is having a homebirth, an abortion, or using criminalised drugs. Women who are most marginalised or reviled by society are the first to be stripped of their rights, but the precedents set can be used against any of us at any time.

References

Abrams, J. (2013). Distorted and diminished tort claims for women. *Cardozo Law Review*, *34*(4), 1955–1997.

American College of Obstetricians and Gynecologists. (2005). Refusal of Medically Recommended Treatment During Pregnancy. Committee of Ethics Opinion No. 321, November.

BBC News Editorial. (2019). Alabama woman charged after losing unborn baby in shooting. *BBC News: USA & Canada*. 3 July. Retrieved from: www.bbc.com/news/world-us-canada-48789836

Bogossian, F. (1998). A review of midwifery legislation in Australia: History, current state and future directions. *ACMI Journal*, *11*(1), 24–31.

Carey, J. (2009a). 'Women's objective – A perfect race': Whiteness, eugenics and the articulation of race. In L. Boucher, J. Carey, & K. Ellinghaus (Eds.), *Re-orienting whiteness* (pp. 183–198). New York, NY: Palgrave.

Carey, J. (2009b). White anxieties and the articulation of race: The women's movement and the making of white Australia, 1910s–1930s. In J. Carey & C. McLisky (Eds.), *Creating white Australia* (pp. 195–213). Sydney: Sydney University Press.

Carey, J. (2012). The racial imperatives of sex: Birth control and eugenics in Britain, the United States and Australia in the interwar years. *Women's History Review*, *21*, 733–752.

Diaz-Tello, F. (2017). Learning the hard way: Lessons on gender and power. *Narrative Inquiry in Bioethics*, *7*, 200–202.

Federici, S. (2018). *Witches, witch-hunting and women*. Oakland, CA: PM Press.

Gaskin, I. M. (2002). *Spiritual midwifery*. Summertown, TN: Book Publishing Co.

If/When/How: Lawyering for Reproductive Justice (2017). Roe's Unfinished Promise: Decriminalizing Abortion Once and For All. Retrieved from: www.ifwhenhow.org/resources/roes-unfinished-promise/.

Kendall, T. (2008). Chapter one: Federation and the geographies of whiteness. In *Within China's orbit? China through the eyes of the Australian Parliament*. Canberra: Commonwealth of Australia, Australian Parliament House.

Keown, J. (1998). *Abortion, doctors and the law: Some aspects of the legal regulation of abortion in England from 1803 to 1982*. Cambridge: Cambridge University Press.

Means, C. C. (1971). The phoenix of abortional freedom: Is a penumbral or ninth-amendment right about to arise from the nineteenth-century legislative ashes of a fourteenth-century common-law liberty? *New York Law Forum*, *17*, 335–410.

Minkoff, H. & Paltrow, L. M. (2004). Melissa Rowland and the rights of pregnant women. *Obstetrics & Gynecology, 104*, 1234–1236.

Ojanuga, D. (1993). The medical ethics of the 'father of gynaecology', Dr J Marion Sims. *Journal of Medical Ethics, 19*, 28–31.

Oparah, J. C. & Bonaparte, A. (Eds.) (2016). *Birthing justice: Black women, pregnancy, and childbirth*. Abingdon: Routledge.

Paltrow, L. M. & Flavin, J. (2013). Arrests of and forced interventions on pregnant women in the United States, 1973–2005: Implications for women's legal status and public health. *Journal of Health Politics, Policy & Law*, *38*, 299–343.

Samuels, T. A., Minkoff, H., Feldman, J., Awonuga, A., & Wilson, T. E. (2007). Obstetricians, health attorneys, and court-ordered cesarean sections. *Womens Health Issues*, *17*, 107–114.

Siegel, R. (1991–1992). Reasoning from the body: An historical perspective on abortion regulation and questions of equal protection. *Stanford Law Review*, *44*, 261–381.

14 The role of the coroner in Australia

Listen to the canary or ignore it?

Bashi Kumar-Hazard

> It follows from the fact that an inquest is a search for truth, that it is neither a witch-hunt nor a whitewash. Inquests are not negligence cases or disciplinary hearings.
>
> (Abernethy, Baker, Dillon, & Roberts, 2010)

About the author

Bashi is a consumer lawyer and Chair of Human Rights in Childbirth. You have read her story in the Introduction to this book and in Chapter 9. Bashi would like to acknowledge Australian lawyer Monica Murffett for her invaluable research and insights during the preparation of this chapter.

Introduction

In 2009, in response to hundreds of consumer submissions seeking access to autonomous midwifery and system-integrated homebirth, the Australian Maternity Services Review (MSR) proposed to support greater scope of practice and autonomy for midwives (including privately practising midwives or PPMs) in primary and cooperative maternity care (Commonwealth of Australia, 2009; Dahlen et al., 2011). To the excitement of consumer advocates, plans were proposed to grant Medicare provider numbers and access to underwritten professional indemnity insurance for PPMs in Australia who had been unable to obtain professional indemnity insurance in Australia since 2002 and the collapse of HIH.

Initial consumer enthusiasm, however, proved short-lived. It soon became apparent there would be no Medicare rebates for birth at home and no insurance coverage for intrapartum care at home. This left midwives and women in the bizarre situation of having no access to financial support or insurance coverage for intrapartum care at home. In addition, PPMs could not obtain hospital visiting rights unless they could enter into a collaborative arrangement with a doctor (which has not been forthcoming). Reports of territorial disputes and collaboration clashes between health professionals only got worse in the years following the MSR (see Chapter 9). Collaboration and integration remains fractious and limited.

Against this background, we examine the coronial inquests into perinatal deaths that occurred at home in the period 2009–2014 in Australia, shortly after the Gillard/Roxon Government announced the first set of changes to affect PPMs and access to homebirth in response to the report of the Maternity Services Review, entitled *Improving Maternity Services in Australia* (Commonwealth of Australia, 2009).

We focus on the homebirth inquests during this period in which women chose, against firm medical advice, to birth within the hospital system, to birth at home, either without any skilled assistance, or with the assistance of an unregistered birthworker or a registered midwife. We consider the coronial response to the evidence given by the women who went to some lengths, during the inquests, to explain their reasons for making seemingly 'extreme' choices in childbirth. We then compared those responses with the coronial investigation and presentation of evidence provided by the medico-legal experts.

Through these examinations we ask two questions. (a) Did the coroner examine the systemic drivers behind the risk-taking behaviours exhibited by the women who chose to homebirth? (b) If not, did the coroner satisfy its mandate to seek the truth and recommend solutions to protect the women from systemic harms?

Controlling the provision of Australian maternity healthcare services ('the coal mine')

Three essential elements are required to support the provision of autonomous midwifery and homebirth in high-income countries. These are:

(a) Consumer demand for homebirth
(b) Skilled careproviders to support women electing homebirth
(c) An integrated emergency care network for home to hospital transfers

While the submissions made during the MSR addressed elements (a) and (b), the crucial third element, which is a requirement for collaboration and system integration, was left to the stakeholders to manage without State oversight. Collaboration is a form of partnership between a multidisciplinary health team which is shown to improve outcomes for birthing women. Recent investigations into Victorian hospitals indicate that poor collaboration leads to an increased threat to perinatal safety for mother and baby (Watkins, Nagle, Kent, & Hutchinson, 2017).

In the context of system-integrated homebirth, collaboration is critical to safe and seamless practice for mothers seeking this model of care. Collaboration, without appropriate State oversight, is beyond the direct control of PPMs. This means that, while PPMs can be held accountable for poor outcomes in homebirth, there were no mechanisms for monitoring or assessing accountability by all the health professionals involved (Heatley & Kruske, 2011). This includes accountability for ambulance service providers, emergency personnel, hospital midwives and visiting medical officers whose engagement was (and is) critical to the success of homebirth integration.

Submissions by medical organisations to the MSR provided early indications that any attempt to integrate homebirth would require proactive state management and oversight. Medical stakeholders used their professional power to both discredit the idea of, and detract public support from, independent midwifery:

> All the medical organisation submissions highlighted adverse outcomes for Australian homebirth … They also ignored the research about the safety of 'new midwifery' in Australia and had minimal reference to international evidence for the safety and effectiveness of midwifery led models of care which they claimed are irrelevant to the Australian context.
>
> (Lane, 2012)

This proved an effective strategy. The submissions did not acknowledge the reported suffering of women at Australian medical facilities. They instead asserted that increased deaths in childbirth would result from the introduction of homebirth. In other words, it didn't matter that women were suffering mistreatment at facility-based care because homebirth was (apparently) much, much worse. As we show below, this strategy was repeatedly deployed during the homebirth inquests and magnified by sensationalist media reporting.

In hindsight, it is clear that many did not anticipate the significant pushback from the medico-legal fraternity, despite the apparent costs to women's health and well-being. Structurally, the incumbent medically dominated maternity healthcare system, together with the lawyers, insurers and government administrators who were operating within it, had long relied on a model of care that is incompatible with the person-centred continuity of care model which midwives are educated at university to provide (De Vries, Benoit, Vam Teijlingen, & Wrede, 2001). For example, Australia's caesarean section rates have continued to exceed 30% (currently 34.6%; AIHW, 2019a), one of the highest in the world, for well over a decade despite no discernible improvements in the maternal or infant mortality rate (*Lancet*, 2018). That rate, and the equally high rates of medical intervention during childbirth, shows no signs of abating.

The negative impact of interdependence between the medical fraternity and a country's legal framework on women's health was expressly discussed as a subset of violence against women in the Report of the Human Rights Council on the issue of discrimination against women in law and in practice:

> The Working Group is concerned that many national laws and policies provide for overmedicalization of certain services that women need to preserve their health without a justified medical reason. These include

> requirements that only doctors can perform certain services, such as pharmaceutical termination of pregnancy or obstetric care. In many countries, women are not given a free choice between different ways of giving birth. Caesarean sections, when medically justified, can be crucial in preventing maternal and perinatal mortality and morbidity. However, studies conducted by WHO demonstrated that performing caesarean sections on more than 10 per cent of women does not lead to improvement in mortality rates. Caesarean section rates of 30 percent in some countries demonstrate overmedicalization of childbirth, with the risks of obstetrical complications and health problems.
>
> (HRC, 2016, para. 74)

Suffice to say, the proposed changes under the MSR were always going to prove challenging to the incumbent stakeholders.

Collaboration following the MSR ('closing the gates')

Territorial disputes in high-income countries are an ongoing problem for midwives and PPMs in a variety of settings: within hospitals, between hospitals and birth centres, and between hospitals and home. In countries seeking to increase the autonomy of midwives and, in particular, PPMs, interprofessional relationships are strained by resistance from incumbent participants used to the subordinate role that midwives have traditionally played (Lewin & Reeves, 2004; Fahy & Parratt, 2006; Smith, 2015; Behruzi, Klam, Dehertog, Jimenez, & Hatem, 2017). Their resistance is attributed to territorial disputes to preserve financial and professional interests and a clash of divergent philosophies (Reiger, 2010; Bradfield, Kelly, Hauck, & Duggan, 2019).

In Australia, within hospitals and between hospitals and birth centres, collaboration clashes intensified following the implementation of the MSR recommendations. While documents were created to support the development of collaborative practice models, limited consideration was afforded to developing concrete mechanisms for the evaluation of, and accountability for, collaboration models and compliance, particularly in relation to the private maternity health sector and homebirth (National Health & Medical Research Council, 2010).

In relation to homebirth, predictable patterns of conflict quickly manifested when PPMs sought hospital transfers for the women in their care. Conflicting views about what constitutes 'woman-centred care' and 'risk' in childbirth resulted in territorial disputes (Beasley, Ford, Tracy, & Welsh, 2012). In reaction to amendments to the National Nurses and Midwives Act 2009 (Cth), which increased the scope of practice and autonomy for midwives, doctors reported fears that the expansion of midwives' scope of practice would result in their eventual exclusion from maternity settings (Lane, 2012). Despite that, to obtain visiting rights to support women in hospitals, midwives were compelled to seek collaborative arrangements with doctors – a requirement which has proved to be a significant barrier to homebirth integration.

Swedish researchers recently provided greater insights into how organisational context can exacerbate both territorial and cultural conflict among doctors and midwives, which is of particular significance to the home to hospital context (Hansson, Lundgren, Hensing, & Carlsson, 2019). In a study comprising focus groups of obstetricians, nurse assistants and hospital managers, open discussions were analysed in response to two questions. (a) What is your opinion of the applicability of a model of woman-centred care provided by midwives? (b) What is your professional role related to woman-centred care? The researchers reported that professionals felt a loss of control and confusion about how midwives worked, calling them 'veiled' in a practice seen as philosophically different to the standardised, process-line type of medical care they knew. The more an organisation, like a major tertiary hospital, aspired to assembly line processes and increasing throughput, the greater the capacity to 'mistrust' midwifery practice. The midwives who aligned themselves to medicalised and standardised care, however, were not mistrusted:

> Veiled midwifery exists in a context that is expressed by the other professions as 'a baby factory' – *a context with an organisation that strives towards an assembly line principle, due to an increasing throughput of 'patient flow,' and a lack of staff*. This baby factory causes a tension and a struggle between the midwives and the context they are working in and this, in turn, affects the other professions. The tension depends on the different objectives the midwives, the other professions and the organisation have regarding labour care. It was described that the midwives aspire to work in a woman-centred way, supporting the woman, being there, beside the woman in the labour room. However, at the same time the midwives have responsibility for several other women, in active labour. The midwives are also supposed to take responsibility and have control over the whole ward's workload. This causes friction and, if the midwife chooses to remain inside the birthing room it is seen as disloyal by the other professions. Furthermore, the midwives are perceived as if they fear to burden others and therefore they do not seek assistance. Consequences like forcing the birth process and leaving the woman by herself occur due to the assembly line's high pace and the ambition to increase the throughput of 'patients'.
>
> (Hansson, 2019, p 83, emphasis added)

Notably, in the 'home to hospital transfer' inquests we examined, the PPMs hired by traumatised women refusing medical care were often transferring from home to a high-throughput tertiary hospital, not unlike the assembly-line context that the focus groups called the 'baby factory context'. The woman, usually already in distress, was expected to transition from a chosen model of care that sits at one end of the spectrum (woman-centred care) to an unwanted model of care on the other (assembly-line care). On any view, government expectations that the divergent philosophies between health professionals would simply and naturally resolve in the best interests of the women who were at the centre of this conflict were without basis.

When women become the casualties of a fractured system ('when the canary sings')

Against this background of collaboration clashes, an independent umpire with the power to investigate systemic causes and recommend accountability mechanisms to help women navigate a fractured system was desperately needed. During the transition period, women, and their babies, had quickly become the casualties of the system.

Consumer complaints about mistreatment in hospitals are not without warrant, or novel. Women have been reporting mistreatment, loss of agency and the harms caused by an overly medicalised hospital maternity care system for several decades (Davis-Floyd, 1994; Reiger, 2001). Well before the MSR, minor improvements in quality of care were coupled with systemic resistance from government and incumbent stakeholders:

> ... impediments towards making services more 'women-friendly' lie not only in the historical location of childbirth management in the medically-driven acute sector but in contemporary neoliberal political and economic pressures that both promote and yet constrain change. Research in selected Victorian hospitals suggests that desirable goals are compromised by working realities in contemporary public hospitals.
>
> (Reiger, 2006, p. 330)

Despite these setbacks, Australian women have refused to be silenced on this enduring dynamic of mistreatment in hospital settings. Many have taken to online forums to describe stories of violating, unwanted, painful and traumatic medical interventions in childbirth. These stories highlight the discord between their desire to birth with as little intervention as possible and their reality of experiencing abusive, unavoidable interventions due to inflexibly applied hospital policies and practices (Cole, LeCouteur, Feo, & Dahlen, 2019). Worse, their many stories are evidence that emotionally and physically injuring healthy mothers-to-be has become a normal, acceptable and foundational component of the hospital maternity healthcare system (Klaas, Berge, Klaas, Klaas, & Noelle Larson, 2014; Byrne, Egan, Mac Neela, & Sarma, 2017; Dikmen-Yildiz, Ayers, & Phillips, 2017). In any other circumstance, such recordings of harm to a significant subset of the population would result in a public inquiry steeped in scandal.

Internationally, the mistreatment of mothers during childbirth in facility-based settings has become a topic of intense public health policy and human rights discussions. In 2014, a growing number of reports of abuse and disrespect of women during childbirth in high-, medium- and low-income countries led the World Health Organisation (WHO) to issue the following statement:

> Many women across the globe experience disrespectful, abusive or neglectful treatment during childbirth in facilities. *This constitutes a violation of trust between women and their health-care providers and can also be a powerful disincentive for women to seek and use maternal health care services.* While disrespectful and abusive treatment of women may occur throughout pregnancy, childbirth and the postpartum period, women are particularly vulnerable during childbirth. *Such practices may have direct adverse consequences for both the mother and infant.*
>
> (WHO, 2014, emphasis added)

It is useful to understand the institutional context in which mistreatment of women in childbirth ordinarily takes place. Hospitals, as institutions created within, and staffed by, any given society, will reflect the social norms, values and hierarchies of that society. In countries like Australia, where structural gender inequality and violence against women is a problem, hospital staff can develop expectations of being in control of women within the facility. They feel entitled to use a range of strategies to achieve this control and punish perceived disobedience (Jewkes et al., 2015). In large tertiary facilities designed to operate like 'baby factories' with a rapid-throughput assembly line, hospital staff develop coping mechanisms which are similar to dehumanisation strategies. In this context, staff have even less inhibition when deploying control and punishment mechanisms (Waytz & Schroeder, 2014). This includes dismissing legal accountability to, and ignoring the rights of, a woman in childbirth (Kruske, Young, Jenkinson, & Catchlove, 2013).

The greater her vulnerability, the more likely that a woman experiences abuse and disrespect in the provision of facility-based care. Unwanted interventions, discriminatory profiling for race, occupation and socio-economic status, loss of control in decision-making, failure to obtain informed consent, and behaviours that involve bullying, badgering and threatening, are commonly reported elements of facility-based abuse and disrespect (Redshaw, Malouf, Gao, & Gray, 2013; Freedman & Kruk, 2014; Bohren, 2015; Holten & De Miranda, 2016; Lee, Ayers, & Holden, 2016; Slaughter-Acey et al., 2016; Rigg, Schmied, Peters, & Dahlen, 2017; Vedam et al., 2017). Pregnant or labouring women easily become overwhelmed by this institutional control and will either acquiesce to, or escape, the power of professionals in this setting.

For some Australian women, choosing to birth at home at any costs has been about avoiding these harmful and overwhelming institutional forms of control which, in their view, is the more extreme choice in childbirth. Their descriptions of feeling betrayed, deceived and dehumanised in facility-based settings are often accompanied by a resulting profound distrust of health professionals and a determination to avoid medical settings, at any cost, in the future (Jackson, Dahlen, & Schmied, 2012; Keedle, Schmied, Burns, & Dahlen, 2015). In the Dignity Survey conducted by Safe Motherhood for All Inc. in 2017, the comments posted by women who had deliberately chosen homebirth highlighted exactly where the risk lay from the woman's perspective:

> I deliberately chose a homebirth against my obstetrically trained gp's advice due to a tremendously devastating experience in a hospital for my second birth. Feel so strongly against the model of current obstetric care I wouldn't send my dog to hospital. There are no choices for women. In order of importance it is doctors/legalities first, baby second, mother last.
>
> (SMAI, 2017, p. 15)

Before the Coroners' Courts ('an opportunity to open the gates')

By reason of their wide-ranging powers, coroners were well-placed to conduct investigations into the systemic concerns expressed by women and to test the evidence put forward by health professionals.

In contrast with the Australian adversarial legal system, the Coroners' Courts have a wide range of statutory powers. To remain independent, members of the judiciary are ordinarily restricted to adjudicative functions: receiving evidence from both sides in court and making determinations of fact and law. By contrast, coroners have wide powers to direct investigations, conduct public hearings and make findings of fact and recommendations in relation to sudden or unexplained deaths (Dillon & Hadley, 2015, p. 173). They are not bound by the usual rules of evidence (unless the material presented is irrelevant) or procedures (except for observing procedural fairness) (Dillon & Hadley, 2015, p. 84). In addition, they can make recommendations to prevent similar deaths from occurring. This preventive role sets the coronial processes apart from any other form of judicially mandated public inquiry (Dillon & Hadley, 2015, p. xiii).

The Coroners' Courts can be a powerful avenue for examining institutions said to be causing harm to individual members of society (Julian Burnside QC in Abernethy et al., 2010, p. xviii). This mandate is so valued that it is often offset against the potential for damage to reputation and the impact a public inquiry can have on family members – particularly through negative media reporting. With such powers, however, the coroner bears a heavy responsibility to use the process responsibly – not to punish or single out individuals, but to lift the veil on institutional malpractice and systemic harms, with the promise of accountability and systemic reform that cannot be achieved in a traditional court of law. The potential for recommending systemic change is significant, particularly in the context of maternity healthcare services and the concerns long held by consumers of maternity services.

Coronial interdependence on the medico-legal framework

Over last decade, however, there have been growing concerns about the tendency for Coroners' Courts to overly rely on established relationships with medical practitioners and police officers (Hogan, Brown, & Hogg, 1988, pp. 121–122; Ranson, 1998; Smith, 2004, para. 7.74). Reports indicate that, when investigating through the lens of the same police, medical and public health personnel, the coronial process can overlook the systemic concealment of sinister practices by hospital staff who know how to circumvent scrutiny. Well-known examples include Harold Shipman (United Kingdom), Michael Swango (United States) and Jayant Patel (Australia); all doctors adept at persuading hospital medical personnel to defend fatal outcomes for a significant period of time (Kinnell, 2000; Stewart, 2000; Smith, 2004; Davies, 2005; Kennedy & Walker, 2007). In Australia, these issues persist. In 2013, two hospitals in the State of Victoria with an alleged 'stillbirth' rate that was 2–3 times the expected State average rate continued to operate for over 3 years without raising administrative concerns (Davey, 2015).

The depth of the interdependence between the Australian Coroners' Courts, and police and medico-legal personnel was evident during the collation and presentation of evidence at the inquests we examined.

The vast majority of perinatal deaths occur in hospitals, where there are well-established and sensitively managed processes for managing them in favour of both families and hospital staff. Following a tragic event, hospital personnel are given time to review their file notes, add comments and internally debrief with management. Following an internal review, the hospital's Director decides whether to notify the coroner or to determine that the death was an unexplained stillbirth (which coroners do not have the legislative power to investigate). More than half the late-term perinatal deaths occurring in hospital are reported as unexplained stillbirths. Only 3–4 of 10 perinatal deaths that occur in hospital are sent to an autopsy (AIHW, 2018, 2019b). Families and staff are offered ongoing bereavement support and counselling.

By contrast, most Australians would be shocked to learn that simply calling an ambulance during a homebirth can trigger police raids and interrogations, media scrutiny and an inquisitorial process that denies families procedural fairness, privacy and dignity (see ACMA Report, 2012). As shown in Chapter 17, police will sometimes attend a homebirth when the ambulance is called and interrogate the PPMs without cautioning them. As you will read in Chapter 11, there have also been cases where ambulance officers have simply lied in reports about the PPM's actions. Women and PPMs transferring from home to hospital report significant difficulties with negative, suspicious attitudes by treating ambulance and hospital personnel (Ball, Hauck, Kuliukas, Lewis, & Doherty, 2016; McLelland, McKenna, Morgans, & Smith, 2016; Fox, Sheehan, & Homer, 2018). On presentation, hospital personnel, particularly midwives, reportedly engage in 'fishing expeditions' or take the PPM's clinical notes, actions which later result in professional misconduct reports to the Australian Health Practitioner and Regulation Agency (AHPRA). Families are placed under police guard and their behaviours monitored and documented for anticipated reporting to child protection services.

The nightmare does not end there. When discharged from hospital, the families are escorted home by police officers who search their home and take evidence *without a warrant*, just hours after the mother has given birth, in the presence of the media. The following is a description given by a young healthy 'low-risk' mother who chose a homebirth which resulted in an unexpected stillbirth:

> When we got out of the ambulance, there were two policemen waiting for us. The hospital didn't have a bed for us, so J and I sat with bub in the staff waiting room, with an armed policeman outside the door. Staff members kept coming in, looking shocked and leaving very quickly until I asked the cop to stop them from coming in. He didn't really care. He just kept rushing us to say goodbye to our baby, telling us that it was late and that he was waiting to send the body to the pathologist as there would be an inquest. I asked why and who decided that, but no one would answer me. All the staff just avoided looking at us. When I had to go to the toilet, I was made to keep the door partially open so the cop could keep an eye on me. We were later 'escorted' home in a police car, and then we stood outside while the police entered the house, took everything as evidence, they searched our fridge, pantry, clothes, bedrooms and collected all these samples. They even raided the garbage bins. They put yellow crime tape around the house as the neighbours watched to mark it as a crime scene. All I wanted to do was climb into bed and cry, but then they questioned us for hours. We were treated like criminals. My punishment for choosing to give birth in the privacy of my home.
>
> (Name withheld, NSW, 2015)

Guilt by association

The failure to afford families due process in these investigations can have serious implications for every member of the family, especially the children. Such investigations constitute a violation of their respective rights to dignity, privacy and due process. Aside from the fact that no crime has been committed, the public nature of these investigations is unduly damaging to the woman's reputation, and they promulgate the misconception, even among members of the legal profession, that pregnant women are not entitled to the same legal rights as everyone else. Finally, and most concerningly, mothers are not informed that the medical and legal information being collected can be used in child protection notifications (Grahame, 2016; MacKenzie, 2016). To be clear, these families are facing the imminent threat of investigations by child protection services, *just for choosing to birth outside a medical facility*. The investigations constitute real threats to already vulnerable families who may well reject any further engagement with health services following such treatment. In any other circumstance – not involving the reputation and livelihoods of women – a failure to afford due process in this manner would simply not be tolerated (see Freckleton, 2015, 2018).

If no crimes have been actually committed, it is reasonable to ask: why are families subjected to such inhumane treatment shortly after the mother has given birth? The answer may lie in the preconceived belief that mothers and midwives share the same ideological (and therefore, illogical) zeal to homebirth at any cost. In Dillon & Hadley's *The Australasian Coroner's Manual*, the authors submit the following views in relation to homebirth:

> The safety of home births is a controversial issue that tends to generate passionate views on both sides of the question. Unfortunately, sometimes, midwives and parents err on the side of 'natural birth' when it is unsafe – even obviously unsafe – to do so.
>
> (Dillon & Hadley, 2015. pp 154–155)

The preconceived judgements about the views of the parents are in themselves of some concern (Nissani, 1994). In addition, as a further guide to all coroners, the authors cite a lengthy extract from a publication by a former obstetrician and a medical ethicist (both white, male, anti-homebirth advocates) who assert that pregnant women have moral obligations towards the unborn, without testing the accuracy of those assertions (de Crespigny & Savulescu, 2014). As we show below, these preconceived views, together with an unquestioning reliance on moral frameworks asserted by medical professionals, had significant implications on the way in which the evidence of mothers about mistreatment in facilities was received.

Listen to the canary or ignore it?

In the rest of this chapter, we examine the coronial inquests into perinatal deaths at home in the period 2009–2014, in circumstances where the families chose to birth at home against medical advice. We examined the inquests in which women chose, against medical advice, to birth at home either without any skilled assistance, or with the assistance of an unregistered birthworker or a registered midwife. We considered the coronial response to the evidence given by the women who went to some lengths during the inquests to try to educate the coroner on their reasons for making seemingly 'extreme' choices in childbirth. We compared this response with the coroner's investigation strategies, presentation of evidence and the findings. Within the confines of this chapter, we limited our discussions below to extracting the common and salient elements in the coroners' overall approaches, which are set out as follows.

Dismissing the mistreatment of mothers as irrelevant

Outside the courtroom of every inquest we examined, the families endured highly polarised media and community opinions, many of which inappropriately targeted the mothers. Conservative pundits and medical professionals crowed that the tragedies were a vindication of unheeded medical provider warnings that homebirth integration would undermine the safety of the

Australian maternity healthcare system. Consumers, on the other hand, sought to draw attention to the lack of homebirth integration and the mistreatment of women in hospital facilities as the driving forces behind their choices which led to tragic outcomes. Midwives who aligned themselves with medicalised childbirth practices openly voiced anger and frustration at their midwifery colleagues who were already being singled out as blameworthy in each inquest, often in disregard to the presence of journalists spruiking for opinions or the impact of those opinions on family members waiting to give evidence.

Media reports and opinions reflected emotive, conflicting and largely misinformed community views speculating about the reasons why the women made these seemingly extreme choices in childbirth (Devine, 2011; McIntyre, Francis, & Chapman, 2011; Mamamia News, 2012; Gartry & Arrow, 2015). The mothers were infantilised and depicted as either foolish, mad, selfish or easily misled, depending on the evidence that was given in court on that day. After all, with the benefit of hindsight, it seemed unthinkable that any mother would knowingly take risks with their unborn infant; it was preferable to assume that they did not what they were doing. Media and medical opinions either falsely maintained the erroneous belief perseverance that mistreatment did not occur in Australian hospitals or reframed women's complaints of mistreatment as the self-indulgent desire to have an enjoyable 'birth experience' (Nissani, 1994). As McIntyre et al. noted:

> As a result, the general public are presented with a conflict, caught between the need for changes that come with the primary maternity model of care and fear that these changes will undermine safe standards. The discourse, 'Australia is one of the safest countries in which to give birth or be born, what is must be best', represents the situation where despite major deficiencies in the system the general public may be too fearful of the consequences to consider a move away from reliance on traditional medical-led maternity care.
>
> (McIntyre et al., 2011, p. 47)

In this space of widespread speculation and confusion, the Coroners' Courts, as seekers of truth, had a precious opportunity to understand, examine and explain the historical and systemic concerns from the perspectives of the families, and to test the medical evidence being put forward. The women were the canaries in the coal mine. Through their views and the analysis of the medical evidence presented, there was an opportunity to make recommendations to improve the quality of maternity care in Australian hospital settings.

It was therefore both surprising and disappointing that no effort was made to investigate the views and experiences of the women who made the choices that sparked the events leading to the inquests – even in the combined inquests where complaints of mistreatment were consistently raised by all the women. In the *Inquests into the deaths of Tate Spencer-Koch, Jahli Hobbs and Tully Kavanagh* in South Australia (Combined Inquests), every mother described prior negative hospital experiences that drove a resulting distrust towards medical advice and their alternative arrangements with an unregistered midwife, despite learning of high-risk factors early in their pregnancies (Schapel, 2012, paras. 10.5, 10.26, 10.46). In the eyes of these mothers, coping with hospital mistreatment *was* the unsafe, exacerbated risk they were desperate to avoid. They knew that hospital mistreatment constituted a real (and known) danger to them and their unborn infant, regardless of outcome. Despite that, there were no discussions about the trauma, postpartum depression or post-traumatic stress disorder that may have contributed to their decisions. Consequently, no efforts were made to understand the systemic issues which point to poor-quality Australian hospital maternity healthcare including, but not limited to, the links between the psychological injuries with poor health outcomes for mothers and babies, the long-term psychological impacts on children and the links to maternal suicide, one of the leading causes of maternal deaths in Australia (Thornton, Schmied, Dennis, Barnett, & Dahlen, 2013; Kendall-Tackett, 2014; Humphrey et al., 2015).

The coroners not only did not investigate the violence and disrespect alleged during prior hospital births, they did not even condemn it in principle. Complaints by mothers and, in some cases, fathers were concisely stated and superseded by lengthy explanations about the undue medical risks the women took, their inability to think for themselves and their capacity to be so easily misled. In the *Inquest into the Death of Joseph Thurgood* (Thurgood Inquest), Kate Thurgood told the Court that she struggled to cope with excessive monitoring during her pregnancies and two unwanted caesarean deliveries in hospital. Coroner Parkinson simply acknowledged that she '*wished*' to avoid medical intervention in her pregnancy, labouring and birth (Parkinson, 2013, p. 22). The surrounding circumstances were, in fact, more complex than just Thurgood's 'wishes'. While she profoundly distrusted the medical advice that she was given to have another repeat caesarean section, Thurgood went to significant lengths to engage with medical professionals to try to minimise the risks to both her and her baby. The coroner did not appear to recognise the trauma and distress that Thurgood was expressing throughout her evidence about attempts to engage with medical care-providers and her frustrations at being deceived and dehumanised in hospital.

Dismissing the views of mothers as misinformed or misled

The lack of consideration given to trauma and the prior harms suffered by the women had serious implications for the court's assessment of the women's choices to homebirth. The coroners' findings dismissed the women's claims as either misinformed or misled by the delusional or ideological mandates of midwives, despite significant evidence to the contrary. In the Thurgood Inquest,

Thurgood's evidence of substantial planning to minimise the risks associated with her homebirth was given limited weight. The coroner concluded that Thurgood, despite experiencing two hospital births, seeing three different obstetricians, receiving unsolicited correspondence from a senior professor of obstetrics strongly advising against homebirth and having the support of two midwives and her family, was not capable of forming her own views and was, in fact, misled into having a homebirth.

Similarly, in the Combined Inquests, Sarah Kerr's attempts to explain to the court that she needed, for her own health and self-preservation, to avoid engaging with the medical system of maternity care was dismissed as ill-informed. Kerr was in her fifth pregnancy, had birthed twice at home without skilled support and was anxious to avoid another traumatic hospital procedure performed without her consent (Schapel, 2012, para. 10.46). The coroner responded by repeating the medical advice she had been given and detailing Kerr's supposed errors of judgement. Seemingly to prove the court's ability to bring common sense back to these 'misguided' mothers, Coroner Schapel cited one discussion with Kerr, where he got her to concede on the record that she had taken a desperate gamble to try and protect her well-being, and lost one of her twin babies in the process (Schapel, 2012, para. 10.76).

In the *Inquest into the Death of Roisin Frazer*, Janet Fraser told the court that she wanted to avoid a repeat of the unduly intrusive treatment by a hospital doctor who caused 'laceration and acute pain' when seeking to rupture her membranes (Mitchell, 2012, para. 31). Her distress motivated her to create and maintain a website advocating against, and reporting on, violence in facility-based childbirth. Coroner Mitchell did not appear to recognise these reports as troubling instances of systemic and enduring violence towards women, at their most vulnerable, during childbirth. Instead, the coroner downplayed Frazer's distress, questioned her pain and suffering, and by using emotive words such as 'proselytise', 'propaganda' and 'convert women', interpreted the website as *a threat to healthcare providers*:

> Another piece appearing on [a birth-related website administered by Ms Fraser] is entitled 'Birthrape, Birthrape, Birthrape, Birthrape, Birthrape'. Here medical and nursing staff are warned – *one might well say threatened*, should they 'shove an arm in a woman who's screaming "no", rupture the membranes because you have to tick the box and comply with "protocol" even when the woman screams "no", slash a woman's vagina with scissors and she's screaming "no".' The piece goes on to say that 'your green gown – your stupid hospital gowns will not protect you' and 'I will charge you'.
>
> (Mitchell, 2012, para. 29, emphasis added)

To sideline the evidence given by these women, some coroners made concerning findings that appeared to disregard pregnant women's human and legal rights to bodily autonomy. In the *Inquest into the Death of Thomas Fremantle* (Fremantle Inquest), Coroner Olle asserted that:

> … the wishes of parents should be considered and where possible, accommodated. However, the safety of the child is paramount, and it follows, in cases of identified high risk, *the wishes of the parents always secondary* to ensuring the safest birthing process.
>
> (Olle, 2014, para. 54, emphasis added)

It is not entirely true that the wishes of both parents – and particularly of the pregnant mother – are always secondary to ensuring the safest birthing process. The human right to bodily autonomy is protected by Australian common law and criminal statutes. Both criminal and tort law prohibit any contact with a person without consent. To be valid, consent has to be free and voluntary, not coerced, pressured or obtained by misleading conduct, deception and manipulation. Well-meaning contact can still constitute assault and battery (White, McDonald, & Willmott, 2014, pp. 130–139). So while it is true that the father's wishes are secondary to the mother's right to bodily autonomy, so too are the wishes and interests of the health services concerned about what constitutes the safest birthing process – even when expressed as notionally altruistic concerns.

It would be tempting to believe, given much of the coronial findings we describe in this chapter, that pregnant women are not entitled to the same human and legal rights as everyone else. That is not the case. Australia's most senior court has made clear that any rights afforded to the unborn, following birth, are mediated by the free will and autonomy of the woman while pregnant. She is the only person with the legal right to decide what happens to her body and her unborn baby before birth (*Harriton v. Stephens*, 2006 per Crennan J; para. 248).

In the Combined Inquests, however, Coroner Schapel dismissed a woman's human right to bodily autonomy as purely an 'opposing philosophy' and said:

> As to the contention that was articulated in a number of quarters during these Inquests that an unborn infant at term has no rights in law, this may be accurate in certain contexts, but one does not have to descend into protracted legal or moral debate as to the overall legitimacy of this contention to realise that the thought processes of those who advance it as an argument in support of the existence of an unrestricted right to place an unborn child at risk of harm or death, are fundamentally flawed. One only has to have regard to the fact that in this State [of South Australia] it remains an offence to terminate the life of an unborn infant at term except in limited and strictly controlled circumstances relating to the preservation of the life of the mother to appreciate that the notion that an unborn infant at term has no rights in law is simply incorrect.

> Moreover, the law regards it as a criminal offence to cause the death of an infant who, following birth, dies as the result of the unlawful infliction of injury in utero. *It is an undeniable fact that to a significant extent the law protects the right to life of the unborn infant at term.*
>
> (Schapel, 2012, para. 3.9, emphasis added)

It is very convenient, with the benefit of hindsight, to simply assert that the women were misinformed or misled, but the evidence presented at each inquest paints a very different, and often overlooked, picture. These women were white, middle-class, educated, experienced in both hospital and homebirths, had prior healthy and unhealthy pregnancies, enjoyed strong family support and, in a few cases, were themselves involved in advocating for women's rights in pregnancy and childbirth. It begs the obvious question: if, in the worldview of the Coroners' Courts, these women were not capable of making their own choices, exactly who in Australia meets this elusive gold standard?

Elevation of hospital protocols over autonomy, choice and quality of care

In all bar one of the inquests we examined, the mothers spoke of repeated attempts to engage with tertiary public hospitals and obstetricians, their disappointment with the dogmatic enforcement of hospitals protocols, their fears about being deceived again and their decision to look outside the medical system. In the Combined Inquests, Naomi Hughes explained that, because of her previous caesarean section, one hospital would not 'allow' her to book in for a natural delivery and another would only 'allow' her to labour naturally for a maximum of eight hours before hospital staff would *insist* on a caesarean section. The Court simply noted that Hughes was definite in her choice not to go back into the hospital system (Schapel, 2012, para. 10.26). Thurgood told the Court that the hospital had refused to engage with her on any of her preferences and that this served as a deterrent to her attending a facility to birth. The coroner noted that:

> There is evidence that the nursing and medical clinicians and administrators were prepared to discuss Ms Thurgood's preferred options, they were not however prepared to compromise patient or baby safety by agreement to processes which were not compatible with good clinical care.
>
> (Parkinson, 2013, para. 207)

Drawing a false equivalence between simply engaging in a discussion about a pregnant woman's preferred options and facilitating a real compromise that serves as an incentive for her to attend hospital unfortunately does not actually make it so. The hospital's behaviour in managing out Thurgood for refusing to accept their terms should not be reframed as an attempt to support Thurgood when it was clearly not the case.

In the *Inquest into the Death of Baby P*, the mother informed the Court that she had opted for a twin homebirth after King Edward Memorial Hospital (KEMH) had refused to accommodate her relatively simple requests for a humanised birth (Linton, 2015). These included water immersion for pain relief, having a known midwife and having the ability to move freely during labour (Linton, 2015, paras. 214–215). This complaint and the context in which it was made were important to the coronial inquiry. In 2001, KEMH faced complaints (Douglas et al., 2001) that:

> KEMH obstetric consultants, like many of their peers elsewhere, devalued much of their routine work at the hospital. Public patients, poor and often Black women, were deemed more 'difficult' and less appreciative and responsive than middle-class private patients.
>
> (Reiger, 2010, p. 10)

In 2008, another inquiry revealed that KEMH was again enforcing protocols which restricted the access sought by public patients to simple quality-of-care measures like water immersion, continuity of midwifery care and movement in labour. These were identified as mechanisms that were driving women away from the hospital (Nicholls, 2011). In 2015, in response to the mother's complaints, Coroner Linton noted that women 'like Baby P's mother' appeared to have forgotten the risks associated with childbirth and may have to 'learn to accept medical advice regardless of the circumstances'. While acknowledging that the mother's basic requests had not been met, the coroner stated:

> That is not, however, a criticism of KEMH or its staff as the risks present in Baby P's mother's case were very real (and sadly realised here) and had to be managed appropriately within the framework [the hospital] had available.
>
> (Linton, 2015, para. 225)

In all three examples, the coroners appeared to openly endorse the dogmatic enforcement of protocols over women's simple quality-of-care requests from large, publicly funded tertiary hospitals for a humanised birth – itself a form of systemic mistreatment. This was not an appropriate management of the provision of public health or in the public interest. It was a constructive refusal by a public facility to provide healthcare to a patient which was turned, during the inquests, into a victim blaming narrative on the mothers. By inflexibly asserting hospital protocols, these well-funded facilities had engaged in the constructive refusal to serve the women, arguably in violation of the women's right to the highest attainable level of physical and mental health. None of these well-funded tertiary facilities were held to account for managing out the mothers.

A recalibration of risk through the dehumanisation of women

The failure to address abuse, disrespect and mistreatment has been referred to as the 'blind spot' in the development of quality maternity healthcare in rich and poor countries alike (Lerberghe et al., 2014). Despite extensive research on this issue, the public examination of the mistreatment of women in childbirth in Australia has also been somewhat limited.

These inquests presented the Coroners' Courts with an opportunity to break the professional impasse that has resulted since the MSR, by paying close attention to the mistreatment that the mothers suffered and challenging the health professionals and systems administrators involved to do better. Some of the questions that needed to be asked were glaringly obvious, such as:

- Why won't the medical profession discuss mistreatment in hospitals?
- If women are feeling deceived by undisclosed restrictive hospital protocols and betrayed by health professionals that bully them into complying with the protocols once in hospital, why are the protocols not disclosed to all women prior to booking so as to facilitate informed choice?
- Why are tertiary public hospitals not responsible for refusing pregnant women access to simple quality-of-care adjustments that could have prevented an infant death?
- If medical stakeholders are so concerned about minimising infant deaths, why won't they attend homebirths or enter into collaborative arrangements with PPMs?
- How difficult would it really be to make arrangements to integrate women who homebirth and PPMs into the system?

None of these questions were considered, let alone examined. The Coroners' Courts determined each inquest by maintaining the 'blind spot', and with it, the interdependence on the medico-legal framework for which the Coroners' Courts have already been soundly criticised.

Maintaining that 'blind spot' created its own set of problems for the coroners in the inquests, including the making of findings that were either inconsistent with, or an exaggeration of, the evidence presented. In the Fremantle Inquest, Forensic Pathologist Dr Baber of the Victorian Institute of Forensic Medicine reported that the tragic outcome *may have been the same had the birth been conducted in a hospital with full medical support.* Coroner Olle agreed, but nevertheless insisted that the risk was higher for homebirth:

> I accept the evidence of Dr Baber. Nonetheless, in all the circumstances, in particular the risks posed in consideration of Katrina's obstetric history, home birth was fraught. It follows, the birth of Thomas should have occurred in a setting which offered immediate and comprehensive emergency medical support, namely a hospital.
>
> (Olle, 2014, para. 33)

This finding essentially asserts that a mother should choose hospital, endure unwanted treatments and suffer trauma, even if her infant would have nevertheless died in childbirth. This would have been a confusing read for the parents who may have assumed, like most of us, that the coroner is concerned for the mother's welfare.

In the Combined Inquests, the court findings inflated the evidence given by medical practitioners in order to support the claim that homebirth was a much, much worse alternative to mistreatment at hospital. The expert testimony asserted that *if* the women had attended hospital and agreed to a *timely* caesarean section, there was a good chance that the infants would have been born alive. It is worth noting that, in the case of twin births, the Australian Institute of Health & Welfare has consistently found that, despite the vast majority of twin births taking place in hospitals, perinatal deaths are between 4 and 11 times more likely to result than for singleton births (AIHW, 2016). Coroner Schapel asserted, however, that '*as a matter of certainty*' the babies would have been *born in a healthy state* if the mothers had agreed to have a caesarean section in hospital (Schapel, 2012, paras. 12.7, 12.16, 12.23). The evidence does not support this simplified assertion (Cheong-See et al., 2016).

In the *Inquest into the death of Bodhi Eastlake-McClure*, the coroner took the unusual step of citing two publications, without testing the biases contained in them, to support his assertion that pregnant women had a moral responsibility to prevent injury to the unborn. This was a case where the mother had transferred from home to hospital ten hours before the infant was delivered deceased by caesarean section and, on the facts, the death appeared to be due to the fact that hospital personnel did not listen when the PPM reported signs of meconium on presentation (Dillon, 2014). The coroner excused hospital staff, but concluded that the PPM had inappropriately pursued an ideological mandate at the mother's expense. He then posited that mothers had a moral obligation to prevent injury to the unborn. The first publication he cited was an opinion piece from a conservative, lifestyle e-magazine about an unrelated case (Mamamia News, 2012). The second was a publication by anti-homebirth advocates which, as we noted earlier, was also cited in *The Australasian Manual for Coroners* (see de Crespigny & Savulescu, 2014, cited in Dillon, 2014, paras. 77–78). There are hidden premises in these extracts that the coroner did not test or question. First, there is a question as to whether a moral obligation even exists and whether it applies to pregnant women alone. Second, even if that moral obligation existed, it does not follow that women are required to endure mistreatment in order to observe it. Indeed, expecting women to endure physical and emotional violence in circumstances that do not apply to men is an endorsement of gender-based violence and discrimination. Third, any moral obligation to protect an unborn infant does not equate with an obligation to attend a hospital. As noted by Professor of Applied Philosophy Hugh Lachlan, who challenged the logic and assumptions underpinning the anti-homebirth publication:

> Their conclusion is highly debatable on two grounds. It is not clear that home deliveries are riskier than hospital ones. Even if they are riskier, it doesn't follow that it is morally wrong for women to choose to have them.
>
> … There might also be particular risks associated with hospital deliveries. For instance, mothers and babies might be more exposed to infectious diseases there. They could also run the risk of injury or death in a road accident on their journey to and from the hospital. These risks are slight but so too are the risks of disability that de Crespigny and Savalescu talk of. It is not clear that it is irrational for a woman to choose to have a baby at home rather than a hospital. *It isn't possible to avoid risk if one chooses to have a baby. And it isn't obvious that one could possibly know that, all things considered, one choice was riskier than the other.*
>
> (Lachlan, 2014, emphasis added)

We highlighted the last sentence to raise a crucially missing aspect in all of the coronial findings we reviewed – an acknowledgment by the coroners and medical practitioners that risk is a subjective, relative concept, and more fundamentally, an inherent aspect of childbirth which simply cannot be eliminated. It is for that very reason that bodily autonomy and the regiment to obtain informed consent *prior* to medical intervention are so important to the human rights and health and welfare of all individuals, including pregnant women.

Conclusion

We deliberately focused in this chapter not on rogue health professional practice or blaming individuals, but on the quality deficiencies in Australia's maternity healthcare system that were repeatedly raised, by women, as a deterrent to seeking hospital-based maternity care. Through the voices of the women at the centre of each inquest, we asked whether the coroner heard their concerns and made recommendations that would facilitate changes to help them in the future. In our view, the coroners did not investigate, let alone condemn in principle, the abuse and mistreatment that was reported as driving the women to seek risky alternatives against medical advice. The coroners maintained the 'blind spot' towards mistreatment of mothers in Australian hospitals, and in so doing, favoured the medico-legal framework which the mothers said had caused them harm. That blind spot resulted in a missed opportunity to listen to mothers and to recommend improvements in quality of maternity care.

At any level, the scale of the controversy mounted around the homebirth tragedies, the sensationalist media reporting, the unduly invasive method of gathering evidence and the attacks (or the attempts to infantilise) the mothers were a sad indictment of Australia's social attitudes towards women. It was not disputed that these mothers were desperately trying to protect their well-being and their families from further harm. Aside from paternalistically sympathising with them for their losses, however, no one really cared enough about these mothers or their well-being to challenge the health systems that forced them into this position in the first place. It was much easier to label the women as mad, selfish or stupid. These mothers were the canaries in the coal mine. They spoke up for all us, and we punished them for it.

The way forward

- Women need to unite under the banner of human rights to protect the full spectrum of reproductive rights for all
- The Australian Government needs to appoint a separate human rights and ethical taskforce to oversee the development and implementation of models of person-centred care and accountability mechanisms in the provision of maternity healthcare
- Courts and lawyers need to develop an understanding of the international discourse around the negative impact an overly interventionist medical culture in pregnancy and childbirth is having on womens' common law, legislated and internationally recognised rights, as well as on their health and well-being

References

Abernethy, J., Baker, B., Dillon, H., & Roberts, H. (2010). *Waller's coronial law and practice in New South Wales*, 4th edn. Chatswood: LexisNexis Butterworths.

Australian Communications and Media Authority (ACMA). (2012). Investigation Report No. 2813 – Channel Nine News Broadcast by NWS. 16 February. File No 2012/722.

Australian Institute of Health & Welfare (AIHW). (2016). *Perinatal deaths in Australia, 1993–2012*. Perinatal deaths series no. 1. Cat. no. PER 86. Canberra: AIHW.

Australian Institute of Health & Welfare (AIHW). (2018). *Perinatal deaths in Australia: 2013–2014*. Cat. no. PER 94. Canberra: AIHW.

Australian Institute of Health & Welfare (AIHW). (2019a). *Australia's Mothers & Babies 2017 – In brief*. Perinatal Statistics Series no. 35. Cat. No. PER 100. Canberra: AIHW.

Australian Institute of Health & Welfare (AIHW). (2019b). *Stillbirths and neonatal deaths in Australia 2015 and 2016: In brief*. Perinatal statistics series no. 36. Cat. no. PER 102. Canberra: AIHW.

Ball, C., Hauck, Y., Kuliukas, L., Lewis, L., & Doherty, D. (2016). Under scrutiny: Midwives' experience of intrapartum transfer from home to hospital within the context of a planned homebirth in Western Australia. *Sexual & Reproductive Healthcare*, *8*, 88–93.

Beasley, S., Ford, N., Tracy, S. K., & Welsh, A. W. (2012). Collaboration in maternity care is achievable and practical, Australia & New Zealand. *Journal of Obstetrics & Gynaecology*, *52*, 576–581.

Behruzi, R., Klam, S., Dehertog, M., Jimenez, V., & Hatem, M. (2017). Understanding factors affecting collaboration between midwives and other health care professionals in a birth center and its affiliated Quebec hospital: A case study. *BMC Pregnancy Childbirth*, *17*, 200.

Bohren, M. A., Vogel, J. P., Hunter, E. C., Lutsiv, O., Makh, S. K., Souza, J., …, Gülmezoglu, M. (2015). The mistreatment of women during childbirth in health facilities globally: A mixed-methods systematic review. *PLoS Medicine*, *12*(6), e1001847. doi:10.1371/journal.pmed.1001847

Bradfield, Z., Kelly, M., Hauck, Y., & Duggan, R. (2019). Midwives 'with woman' in the private obstetric model: Where divergent philosophies meet. *Women and Birth, 32*, 157–167.

Byrne, V., Egan, J., Mac Neela, P., & Sarma, K. (2017). What about me? The loss of self through the experience of traumatic childbirth. *Midwifery*, 51, 1–11.

Cheong-See, F., Schuit, E., Arroyo Manzano, D., Khalil, A., Barrett, J., Joseph, K. S., … Thangaratinam, S. (2016). Prospective risk of stillbirth and neonatal complications in twin pregnancies: Systematic review and meta-analysis. *BMJ, 354*, i4353.

Cole, L., LeCouteur, A., Feo, R., & Dahlen, H. (2019). 'Trying to give birth naturally was out of the question': Accounting for intervention in childbirth. *Women and Birth*, 32(1), e95–e101.

Commonwealth of Australia. (2009). *Improving Maternity Services in Australia: The Report of the Maternity Services Review*. Canberra: Commonwealth of Australia.

Dahlen, H., Schmied, V., Tracy, S. K., Jackson, M., Cummings, J., & Priddis, H. (2011). Home birth and the National Australian Maternity Services Review: Too hot to handle? *Women & Birth, 24*(4), 148–155.

Davey, M. (2015). Review finds deaths of seven babies due to 'key failings' at Melbourne hospital. *The Guardian News.* 16 October. Retrieved from: www.theguardian.com/australia-news/2015/oct/16/review-finds-deaths-of-seven-babies-due-to-key-failings-at-melbourne-hospital [accessed 5 July 2019].

Davies, G. (2005). *Queensland Public Hospitals Inquiry Report*. Brisbane: Govt Printer. Retrieved from: www.qphci.qld.gov.au/final-report/Final-Report.pdf [accessed 11 December 2019].

Davis-Floyd, R. (1994). The technocratic body: American childbirth as cultural expression. *Social Science and Medicine*, *38*, 1125–1140.

de Crespigny, L. & Savulescu, J. (2014). Home birth and the future child. *Journal of Medical Ethics*, doi:10.1136/medethics-2012-101258. Retrieved from: http://jme.bmj.com/content/40/12/807 [accessed 8 January 2020].

De Vries, R., Benoit, C., Van Teijlingen, E., & Wrede, S. (Eds.). (2001). *Birth by design: Pregnancy, maternity care, and midwifery in North America and Europe*. New York, NY: Routledge.

Devine, M. (2011). Mums who birth at home are mad. *Sunday Herald Sun.* 23 October 2011. Retrieved from: www.heraldsun.com.au/news/opinion/mums-who-birth-at-home-are-mad/news-story/1e9a5ebd78f0988aa192418a12fdbcf [accessed 8 January 2020].

Dikmen-Yildiz, P., Ayers, S., & Phillips, L. (2017). Factors associated with post-traumatic stress symptoms (PTSS) 4–6 weeks and 6 months after birth: A longitudinal population-based study. *Journal of Affective Disorders*, *221*, 238–245.

Dillon, H. (2014). *Inquest into the death of Bodhi Eastlake-McClure.* State Coroner's Court of New South Wales, Glebe.

Dillon, H. & Hadley, M. (2015). *The Australasian coroner's manual.* Leichardt: The Federation Press.

Douglas, N., Robinson, J., & Fahy, K. (2001). *Inquiry into obstetric and gynaecological services at King Edward Memorial Hospital 1990–2000. Final report.* Perth: Government of Western Australia.

Fahy, K. M. & Parratt, J. A. (2006). Birth territory: A theory for midwifery practice. *Women and Birth*, *19*(2), 45–50

Fox, D., Sheehan, A., & Homer, C. (2018). Birthplace in Australia: Processes and interactions during the intrapartum transfer of women from planned homebirth to hospital. *Midwifery*, *57*, 18–25.

Freckleton, I. (2015). The privilege against self-incrimination in coroners' inquests. *Journal of Law and Medicine*, *22*, 491–505.

Freckleton, I. (2018). Procedural fairness and the coroner. *Journal of Law and Medicine*, *26*, 7–22.

Freedman, L. P. & Kruk, M. E. (2014). Disrespect and abuse of women in childbirth: Challenging the global quality and accountability agendas. *Lancet*, *384*, e42–44. doi:10.1016/S0140-6736(14)60859-X

Gartry, L. & Arrow, B. (2015). Women ignoring medical advice on homebirth 'selfish': Peak medical body says. *ABC News*. Retrieved from: www.abc.net.au/news/2015-06-18/women-choosing-homebirths-selfish-peak-medical-groups-says/6555662 [accessed 8 January 2020].

Grahame, H. (2016). *Inquest into the death of NA File number*: 2015/60842 NSW Coroner's Court (Deputy State Coroner Harriet Grahame). 14 September.

Hansson, M., Lundgren, I., Hensing, G., & Carlsson, I. (2019). Veiled midwifery in the baby factory – A grounded theory study. *Women and Birth*, *32*(1), 80–86.

Harriton v. Stephens (2006). 226 CLR 52.

Heatley, M. & Kruske, S. (2011). Defining collaboration in Australian maternity care. *Women & Birth*, *24*(2), 53–57.

Hogan, T., Brown, D., & Hogg, R. (Eds.) (1988). *Death in the hands of the State*. Sydney: Redfern Legal Centre Publishing.

Holten, L. & de Miranda, E. (2016). Women's motivations for having unassisted childbirth or high-risk homebirth: An exploration of the literature on 'birthing outside the system'. *Midwifery*, *38*, 55–62.

Human Rights Council. (2016). *Report of the Working Group on the issue of discrimination against women in law and in practice*. 8 April. A/HRC/32/44. Geneva: UN General Assembly.

Humphrey, M. D., Bonello, M. R., Chughtai, A., Macaldowie, A., Harris, K., & Chambers, G. M. (2015). *Maternal deaths in Australia 2008–2012* (AIHW Cat. No. PER 70; Maternal Deaths Series No. 5). Canberra: Australian Institute of Health and Welfare.

Jackson, M., Dahlen, H., & Schmied, V. (2012). Birthing outside the system: Perceptions of risk amongst Australian women who have freebirths and high risk homebirths. *Midwifery*, *28*, 561–567.

Jewkes, R. & Penn-Kekana, L. (2015). Mistreatment of women in childbirth: Time for action on this important dimension of violence against women. *PLoS Medicine*, *12*(6), e1001849.

Keedle, H., Schmied, V., Burns, E., & Dahlen, H. G. (2015). Women's reasons for, and experiences of, choosing a homebirth following a caesarean section. *BMC Pregnancy and Childbirth*, *15*, 206.

Kendall-Tackett, K. A. (2014). Childbirth-related posttraumatic stress disorder: Symptoms and impact on breastfeeding. *Clinical Lactation*, *5*(2), 51–55.

Kennedy, V. & Walker, D. (2007). *Dancing with Dr Death*. Sydney: New Holland.

Kinnell, H. (2000). Serial homicide by doctors: Shipman in perspective. *British Medical Journal*, *321*, 1594.

Klaas, P. B., Berge, K. H., Klaas, K. M., Klaas, J.P., & Noelle Larson, A. (2014). When patients are harmed, but are not wronged: Ethics, law, and history. *Mayo Clinic Proceedings*, *89*, 1279–1286.

Kruske, S., Young, K., Jenkinson, B., & Catchlove, A. (2013). Maternity care providers' perceptions of women's autonomy and the law. *BMC Pregnancy and Childbirth*, *13*, 84. Retrieved from: www.biomedcentral.com/1471-2393/13/84 [accessed 8 January 2020].

Lachlan, H. (2014). There is no moral imperative for women to give birth in hospital. *The Conversation*. 8 February. Retrieved from: https://theconversation.com/there-is-no-moral-imperative-for-women-to-give-birth-in-hospital-22732 [accessed 11 December 2019].

Lancet Editorial. (2018). Stemming the global caesarean section epidemic. *The Lancet*, *392*(10155), 1279.

Lane, K. (2012). When is collaboration not collaboration? When it's militarized. *Women and Birth*, *25*(1), 29–38.

Lee, S., Ayers, S., & Holden, D. (2016). How women with high risk pregnancies perceive interactions with healthcare professionals when discussing place of birth: A qualitative study. *Midwifery*, *38*, 42–48. doi:10.1016/j.midw.2016.03.009

Lerberghe, W. V., Matthews, Z., Achadi, E., Ancona, C., Campbell, J., Channon, A., …, Turkmani, S. (2014). Country experience with strengthening of health systems and deployment of midwives in countries with high maternal mortality. *Lancet*, *384*, 1215–1225. doi:10.1016/S0140-6736(14)60919-3

Lewin, S. & Reeves, S. (2004). Interprofessional collaboration in the hospital: Strategies and meanings. *Journal of Health Services Research & Policy*, *9*, 218–225.

Linton, Inquest into the death of Baby P (681/2011) (2015). WA Coroner's Court (Coroner Linton). 8 June.

MacKenzie, B. (2016). Concerns about plans for high-risk home birth not acted on: Inquest. *ABC News*. 27 June.

Mamamia News. (2012). Homebirths killed three babies. It's official. *Mamamia*. 10 June. Retrieved from: www.mamamia.com.au/home-birth-killed-three-babies-coroner-says-they-could-have-lived [accessed 8 January 2020].

McIntyre, M. J., Francis, K., & Chapman, Y. (2011). Shaping public opinion on the issue of childbirth: A critical analysis of articles published in an Australian newspaper. *BMC Pregnancy Childbirth*, *11*(1), 47.

McLelland, G., McKenna, L., Morgans, A., & Smith, K. (2016). Paramedics' involvement in planned home birth: A one-year case study. *Midwifery*, *38*, 71–77.

Mitchell (2012). *Inquest into the Death of Roisin Frazer*. File No 0817/2009 NSW Coroner's Court (Deputy State Coroner Mitchell). 28 June.

National Health and Medical Research Council. (2010). National Guidance on Collaborative Maternity Care. Retrieved from: www.nhmrc.gov.au/_files_nhmrc/publications/attachments/CP124.pdf.

Nicholls, M. (2011). Jumped or pushed? *O&G Magazine*, *13*(4), 34.

Nissani, M. (1994). Conceptual conservatism: An understated variable in human affairs? *The Social Science Journal*, *31*, 307–318. doi:10.1016/0362-3319(94)90026-4

Ojanuga, D. (1993). The medical ethics of the 'father of gynaecology', Dr J Marion Sims. *Journal of Medical Ethics*, *19*, 28–31.

Olle, J. (2014). *Inquest into the Death of Thomas Fremantle*. 8 April. COR 2010 4201 Vic Coroner's Court (Coroner J. Olle).

Parkinson. (2013). *Inquest into the Death of Joseph Thurgood-Gates* (COR 2010 04851). Coroner's Court Victoria (Coroner Parkinson).

Ranson, D. (1998). *How effective? How efficient? The coroner's role in medical treatment related deaths. Alternative Law Journal, 23*, 284.

Redshaw, M., Malouf, R., Gao, H., & Gray, R. (2013). Women with disability: The experience of maternity care during pregnancy, labour and birth and the postnatal period. *BMC Pregnancy and Childbirth, 13*, 174.

Reiger, K. M. (2001).*Our bodies, our babies*. Melbourne: Melbourne University Press.

Reiger, K. M. (2006). A neoliberal quickstep: Contradictions in Australian maternity policy. *Health Sociology Review, 15*(4).

Reiger, K. M. (2010). 'Knights' or 'knaves'? Public Policy, professional power, and reforming maternity services. *Health Care for Women International, 32*(1), 2–22.

Rigg, E. C., Schmied, V., Peters, K., & Dahlen, H. G. (2017). Why do women choose an unregulated birth worker to birth at home in Australia: A qualitative study. *BMC Pregnancy and Childbirth, 17*(1), 99. doi:10.1186/s12884-017-1281-0

Safe Motherhood for All Inc. (SMAI). (2017) .Women's Experiences of Birth Care in Australia The Birth Dignity Survey 2017. Safe Motherhood for All Inc. 15 May. Retrieved from: www.safemotherhoodforall.org.au/wp-content/uploads/2017/05/Dignity-Survey-Safe-Motherhood-for-All-Circulated.pdf [accessed 8 January 2020].

Samuels, T. A., Minkoff, H., Feldman, J., Awonuga, A., & Wilson, T. E. (2007). Obstetricians, health attorneys, and court-ordered cesarean sections. *Womens Health Issues, 17*(2),107–114.

Savulescu, J. & de Crespigny, L. (2014). Should it be a crime to harm an unborn child. *The Conversation*. 21 March. Retrieved from: https://theconversation.com/should-it-be-a-crime-to-harm-an-unborn-child-24407 [accessed 8 January 2020].

Schapel. (2012). *Inquest into the deaths of Tate Spencer-Koch, Jahli Hobbs and Tully Kavanagh*. File Number 17/2010 (0984/2007, 0703/2009) & 45/2011 (1628/2011) Coroners' Courts of SA.

Slaughter-Acey, J. C., Sealy-Jefferson, S., Helmkamp, L., Caldwell, C. H., Osypuk, T. L., Platt, R. W., … Misra, D. P. (2016). Racism in the form of micro aggressions and the risk of preterm birth among black women. *Annals of Epidemiology, 26*(1), 7–13.e1.

Smith, D. C. (2015). Midwife–physician collaboration: A conceptual framework for interprofessional collaborative practice. *Journal of Midwifery and Womens' Health, 60*(2), 128–139.

Smith, J. (2004). *Third report: Death certification and the investigation of death by coroners*. Cmnd 5834.

Stewart, J. B. (2000). *Blind eye: The terrifying story of a doctor who got away with murder*. New York, NY: Touchstone/Simon and Schuster.

Thornton, C., Schmied, V., Dennis, C., Barnett, B., & Dahlen, H. G. (2013). Maternal deaths in NSW (2000–2006) from nonmedical causes (suicide and trauma) in the first year following birth. *BioMed Research International, 2013*, Article ID 623743.

Vedam, S., Stoll, K., Rubashkin, N., Martin, K., Miller-Vedam, Z., Hayes-Klein, H., … CCinBC Steering Council. (2017) The Mothers on Respect (MOR) index: Measuring quality, safety, and human rights in childbirth. *SSM – Population Health, 3*, 201–210.

Watkins, V., Nagle, C., Kent, B., & Hutchinson, A. M. (2017). Labouring together: Collaborative alliances in maternity care in Victoria, Australia – Protocol of a mixed-methods study. *BMJ Open, 7*(3), e014262.

Waytz, A. & Schroeder, J. (2014). Overlooking others: Dehumanisation by omission and commission. *Testing, Psychometrics, Methodology in Psychology, 21*(3), 1–16.

White, B., McDonald, F., & Willmott, L. (2014). *Health law in Australia*, 2nd edn. Pyrmont: Lawbook Co.

World Health Organisation (WHO). (2014). *The prevention and elimination of disrespect and abuse during facility-based childbirth*. Geneva: Department of Reproductive Health and Research.

15 Keeping the canary singing

Maternity care plans and respectful homebirth transfer

Bec Jenkinson and Deborah Fox

> It's time to look beyond mortality and morbidity, and recognise the harm done to women, babies, families and society through disrespect and abuse in maternity care. It's worth getting respectful maternity care right, it just might keep the canary singing.
>
> (Bec Jenkinson)

About the authors

I (Bec Jenkinson) chose to birth my three children at home with the care of privately practising midwives (PPMs) in 2007, 2009 and 2011. In Australia, my choice is an uncommon one; it reflected my belief that birthing at home would afford me the greatest degree of autonomy. I was concerned that if I birthed in hospital it would be more difficult, if not impossible, to have my choices respected. This view is widely shared by the homebirth community. These concerns can deter women (and their midwives) from hospital birth, even if they develop risk factors that may make hospital birth safer for them, at least in the biomedical sense. My doctoral research was therefore overtly activist: I set out to support women's autonomy in hospital maternity care by asking whether a structured documentation and communication process could support women's rights to decline recommended maternity care. My view was that such strategies are both needed and important for the safety (not just in the biomedical sense) of women and their babies.

My (Deborah Fox) research on intrapartum transfers from planned homebirth emerged from a larger research focus upon the care of women who have unexpected outcomes during their childbearing experience. I am especially interested in healthy women planning a normal birth with little or no intervention who experience a change in clinical circumstances that may result in the need for increased monitoring and intervention. This change of circumstances includes women planning a homebirth who are transferred to hospital during labour. I am also interested in how women with pregnancy-related complications may be pathologised by the healthcare system, and the ways in which midwives may support their desire to optimise physiological processes.

Supporting women's autonomy in maternity care

Bec Jenkinson

Pregnant women enjoy the same rights as their non-pregnant peers, including the right to refuse recommended maternity care. Despite the apparent legal clarity and Australian health policy, which emphasises woman-centredness and informed decision-making, affording women meaningful control over decision-making in their maternity care remains challenging, and this is reflected in evidence from other countries (Thompson & Miller, 2014; Bohren et al., 2015; Declercq, Cheng, & Sakala, 2018). Being able to decline recommended care is an acid test of woman-centred care, as midwives and obstetricians wrestle with the ethical turmoil related to protecting the foetus which, in turn, is compounded by professional and medico-legal fears. As discussed in other chapters, for some women, the perception that their decisions will not be respected by hospital clinicians leads them to disengage from mainstream maternity care or engage in selective telling (Keedle, Schmeid, Burns, & Dahlen, 2015; Holten & de Miranda, 2016).

The chapters in this book paint a daunting picture of a broken and inflexible system, replicated across the globe, from which women are increasingly opting out. When women birth at home, with or without skilled care providers, because the system is not meeting their needs, it is not an expression of autonomy. It is an act of last resort and a sad indictment on the realities of mainstream maternity care. If their actions are akin to the proverbial canary in the coal mine, how do we keep the canary singing? What can be done to enable more responsive and flexible maternity care for those that need it?

The findings of my doctoral study have been reported in detail (Jenkinson et al., 2015, 2016; Jenkinson, Kruske, & Kildea, 2017). A summary is provided below. I reviewed cases involving refusal of recommended maternity care and interviewed the women, midwives and obstetricians involved in each case. The clinical outcomes of the women were unremarkable. About half birthed as they intended; the other half consented to more intervention than they had planned, usually on the basis of specific clinical indications during their labour and birth. All the women and babies were physically well after their births. I say this not to vindicate the women's choices as being 'safe', but to highlight that clinicians were able to respond to evolving clinical situations, advise women accordingly and intervene in timely ways, as medically indicated and with informed consent.

Interviews with the women, midwives and obstetricians, however, produced a somewhat different picture. Whether a woman experienced supportive care that valued her journey, or disrespectful and abusive maternity care, depended on whether the woman's refusal was perceived by individual clinicians' as crossing their own 'line in the sand'. The location of this 'line' appeared to depend on characteristics of the clinician, the woman and the situation, and shifted over time. This left women in a very difficult situation, as the responses of care providers to their birth intentions were unpredictable, especially in the context of fragmented care.

I encountered numerous examples of women who experienced this unpredictability. One woman, Jane, recounted her experience of seeking a normal birth. She expressed a desire, early in her pregnancy, to go into labour spontaneously even if that meant continuing past her due date. Jane initially felt that her care providers respected her choice and understood its importance to her. Late in pregnancy, however, that support diminished rapidly. A succession of increasingly senior clinicians called upon and counselled Jane, eventually pulling the 'dead baby card' when Jane refused intervention. Jane recalled being told that she was prioritising a birth experience over a healthy baby. Jane reluctantly agreed to a 'stretch and sweep',[1] during which her waters broke. She then felt trapped, as she wasn't 'allowed' to leave hospital even to retrieve her bags from home. Clinicians continued to badger Jane about interventions she had declined, such as continuous foetal heart monitoring. Jane felt it would interfere with her ability to labour. Her baby was later born by caesarean section. Still, Jane endured derogatory comments from clinicians, along the lines of 'we told you so'. Jane was left with a feeling of having lost the battle: the battle to be treated respectfully.

Jane's experience highlights how declining induction of labour is a particularly challenging situation for women and clinicians to negotiate. It brings together a constellation of circumstances that appear very likely to cross the clinician's 'line in the sand', including:

- Highly routinised intervention perceived to carry little risk to the woman. The more routine interventions become, the less likely women are to be informed and involved in the decision-making about them (Thompson & Miller, 2014);
- Small increases in the absolute risk of stillbirth (Gülmezoglu, Crowther, Middleton, & Heatley, 2012) that sound more provocative when expressed in relative terms (Minkoff & Marshall, 2016);
- Full-term baby perceived by clinicians to be deserving of full legal personhood (Edvardsson, Small, Lalos, Persson, & Mogren, 2015), aside from the 'technicality' of being contained in the woman's (increasingly dangerous and inadequate) body;
- Woman remains 'out of hospital' and therefore beyond the scrutiny of clinicians, who fear that the next time she presents for care her baby will have died *in utero*.

While Maternity Care Plans (MCPs) are commonly used in countries like the UK (see Chapter 17), they are relatively new in Australia. In my doctoral research, the hospital's MCP process was an important symbol of institutional respect for women's autonomy. MCPs were used to support communication and documentation in situations where women declined recommended maternity care. The process required a consultant obstetrician to meet with the woman during the antenatal period to discuss and document her birth intentions, as well as the risks and benefits of all available options. The completed MCP was then circulated to obstetric and midwifery leaders, who could discuss and clarify issues with the consulting obstetrician. A copy was placed with the woman's record and an alert added to the electronic patient management system to ensure that clinicians involved in the woman's care were aware and, hopefully, to reduce the frequency with which the woman must retell her story. Most importantly, the policy defining the MCP process explictly recognised the woman's right to refuse and committed the hospital to providing ongoing care – even if outside hospital policy.

Hospital clinicians valued the MCP process, at least in part, because it endowed the women's birth intentions with the perception of having been authorised. This perceived authorisation reassured clinicians, which protected the woman's access to care and may have reduced efforts to coerce compliance. I theorised that a structured documentation and communication process could serve to expand a clinician's 'comfort zone', push back their 'line in the sand' and perhaps minimise recourse to disrespectful practices. This may be particularly true for midwives and junior doctors in hierarchical institutions, who are more likely assured by obstetric authorisation.

The master's tools

My view that MCPs can be effective at disrupting obstetric dominance and the medicalisation of birth is not without critics. Audre Lorde (1983) famously argued that 'the master's tools will never dismantle the master's house. They may allow us temporarily to beat him at his own game, but they will never enable us to bring about genuine change'. In other words, merely adding women to patriarchal structures does not transform those structures. Her point is salient in the mainstream hospital maternity care context, which has long been the subject of feminist and midwifery critique for its patriarchal structure. Guidelines and processes that seek to increase hospital and clinician flexibility in accommodating women's birth intentions sit within this patriarchal structure. They do not necessarily challenge the underlying values or power structures that exclude women from decision-making about their maternity care, and may perpetuate the perception of women needing permission. In essence, hospital policies and guideline are the master's tools, and by Lorde's logic, will not lead to more woman-centred maternity care.

Reappropriating clinical documentation and communication for woman-centred ends

By contrast, Robin James (2009) argues that we should not so quickly dismiss 'the master's tools' or the benefits that may accrue from their use: 'Appropriately hacked, the master's tools in certain situations and under certain criteria might even be very effective tools for feminist, anti-racist work' (James, 2009, p. 78). The successful reappropriation of the master's tools relies on two conditions: (a) that 'nothing else does quite what the master's tools do'; and (b) that the reappropriation 'collapses the insider/outsider or master/marginalized distinction' (James, 2009, p. 78).

Structured documentation and communication processes, like MCPs, can deliver such a reappropriation (see also: Jenkinson, Kruske, & Kildea, 2018). I have also worked closely with Queensland Health since 2017 to develop the *Guideline: Partnering with the woman who declines recommended maternity care* (Queensland Health, 2019). I describe below the key requirements for creating an effectively structured documentation and communication process for women who decline recommended maternity care.

Including the woman's voice

Many women write a birth plan to communicate their intentions to their care providers. Hélène Cixous's (1976) description of *écriture feminine* ('feminine writing'), developed in the context of literary forms of fiction, seems a fitting description for birth plans: feminine writing can 'foresee the unforeseeable' (Cixous, 1976, p. 875) and 'write the non-existent into existence' (as quoted in Tong, 2008, p. 276). Cixous calls for 'woman to write her self … By writing her self, woman will return to the body which has been more than confiscated from her' (Cixous, 1976, p. 880). Similarly, the popularity of birth plans has grown concurrently with the effort to reclaim childbirth as valuable, even sublime experience (Lintott, 2013). That is, birth plans have, as Cixous suggested in the context of feminine writing, served 'as a springboard for subversive thought, the precursory movement of a transformation of social and cultural structures' (Cixous, 1976, p. 879).

As subversive thought and social transformation provoked opposition, so too birth plans are greeted with hostility in some settings (Lothian, 2006; White-Corey, 2013). The proliferation of online birth plan templates has, in some cases, reduced the concept to a list of checkboxes, perhaps in an attempt to render them acceptable to a medical audience (Lothian, 2006); such birth plans bear little resemblance to Cixous's feminine writing. However, when a woman's own textual account of her aspirations for birth is made part of her clinical record, she writes herself into that record, thereby disrupting the 'insider/outsider hierarchy' (James, 2009, p. 95) which usually excludes her from decision-making. The clinical record no longer consists of only clinician accounts (i.e. insiders). Through MCPs, the woman can seize 'the occasion to speak' (Cixous, 1976, p. 880).

According to Cixous (as quoted in Tong, 2008, p. 276), unlike feminine writing, male writing is 'stamped with the official seal of social approval' and contained within sharply defined and rigidly imposed structures. This is an apt description of a clinical form! That said, this seal of approval may be useful to women: when MCPs are (as in my study) authored by consultant obstetricians, the women's birth preferences were endowed with a perception of authorisation. This perceived obstetric authorisation benefits the woman because it reassures the clinicians and the health service about their own medico-legal, reputational and professional exposure. While women (rightly) may not share the view that they need 'permission' to decline recommended care (Pascucci, 2014), clinicians working in hierarchical hospital settings are concerned that *they* need permission to deviate from local protocols. Without robust documentation and the medico-legal protection it provides to the health service and its employees, clinicians expect professional censure if their practice deviates from local policies.

James' (2009) view that the master's tools can be appropriately hacked for feminist ends supports the approach we took within Queensland. Because 'all agency arises from one's insertion in networks of power relations, the process must be "recognizable" to the "master's" system(s) in order to participate in the working(s) of power in the first place' (James, 2009, p. 84). Birth plans do not participate in the workings of power within a hospital in the same way that an MCP can. They are not recognisable to the master's system, whereas an MCP is. To effectively 'hack' a care plan, however, the woman's voice must be included. This satisfies James' criteria and mindfully deploys the master's tools to secure more respectful woman-centred care.

Widely promoted

A prerequisite to the MCP process must be raising awareness among women of their right to refuse recommended care (along with their other healthcare rights) and of the availability of an MCP process. Some women hesitate to refuse recommended care, for fear of repercussions like neglect or being refused care. Broadly informing them about their right to refuse recommended care is important so they do not decide to either avoid care (Ireland, Wulili Narjic, Belton, & Kildea, 2011) or engage in 'selective telling' (Keedle et al., 2015, p. 1), each of which can diminish the quality and safety of maternity care. Just the existence of a structured process for documenting and communicating the refusal of recommended care can shift the balance of power in the provision of maternity care. It assures the woman that she will not be refused access to care at the hospital. It opens the door to a conversation about the risks and benefits of birth intentions, the woman's reasons for those birth intentions, and if relevant, provides an opportunity for clinicians to make proactive plans for a safe birth. It does not mean that clinicians change their advice and 'agree' with a 'risky' birth intention; it means they disagree *and* provide care anyway. The MCP is about harm minimisation, rather than prohibition, 'mak[ing] and support [ing] options that may make certain behaviours less risky, even if not risk free or recommended' (Ecker & Minkoff, 2011, p. 1182).

Scaffolded

A structured documentation approach uses clinical forms to scaffold balanced and sensitive conversations with women, as well as high-quality documentation of those conversations. It is appropriate to investigate why a woman is declining a procedure, and to supply information that fills a knowledge gap or addresses a misconception. However, the line between informing, maybe even respectfully persuading, and pressuring or coercion is difficult to locate. Shaw and Elger (2013) identify three different types of persuasion, only the first of which is always appropriate: the removal of biases, recommending a particular course of action and providing evidence and reasons in favour of it, and the creation of new biases. The latter of these, involving for example the manipulation of information to overstate benefit or understate risk, is 'unacceptable' (Shaw & Elger, 2013, p. 1689).

By communicating appropriate, unbiased information about the risks *and* benefits to *both* the woman and her baby of recommended care *and* its alternatives (and there are always alternatives), clinicians can inform the woman (removing bias) without creating new biases. Where there is clear evidence in favour of a particular course, where the benefits clearly outweigh the risks, clinicians are justified in recommending that course (Kotaska, 2017), but giving information so relentlessly that, eventually, the woman is 'bulldozed' into compliance is unacceptable. Where the evidence is equivocal or difficult to apply to the woman's unique individual circumstances or where the clinician judges the risks and benefits to be of similar weight, more tentative advice is appropriate: offering, rather than recommending (Kotaska, 2017). This balanced approach may be challenging to deliver, especially in the maternity context (Minkoff & Marshall, 2016), and therefore needs to be scaffolded by appropriate guidance and clinical forms which offer discussion prompts and reminders to clinicians.

The women in my study encountered unacceptable forms of persuasion including, at the least intrusive end, (over)emphasising risks to the foetus and downplaying risks to the woman to favour intervention for foetal benefit. Such approaches overlook considerations the woman may prioritise, be they current and future biomedical risks or psychological, social, cultural and spiritual risks (Barclay et al., 2016). It also sets up the so-called 'maternal–foetal conflict': pitting the woman against her foetus and creating an erroneous perception that women who decline recommended maternity care are pursuing a particular experience 'at any cost' (Edwards & Murphy-Lawless, 2006).

Refusal of recommended maternity care is more appropriately conceptualised as a conflict between the woman's autonomy and her care provider's judgement about foetal interests (Oberman, 2000). The conventional construction of the pregnant woman as a threat to her foetus which requires rescuing by paternalistic clinicians is unhelpfully narrow (Harris, 2000, p. 789). By understanding the social and family relationships, context and constraints on a woman's decision-making, the pregnant woman and foetus retain their status as a single unit, with foetal well-being best protected by supporting maternal well-being (Laufer-Ukeles, 2011). This reflects feminist understandings of autonomy as a relational, rather than individualistic, construct and underpins a broad, comprehensive and bias- and conflict-aware account of refusal (Laufer-Ukeles, 2011).

Understanding the woman's perspective was a key component of supportive care interactions for both women and clinicians in my doctoral research, but it was apparently rarely the focus of communication. An effective structured document and communication process would therefore scaffold opportunities for clinicians to develop this understanding. Doing so may support clinicians to maintain respectful care practices (Minkoff & Paltrow, 2007; Scott, 2007) as they listen more closely to women's knowledge, experiences and anxieties (Edwards & Murphy-Lawless, 2006).

Flexible initiation

It is also important that a wide range of stakeholders, including women, are able to initiate the structured documentation and communication process. In the MCP process, the benefits of obstetric authorisation particularly accrued to junior doctors and midwives who felt protected from professional censure, yet these clinicians were unable to initiate the process directly. Likewise, women frequently didn't know that a care plan had been created for them, or what this meant. Other women who might have valued that additional discussion and communication had no way of making it happen. By making the clinical forms available to women, a radical power shift could occur: rather than relying only on clinicians to identify women on the basis of their own 'comfort zone', a woman could initiate the process as a way of seeking additional discussion and shoring up support for her anticipated birth.

It is also important that an MCP is developed as soon as a woman indicates her intention to decline recommended care. Clinicians are understandably keen to avoid the additional documentation requirements of an early MCP, but delays have unintended consequences. In my doctoral study, MCPs were only initiated late in pregnancy; the women were still exposed to repeated rounds of counselling about risk, which women and midwives perceive to be 'badgering'. Late care plans affect the opportunity to plan steps to maximise the chances of good outcomes, such as in the care of women who decline blood products (Belaouchi et al., 2016; Kidson-Gerber et al., 2016). A woman-centred approach to the process will require an early discussion whenever a woman signals her intention to decline recommended care.

It is clear that women want to discuss the management of their labour and birth. Women regularly use social media to ask whether a particular hospital will 'allow' them to labour and birth in a particular way. They also describe experiences of being told they are 'not allowed' to birth in a particular way. In some cases, the comments that follow or the woman's question itself point to using homebirth as an escape from inflexible hospital policies. For the woman who prefers hospital birth, a structured documentation and communication process that enabled her to initiate a conversation with her care providers may be more effective. In Queensland, where the *Guideline: Partnering with the woman who declines recommended maternity care* (Queensland Health, 2019) is now available online and has recently been trialled in several hospitals, offering a pathway for the woman to initiate the care plan, the MCP is becoming a reality.

A shared, living document

Regardless of how it is initiated, an MCP should be circulated to all clinicians likely to be involved in the woman's care. Appropriately informing clinicians about the woman's circumstances and decisions may help to establish a respectful atmosphere in future clinical encounters and prevent the woman from having to 'tell her story' repeatedly (Zeybek et al., 2016). It is also an opportunity for constructive discussion among clinicians, which is respectful of each clinician's autonomy, while still protecting the woman's access to care. It may also contribute to improving the quality of documentation over time.

The woman's care plan must be a 'living' document. That is, it can and should be reviewed at the onset of labour or if the woman's intentions or clinical indications change. Women who decline recommended maternity care are not seeking a birth experience at the expense of (physical) safety (Edwards & Murphy-Lawless, 2006; Downe, 2015). They want to discuss alternatives in the event of changes to their clinical indications. This kind of responsiveness to changing indications serves as a safety net.

A failsafe[2]

Sound MCPs require a failsafe or back-up plan in the event of a dispute. Structured documentation and communication processes do not guarantee respectful care, nor protect clinicians entirely from criticism and professional censure. A Respectful Maternity Care Advocate (RMCA) should be established to mediate conflict.

The concept of an RMCA borrows from the UK's Supervisor of Midwives (SoM) role, which provided (among other functions) supported midwives and women when women declined recommended care (Carr, 2008; Read & Wallace, 2014), but with some important distinctions. The establishment of SoMs in Australia was recommended by a review of midwifery professional indemnity insurance arrangements in Australia (Price Waterhouse Coopers Australia, 2013), but has not gained political support. This may be because the term 'supervision' has multiple meanings and a history of surveillance, assessment and misuse of power (Lennox, Skinner, & Foureur, 2008). The UK SoM model also recently faced significant changes (Department of Health, 2016) in response to concerns expressed about overlap with regulatory processes (Baird, Murray, Seale, Foot, & Perry, 2015; Murphy, 2016) and between managerial and clinical supervision in employed practice contexts

(Nipper & Roseghini, 2014). The RMCA role proposed here should be independent of both Australian medical and midwifery regulatory authorities and health services.

Another important distinction is the wider role played by RMCAs. The RMCA should provide on-call, real-time support and mediation at any stage of care, even if that be by telephone, to clinicians, women and health services, in situations of maternal refusal. The proposed role's focus is on supporting all parties in the practice of respectful maternity care, debriefing and reflecting on their experiences and supporting the health service by providing a quality-assurance mechanism.

Conclusion

Woman-centred care is the widely touted tenet of progressive maternity services policy in Australia (and abroad), but refusal represents something of an 'acid test' to that mantra. When women decline recommended care, clinicians are required to provide care on the woman's terms, even where that carries an increased risk and is at odds with evidence-based clinical guidelines. Woman-centred care in the current hospital context is difficult to achieve, particularly where beliefs about foetal rights are not disclosed. The challenge is amplified by hierarchical, medicalised maternity services, where concerns about medico-legal exposure and professional censure drive practice.

Midwives and obstetricians regularly espouse respect for women's rights to refuse and strive to provide respectful maternity care. Knowing the right thing to do is necessary, but not sufficient, for actually doing it. It is time to look beyond mortality and morbidity, and recognise the harm done to women, babies, families and society by disrespect and abuse in maternity care. It is worth getting respectful maternity care right as it may just keep the canary singing.

The way forward

- Build strategic maternity policy on the foundation of *Respectful maternity care: The Universal right of childbearing women* (White Ribbon Alliance, 2011)
- Support the development and implementation of structured documentation and communication processes for use when women decline recommended maternity care. These need to be 'appropriately hacked' to deliver a woman-centred approach by
  - Directly including the woman's voice
  - Being widely promoted and accessible to women
  - Scaffolding high-quality, balanced and respectful discussions between women and clinicians, and thorough documentation thereof
  - Embedding flexible pathways for the initiation of the process

- Yielding a shared living document for reference throughout the woman's maternity care
- Establishing and funding a new role in maternity services to act as a fail-safe: the Respectful Maternity Care Advocate, to provide on-call, real-time support and mediation at any stage of care to clinicians, women and health services

Principles for handover in the homebirth transfer context

Deborah Fox

> Homebirth transfer is a complex social process that disrupts and challenges the status quo for everyone involved, not just the woman and the homebirth midwife.
>
> (Deborah Fox)

Planned homebirth is safe for healthy women with low-risk pregnancies when professional midwifery care and collaborative arrangements for medical referral and transfer are in place (Catling-Paull, Coddington, Foureur, & Homer, 2013; Keirse, 2014; de Jonge et al., 2013; Hutton et al., 2016). Sometimes, women and the midwives caring for them at home make the decision to transfer to hospital during labour. Transfer most often occurs for non-urgent indications, such as delayed progress in labour, or a woman's request for pharmacological pain management. Very small numbers of women are transferred due to emergencies (Amelink-Verburg et al., 2008; Lindgren, Hildingsson, Christensson, & Rådestad, 2008; Rowe et al., 2013; Blix et al., 2016). Women and newborns are also transferred soon after birth at home in smaller numbers, but the focus of our study was upon interactions that occurred when a woman is transferred during labour.

Timely referral, consultation and transfer, and smooth collaboration between caregivers is important for the safety and well-being of women and their babies when place of birth and caregivers change (Downe, Finlayson, & Fleming, 2010). The quality of the handover communication has the capacity to influence the level of collaborative interactions and processes that ensue.

Handover communication between multidisciplinary health professionals can be problematic because of the different perspectives and priorities held within each discipline. In the absence of policy, successful handovers often occur simply due to the presence of trust and mutual respect between health professionals who may be familiar (Cyna, Andrew, Tan, & Smith, 2011). In the homebirth transfer context, handover interactions have the capacity to support collaboration between women, and homebirth and hospital caregivers, by establishing the patterns of communication that follow. High-quality transfer processes are a crucial element of the provision of safe and woman centred homebirth services (Cheyney & Everson, 2009; Vedam et al., 2012, 2014; McLachan et al., 2016; Fox, Sheehan, & Homer, 2018a).

This next section was adapted from a larger qualitative research study exploring the processes and interactions involved in the intrapartum transfer of a woman from planned homebirth to hospital (Fox et al., 2018a). We interviewed 36 women, midwives and obstetricians who worked in a variety of contexts including in publicly funded homebirth programmes, through private midwifery practices and in public hospitals which receive transferred women. Handover processes were especially challenging for midwives in private practice and the women they care for. When a privately practising midwife (PPM) transferred with a woman to a public hospital in which the midwife did not have visiting rights, they were expected to provide a professional handover at the time they simultaneously lost their clinical rights to practice. Due to the absence of guidelines and the perceived lesser status of the PPM, individual hospital staff were left to choose whether to take any notice of the handover or not. This was more likely to occur if the PPM was not known to hospital staff. When PPMs felt that their handover was disregarded, they were concerned about the potential impact on the woman's care. Poorly managed interactions during the handover of care of a woman transferred to hospital from planned homebirth have the capacity to delay care and increase levels of uncertainty for hospital staff, which may impact upon the health, safety and well-being of the woman and her baby.

Detailed findings of the studies that lay the foundation for these handover principles are published elsewhere (Vedam et al., 2014; Fox et al., 2018a; 2018b). We provide a summary below, as background to the development of the 'Principles for handover in the homebirth transfer context'.

Transferring out of the comfort zone

When transferring, women made the journey to hospital as well as making a psychological journey out of their comfort zone. While hospitals often wanted to immediately expedite their labour, the women valued having time to process their psychological journey, adjust to a new environment, think about their options and manage their changing expectations for the birth of their baby.

Hospital staff reported that women often resisted monitoring and intervention after transfer and perceived them to be 'difficult' to care for. The women reported simply buying time to process and adapt to what was happening for them. Most transferred women felt pressured and 'on the clock' as soon as they entered the hospital.

Midwives also often felt as if they were transferring out of their comfort zone. Transfer events result in a convergence of women, midwives and obstetricians, each of whom possesses conflicting paradigms of childbearing derived from educational, professional and life experiences. This issue has the capacity to reconstruct women's labour and birth experiences into complex and unique clinical circumstances.

The power of the midwife–woman partnership

Strong relationships based on trust develop between women and their homebirth midwives during pregnancy, often referred to as the 'midwife–woman partnership' (Boyle, Thomas, & Brooks, 2016). One woman described what this meant for her:

> It was good to know that she would always be there and be our advocate … she could stand up for us … she was the support structure for us and knowing she would be with us … in the hospital, was brilliant.
>
> (Homebirth woman)

Reciprocal trust was a key element of the partnership for participants. Women planning a homebirth invested time and energy into making informed decisions about their care and place of birth, with their midwives. Women trusted their midwives to transfer them when necessary, and to *not* suggest transferring them unless it *was* necessary. Knowing that her decision-making was guided by her known midwife was important:

> I didn't mind others advising me if I had a relationship of trust with them. That was the critical thing with me.
>
> (Homebirth woman)

In Australia, at the time of writing, PPMs lose their rights to practise in most hospitals. During transfer, they are relegated to the role of a support person. Despite this, they continue to provide emotional and physical support, and advocacy. Our research clearly showed that the midwife–woman partnership had a powerful capacity to support women through their changing expectations for birth and the uncertainty of transfer.

The midwife–woman partnership, despite its value, had the capacity to create barriers to collaboration when hospital midwives felt unsure how to fit into the dynamic. Some sought to avoid it if possible, for example:

> I have tried to avoid being allocated to 'these women' … If I could avoid a homebirth transfer I would.
>
> (Hospital midwife)

The presence of the powerful midwife–woman partnership and the conflicting paradigms were some of the social processes that contributed to an 'us and them' dynamics.

Encountering 'us and them'

Midwives often encountered 'us and them' dynamics in the birthing room of a transferred woman. 'Us and them' behaviours include stereotyping, resisting, blaming and taking over. A lack of clarity around respective roles and responsibilities had the potential to cause conflict between midwives. Hospital midwives often perceived the need to take over, while PPMs were striving to continue to support and advocate for the woman.

For PPMs unable to practise in hospital, negotiating their role in the birth space was especially complex when hospital policy required staff to take over the woman's care, clinically and emotionally. One hospital midwife explained this by saying:

> The hospital protocol was that they [privately practising midwives] were there as support person only … we were then responsible for that mother and baby.
>
> (Hospital midwife)

Hospital midwives had different perspectives on what constituted 'taking over'. Some were adamant that their role was to take over the woman's care in every sense. This reflected their routine experience of receiving the care of a woman at a change of shift, by taking over from another midwife who would leave her to continue the care. Others felt this was an unfortunate approach that led to breakdown in trust and cooperation:

> The [privately practising] midwives that are coming in are just pushed to the side, they are not allowed to do anything … there's no discourse of communication … that I'd have with a midwife, normally … with my colleagues on a shift. So, they're not even given a say, so I don't think trust can be built in that setting, whatsoever.
>
> (Hospital midwife)

Understanding the social process driving problematic interactions between midwives in the homebirth transfer context

Our findings about the power of the midwife–woman partnership and conflicting paradigms of childbearing in the birthing room of a transferred woman build upon Melissa Cheyney's (see Chapter 18) concept of a 'contested space' (Cheyney, Everson, & Burcher, 2014, p. 451). The barriers to collaboration in the homebirth transfer context extend further, to the influences of 'us and them' dynamics. The social dynamics between professional groups add another layer to the psychological and cultural influences that drive individual behaviours. All this can be assessed through a social psychology lens known as the theory of 'intergroup conflict'.

Intergroup conflict theory analyses human interaction by situating individuals within social processes and making distinctions between personal identity and group identity (Hogg & Abrams, 2001; Hogg, 2015). To increase confidence and self-esteem, humans align themselves with groups of like-minded individuals. Seeking a group identity is known to be an effective way to reduce feelings of uncertainty because it enables individuals to predict the behaviours of others and plan their actions accordingly. Common examples include the way in which we identify with those who have similar political or religious views. In situations of uncertainty, we boost the perceived status of our in-group and discriminate against the 'other' out-group. That discrimination motivates individuals to adopt negative behaviours such as stereotyping, blaming and trying to control others. What follows is an 'us and them' situation. In settings where high levels of collaboration are required, the presence of intergroup conflict creates a barrier to the flow of communication and to understanding the perspectives of others. The homebirth transfer context may be one such setting.

Intergroup conflict theory is particularly helpful for analysing birth room interactions given the influence that oxytocin has on intergroup behaviours. The evidence that oxytocin released endogenously in women's bodies during labour and birth influences intergroup behaviours is well established (de Dreu et al., 2010; Bartz, Zaki, Bolger, & Ochsner, 2011; Van IJzendoorn & Bakermans-Kranenburg, 2012). Seminal research by Kosfeld et al. (2005) demonstrated that oxytocin administered exogenously via intranasal spray increased levels of trust felt by humans. More recently, however, studies note this effect to be dependent upon the social context and the level of connection between the interacting people. Oxytocin enhances group identification with the familiar (Van IJzendoorn & Bakermans-Kranenburg, 2012), for example, a known midwife, thereby increasing trust and cooperation (de Dreu et al., 2010; Bartz et al., 2011; Van IJzendoorn & Bakermans-Kranenburg, 2012). Conversely, oxytocin elevates defensive behaviour toward an out-group and decreases out-group cooperation (de Dreu et al., 2010).

Ameliorating 'us and them' dynamics in the transfer context

During pregnancy, midwives deployed some strategies to help prepare women for the possibility of transfer, including booking a back-up hospital, ensuring women had ambulance cover, making a transfer birth plan and packing a bag for hospital 'just in case' it is needed. Midwives who experienced respectful interactions during homebirth transfers described those that were key to helping create a woman-centred approach. These include sharing the care, communicating in a way that demonstrates mutual respect and supporting the midwife–woman partnership:

> We tried to work very much with her [homebirth midwife], without getting in her way ... the homebirth midwife did one set of obs ... then the hospital midwife did another set of obs. You were then building up that rapport with the woman, that we were both caring for her in this setting where she wasn't necessarily expecting to be.
>
> (Hospital midwife)

> To have the [hospital midwives] respect [my midwife] and respect our relationship with her was amazing, it was unexpected, it was so wonderful, it just provided a seamless passage … I still felt loved and supported in a really hard time and that was great.
>
> (Homebirth woman)

> My job is to support her emotionally once we go into that environment and I admire the [hospital] midwife that gets that. So, she doesn't spend time when she's in the room trying to connect with the woman, because that's my job. Her job is to come in, do her observations, and liaise with us all as a team of people looking after her, on what the next step is or isn't.
>
> (Homebirth midwife)

> Hospital midwives should be functioning as a support for the midwife and the woman, really, and there should be a team approach … we should be really involving independent midwives when women are transferred into hospital because we need the relationship that they have. That sustains women and that that helps them through the experience and it means that their outcomes are better … [The] medical role is very much the tricky complicated stuff [doctors] will deal with and the normal and the relationship stuff is what the midwife's role is … Independent midwives are much more likely to have that ongoing, through their continuity and through the sort of care they give with women and we should be harnessing it … using it … [in working as] a good team.
>
> (Hospital midwife)

Shared goals can enhance collaboration when the goal of 'healthy mother and healthy baby' is based upon what is important to each individual childbearing woman. The goal of 'a healthy mother and a healthy baby' was shared by all who participated in our study. 'Healthy' is commonly defined as 'physically alive and well'; however, for women giving birth to their babies, 'healthy' may encompass deeper meanings that emerge from psychological, emotional, social, cultural and spiritual domains. These participants below expressed the importance of a woman-centred approach:

> [The] outcome hopefully … is a live mother and a live baby, but at the same time you also want to have experiences where the women feel ok about the whole thing.
>
> (Hospital midwife)

> This woman's made the choice [to plan a homebirth]. So, this [transfer] is what's happened, let's go on and help her to have a nice baby now … and a birth as great as we can give … and a safe mother and baby at the end of it.
>
> (Hospital midwife)

> What I perceive as risk, and what I perceive as an adverse outcome, will be different to you, will be different to everybody else. And at the end of the day the person who's taking that risk of having that adverse outcome is the woman who's having a baby.
>
> (Obstetrician)

Why is homebirth transfer unique?

Homebirth transfer is a complex social process that disrupts and challenges the status quo for everyone involved, and does not only affect the woman and the homebirth midwife. Handover guidelines from other clinical contexts cannot be easily adapted because the transfer of a woman from a planned homebirth with a PPM is unlike any other clinical situation. The reasons why homebirth transfer is so unique are listed in Box 15.1).

Box 15.1 The reasons why homebirth transfer is a unique clinical situation

- Women who choose to give birth outside the system are well-informed and aware of their rights to make informed decisions; however, somewhat paradoxically, they are viewed as naïve and ignorant by those who assume homebirth is dangerous.
- Women who plan to give birth outside the mainstream system are stereotyped as 'alternative', potentially leading to negative or discriminatory attitudes and behaviours being displayed towards them.
- Women planning a homebirth desire to labour and give birth without medical intervention or pharmacological pain management. While there is no possibility of these events occurring at home, her expectations are significantly challenged in the event of a transfer where there is a high likelihood of technological monitoring and medical intervention.
- Homebirth transfer brings high levels of uncertainty around practising rights, expectations for the labour and birth, social and environmental unfamiliarity, conflicting paradigms of risk and safety in childbearing, different philosophies of care, different views about place of birth, different approaches to time and progress in labour, differing styles of handover communication and documentation, allegiance to conflicting professional guidelines and/or divergent views of accountability to the woman or the institution. In the face of this uncertainty, women need time to adjust to their changing expectations and process what is occurring; however, hospital staff may be more accustomed to expediting the progress of labour and birth.

- The paradigms that underpin homebirth midwifery as compared with obstetric-led hospital care contrast the way risk and safety are assessed. The parameters of risk and safety in a hospital are biomedically driven. The parameters of risk and safety in a homebirth setting stem from physiological expectations and have clinical, emotional, psychological and social dimensions.
- The midwife–woman partnership is a unique relationship in the healthcare setting, which may not sit comfortably with mainstream care. A woman planning a homebirth usually has a strong, pre-existing relationship with her homebirth midwife. The partnership is based on reciprocal trust and shared understanding. It has different characteristics from the traditional therapeutic relationship with which many health professionals are familiar. This partnership is more powerful than the rapport that can develop between birthing women and caregivers in traditional fragmented models of hospital maternity care. Conversely, traditional fragmented models of care rely on notions of caregiver expertise and expectations of compliance from women.
- Interactions between midwives in the birthing room of a transferred woman are complex. Hospital midwives find the strength of the homebirth midwife–woman partnership challenging – both in relation to the ability to develop rapport with women and to their practice as hospital midwives. When women look to their homebirth midwife for support and advocacy, hospital midwives are left wondering how and where they fit, and how they can manage the social dynamics in the room.
- The woman's homebirth midwife is her primary caregiver throughout pregnancy up until the time of transfer; however, they may not be allowed into the hospital in her capacity as the primary caregiver. The homebirth midwife is usually denied clinical access upon transfer, even though, paradoxically, the PPM is expected to provide a professional handover after losing such clinical rights and responsibilities.

The way forward

The following best-practice principles (Box 15.2) have been adapted from a model for handover between anaesthetists and other health professionals in the operating theatre setting (Cyna et al., 2011) and are informed by the findings of Fox, Sheehan and Homer (2014, 2018a, 2018b) and those of the United States Home Birth Consensus Summits (Vedam et al., 2014).

Box 15.2 Best practice principles for handover in the context of homebirth transfer

Handover occurs in the presence of the woman, partner/support team, her transferring homebirth midwife, receiving hospital midwife and obstetric staff, and includes the following:

- In the event of a clinical emergency, a clear verbal summary of clinical details is given immediately, to address physical safety concerns for the woman and baby.
- In the absence of an emergency, handover requires the provision of:
  - A summary of what is important to the woman, including handover of a written transfer birth plan if available, which acknowledges the woman's emotional, psychological, cultural, spiritual and environmental needs;
  - Written and verbal clinical information, such as the woman's hand-held pregnancy record and/or a written antenatal and intrapartum history;
  - A summary of the decision-making process leading up to the transfer, and a discussion with the woman about her emotional and/or psychological readiness to accept medical intervention;
  - A discussion of the roles of the midwives who will provide ongoing care of the woman, where hospital staff respect and support the midwife–woman partnership and homebirth midwives respect and support the clinical responsibilities and duties of the hospital staff;
  - In the absence of clinical access, homebirth midwives remain with the woman in the hospital setting in a support and advocacy role. If the midwife is not available due to fatigue, her back-up midwife (known to the woman) will step in if possible. If not, the homebirth midwife spends 30 minutes in the hospital with the woman to complete handover and assist her to make the transition to hospital care.

Deborah Fox would like to acknowledge Associate Professor Athena Sheehan (Western Sydney University, Australia) and Associate Professor Saraswathi Vedam (University of British Columbia, Canada) for their contribution to this section of the chapter.

Notes

1 Although not supported by strong evidence, a 'stretch and sweep' is sometimes used to try to initiate labour. It involves the clinician inserting their index finger into the woman's cervix and sweeping around to separate the amniotic membrane from the cervix.

2 The term failsafe is not intended to imply infallibility. Rather, it means a system that is intended to 'counteract the effect of an anticipated possible source of failure' (Merriam-webster.com, 2017).

References

Amelink-Verburg, M. P., Verloove-Vanhorick, S. P., Hakkenberg, R. M. A., Veldhuijzen, I. M. E., Bennebroek Gravenhorst, J., & Buitendijk, S. E. (2008). Evaluation of 280 000 cases in Dutch midwifery practices: A descriptive study. *British Journal of Obstetrics & Gynaecology, 115*, 570–578.

Baird, B., Murray, R., Seale, B., Foot, C., & Perry, C. (2015). Midwifery regulation in the United Kingdom. Retrieved from: www.nmc.org.uk/globalassets/sitedocuments/councilpapersanddocuments/council-2015/kings-fund-review.pdf

Barclay, L., Kornelsen, J., Longman, J., Robin, S., Kruske, S., Kildea, S., … Morgan, G. (2016). Reconceptualising risk: Perceptions of risk in rural and remote maternity service planning. *Midwifery, 38*, 63–70. doi:10.1016/j.midw.2016.04.007

Bartz, J. A., Zaki, J., Bolger, N., & Ochsner, K. N. (2011). Social effects of oxytocin in humans: Context and person matter. *Trends in Cognitive Sciences, 15*, 301–309.

Belaouchi, M., Romero, E., Mazzinari, G., Esparza, M., García-Cebrían, C., Gil, F., & Muñoz, M. (2016). Management of massive bleeding in a Jehovah's Witness obstetric patient: The overwhelming importance of a pre-established multidisciplinary protocol. *Blood Transfusion, 14*, 541. doi:10.2450/2016.0229–15

Blix, E., Kumle, M. H., Ingversen, K., Huitfeldt, A. S., Hegaard, H. K., Ólafsdóttir, Ó. Á., Øian, P., & Lindgren, H. (2016). Transfers to hospital in planned home birth in four Nordic countries – A prospective cohort study. *Acta Obstetrica et Gynecologica Scandinavica, 95*, 420–428.

Bohren, M. A., Vogel, J. P., Hunter, E. C., Lutsiv, O., Makh, S. K., Souza, J. P., … Gülmezoglu, A. M. (2015). The mistreatment of women during childbirth in health facilities globally: A mixed-methods systematic review. *PLoS Medicine, 12*(6), e1001847. doi:10.1371/journal.pmed.1001847

Boyle, S., Thomas, H., & Brooks, F. (2016). Women's views on partnership working with midwives during pregnancy and childbirth. *Midwifery, 32*, 21–29. doi: 10.1016/j.midw.2015.09.001

Carr, N. J. (2008). Midwifery supervision and home birth against conventional advice. *British Journal of Midwifery, 16*, 743–745. doi:10.12968/bjom.2008.16.11.31617

Catling-Paull, C., Coddington, R., Foureur, M. J., & Homer, C. S. E. (2013). Publicly funded homebirth in Australia: A review of maternal and neonatal outcomes over 6 years. *Medical Journal of Australia, 198*, 616–620.

Cheyney, M. & Everson, C. (2009). Narratives of risk: Speaking across the hospital/homebirth divide. *Anthropology News, 50*, 7–8.

Cheyney, M., Everson, C., & Burcher, P. (2014). Homebirth transfers in the United States: Narratives of risk, fear, and mutual accommodation. *Qualitative Health Research, 24*, 443–456.

Cixous, H. (1976). The laugh of the Medusa. *Signs, 1*, 875–893.

Cyna, A. M., Andrew, M. I., Tan, S. G. M., & Smith, A. F. (Eds.) (2011). *Handbook of communication in anaesthesia and critical care: A practical guide to exploring the art.* Oxford: Oxford University Press.

Declercq, E. R., Cheng, E. R., & Sakala, C. (2018). Does maternity care decision-making conform to shared decision-making standards for repeat cesarean and labor induction after suspected macrosomia? *Birth, 45*, 236–244. doi:10.1111/birt.12365

Department of Health. (2016). Changes to midwife supervision in the UK. Retrieved from: www.gov.uk/government/publications/changes-to-midwife-supervision-in-the-uk

Downe, S. (2015). Beliefs and values moderate evidence in guideline development. *British Journal of Obstetrics and Gynaecology, 123*, 383. doi:10.1111/1471–0528.13634

Downe, S., Finlayson, K., & Fleming, A. (2010). Creating a collaborative culture in maternity care. *Journal of Midwifery and Women's Health, 55*, 250–254.

de Dreu, C. K. W., Greer, L. L., Handgraaf, M. J. J., Shalvi, S., Van Kleef, G. A., Baas, M., … Feith, S. W. W. (2010). The neuropeptide oxytocin regulates parochial altruism in intergroup conflict among humans. *Science, 328*(5984), 1408–1411.

de Jonge, A., Mesman, J. A. J. M., Mannien, J., Zwart, J. J., Van Dillen, J., & Van Roosmalen, J. (2013). Severe adverse maternal outcomes among low risk women with planned home versus hospital births in the Netherlands: Nationwide cohort study. *British Medical Journal, 346*(f3263). http://dx.doi.org/10.1136/bmj.f3263.

Ecker, J. & Minkoff, H. (2011). Home birth: What are physicians' ethical obligations when patient choices may carry increased risk? *Obstetrics & Gynecology, 117*, 1179–1182. doi:10.1097/AOG.0b013e3182167413

Edvardsson, K., Small, R., Lalos, A., Persson, M., & Mogren, I. (2015). Ultrasound's 'window on the womb' brings ethical challenges for balancing maternal and fetal health interests: Obstetricians' experiences in Australia. *BMC Medical Ethics, 16*(1), 31.

Edwards, N. P. & Murphy-Lawless, J. (2006). The instability of risk: Women's perspectives on risk and safety in birth. In A. Symon (Ed.), *Risk and choice in maternity care: An international perspective* (pp. 1–12). Edinburgh: Churchill Livingstone Elsevier.

Fox, D., Sheehan, A., & Homer, C. S. E. (2014). Experiences of women planning a homebirth who require intrapartum transfer to hospital: A meta-synthesis of the qualitative literature. *International Journal of Childbirth, 4*, 103–119.

Fox, D., Sheehan, A., & Homer, C. (2018a). Birthplace in Australia: Processes and interactions during the intrapartum transfer of women from planned homebirth to hospital. *Midwifery*, 57, 18–25.

Fox, D., Sheehan, A., & Homer, C. (2018b). Birthplace in Australia: Antenatal preparation for the possibility of transfer from planned homebirth. *Midwifery, 66*, 134–140.

Gülmezoglu, A. M., Crowther, C. A., Middleton, P., & Heatley, E. (2012). Induction of labour for improving birth outcomes for women at or beyond term. *Cochrane Database of Systematic Reviews,* 2012(6). doi:10.1002/14651858.CD004945.pub3

Harris, L. H. (2000). Rethinking maternal–fetal conflict: Gender and equality in perinatal ethics. *Obstetrics & Gynecology, 96*, 786–791.

Hogg, M. A. (2015). Constructive leadership across groups: How leaders can combat prejudice and conflict between subgroups. *Advances in Group Processes, 32*, 177–207.

Hogg, M. A. & Abrams, D. (Eds.) (2001). *Intergroup relations: Essential readings.* Philadelphia, PA: Psychology Press.

Holten, L. & de Miranda, E. (2016). Women's motivations for having unassisted childbirth or high-risk homebirth: An exploration of the literature on 'birthing outside the system'. *Midwifery,* 38, 55–62. doi:10.1016/j.midw.2016.03.010

Hutton, E. K., Cappelletti, A., Reitsma, A. H., Simioni, J., Horne, J., McGregor, C., & Ahmed, R. J. (2016). Outcomes associated with planned place of birth among women with low-risk pregnancies. *Canadian Medical Association Journal, 188*(5), e80–e90.

Ireland, S., Wulili Narjic, C., Belton, S., & Kildea, S. (2011). Niyith Nniyith Watmam (the quiet story): Exploring the experiences of Aboriginal women who give birth in their remote community. *Midwifery, 27*, 634–641. doi:10.1016/j.midw.2010.05.009

James, R. M. (2009). Autonomy, universality, and playing the guitar: On the politics and aesthetics of contemporary feminist deployments of the 'Master's Tools'. *Hypatia, 24*(2), 77–100. doi:10.1111/j.1527–2001.2009.01033.x

Jenkinson, B., Kruske, S., Stapleton, H., Beckmann, M., Reynolds, M., & Kildea, S. (2015). Maternity Care Plans: A retrospective review of a process aiming to support women who decline standard care. *Women & Birth, 28*, 303–309. doi:10.1016/j.wombi.2015.05.003

Jenkinson, B., Kruske, S., Stapleton, H., Beckmann, M., Reynolds, M., & Kildea, S. (2016). Women's, midwives' and obstetricians' experiences of a structured process to document refusal of recommended maternity care. *Women & Birth, 29*, 531–541. doi:10.1016/j.wombi.2016.05.005

Jenkinson, B., Kruske, S., & Kildea, S. (2017). The experiences of women, midwives and obstetricians when women decline recommended maternity care: A feminist thematic analysis. *Midwifery, 52*, 1–10. doi:10.1016/j.midw.2017.05.006

Jenkinson, B., Kruske, S., & Kildea, S. (2018). Refusal of recommended maternity care: Time to make a pact with women? *Women & Birth, 31*, 433–441. doi:10.1016/j.wombi.2018.03.006

Keedle, H., Schmeid, V., Burns, E., & Dahlen, H. (2015). Women's reasons for, and experiences of, choosing a homebirth following a caesarean. *BMC Pregnancy and Childbirth, 15*. doi:10.1186/s12884–015–0639–4

Keirse, M. J. N. C. (2014). Cohort study: Healthy women with a normal singleton pregnancy at term are not likely to be harmed by planning a home birth. *Evidence Based Medicine, 19*(2), 69.

Kidson-Gerber, G., Kerridge, I., Farmer, S., Stewart, C. L., Savoia, H., & Challis, D. (2016). Caring for pregnant women for whom transfusion is not an option. A national review to assist in patient care. *Australian and New Zealand Journal of Obstetrics and Gynaecology, 56*, 127–136. doi:10.1111/ajo.12420

Kosfeld, M., Heinrichs, M., Zak, P. J., Fischbacher, U., & Fehr, E. (2005). Oxytocin increases trust in humans. *Nature, 435*(7042), 673–676.

Kotaska, A. (2017). Informed consent and refusal in obstetrics: A practical ethical guide. *Birth, 44*, 195–199. doi:10.1111/birt.12281

Laufer-Ukeles, P. (2011). Reproductive choices and informed consent: Fetal interests, women's identity, and relational autonomy. *American Journal of Law and Medicine, 37*, 567–623.

Lennox, S., Skinner, J., & Foureur, M. (2008). Mentorship, preceptorship and clinical supervision: Three key processes for supporting midwives. *New Zealand College of Midwives Journal, 39*.

Lindgren, H. E., Hildingsson, I. M., Christensson, K., & Rådestad, I. J. (2008). Transfers in planned homebirths related to midwife availability and continuity: A nationwide population-based study. *Birth: Issues in Perinatal Care, 35*(1), 9–15.

Lintott, S. (2013). The sublimity of gestating and giving birth: Towards a feminist conception of the sublime. In S. Lintott & M. Sander-Staudt (Eds.), *Philosophical inquiries into pregnancy, childbirth, and mothering: Maternal subjects* (pp. 237–250). New York, NY: Routledge.

Lorde, A. (1983). The master's tools will never dismantle the master's house. In C. Moraga & G. Anzaldua (Eds.), *This bridge called my back: Writings by radical women of color* (Vol. 25, pp. 94–101). New York, NY: Kitchen Table Press.

Lothian, J. (2006). Birth plans: The good, the bad, and the future. *Journal of Obstetrics, Gynecology and Neonatal Nursing, 35*, 295–303. doi:10.1111/j.1552–6909. 2006.00042.x

McLachlan, H., McKay, H., Powell, R., Small, R., Davey, M., Cullinane, F., … Forster, D. (2016). Publicly-funded home birth in Victoria, Australia: Exploring the views and experiences of midwives and doctors. *Midwifery, 35*, 24–30.

Merriam-webster.com. (2017). Definition of FAIL-SAFE. [Online.] Retrieved from www.merriam-webster.com/dictionary/fail-safe

Minkoff, H., & Marshall, M. F. (2016). Fetal risks, relative risks, and relatives' risks. *American Journal of Bioethics, 16*(2), 3–11. doi:10.1080/15265161.2015.1120791

Minkoff, H., & Paltrow, L. M. (2007). Obstetricians and the rights of pregnant women. *Womens Health, 3*, 315–319. doi:10.2217/17455057.3.3.315

Murphy, M. (2016). Looking to the future of supervision. *British Journal of Midwifery, 24*, 309–309. doi:10.12968/bjom.2016.24.5.309

Nipper, B., & Roseghini, M. (2014). Full-time supervisor of midwives: Is this the future for supervision? *British Journal of Midwifery, 22*(1), 46–52. doi:10.12968/bjom.2014.22.1.46

Oberman, M. (2000). Mothers and doctors' orders: Unmasking the doctor's fiduciary role in maternal–fetal conflicts. *Northwest University Law Review, 94*, 451–501.

Pascucci, C. (2014). You're not allowed to not allow me. Retrieved from: http://birthmonopoly.com/allowed/

Price Waterhouse Coopers Australia. (2013). Professional indemnity insurance for midwives research. Retrieved from: www.nursingmidwiferyboard.gov.au/News/2013–12–06-media-statement.aspx

Queensland Health. (2019). Partnering with the woman who declines recommended maternity care. Retrieved from: www.health.qld.gov.au/consent/html/pwdrmc

Read, J. & Wallace, V. (2014). Supervision in action: An introduction. *British Journal of Midwifery, 22*, 196–199. doi:10.12968/bjom.2014.22.3.196

Rowe, R. E., Townend, J., Brocklehurst, P., Knight, M., MacFarlane, A., McCourt, C., … Hollowell, J. (2013). Duration and urgency of transfer in births planned at home and in freestanding midwifery units. *BMC Pregnancy and Childbirth, 13*(1), 1.

Scott, R. (2007). Maternal–foetal conflict. In R. E. Ashcroft, A. Dawson, H. Draper, & J. McMillan (Eds.), *Principles of health care ethics* (pp. 401–407). Chichester: Wiley.

Shaw, D. & Elger, B. (2013). Evidence-based persuasion: An ethical imperative. *JAMA, 309*, 1689–1690.

Thompson, R. & Miller, Y. (2014). Birth control: To what extent do women report being informed and involved in decisions about pregnancy and birth procedures? *BMC Pregnancy & Childbirth, 14*(1), 62. doi:10.1186/1471–2393–14–62

Tong, R. (2008). *Feminist thought: A more comprehensive introduction.* Retrieved from: http://UQL.eblib.com.au/patron/FullRecord.aspx?p=709031

Van Ijzendoorn, M. H. & Bakermans-Kranenburg, M. J. (2012). A sniff of trust: Meta-analysis of the effects of intranasal oxytocin administration on face recognition, trust to in-group, and trust to out-group. *Psychoneuroendocrinology, 37*, 438–443.

Vedam, S., Schummers, L., Stoll, K., Rogers, J., Klein, M.C., Fairbrother, N., ... Kaczorowski, J. (2012). The Canadian Birth Place Study: Describing maternity practice and providers' exposure to home birth. *Midwifery, 28*, 600–608.

Vedam, S., Cheyney, C., Fisher, T. J., Kane Low, L., Leeman, L., Myers, S., & Ruhl, C. (2014). Transfer from planned home birth to hospital: Improving inter-professional collaboration. *Journal of Midwifery & Women's Health, 59*, 624–634.

White-Corey, S. (2013). Birth plans: Tickets to the OR? *MCN: The American Journal of Maternal/Child Nursing, 38*, 268–273.

White Ribbon Alliance. (2011). Respectful Maternity Care: The universal rights of childbearing women. Retrieved from: http://whiteribbonalliance.org/wp-content/uploads/2013/10/Final_RMC_Charter.pdf

Zeybek, B., Childress, A. M., Kilic, G. S., Phelps, J. Y., Pacheco, L. D., Carter, M. A., & Borahay, M. A. (2016). Management of the Jehovah's Witness in obstetrics and gynecology: A comprehensive medical, ethical, and legal approach. *Obstetrical and Gynecological Survey, 71*, 488–500. doi:10.1097/OGX.0000000000000343

16 Why Aboriginal women want to avoid the biomedical system

Aboriginal and Torres Strait Islander women's stories

Donna Hartz, Melanie Briggs, Sue-anne Cutmore, Dea Delaney-Thiele and Cherisse Buzzacott

> The bio-medical model is birthing outside of *our system*. For many non-Aboriginal people, they just can't believe it, because they can't fathom it. And I'm like, 'Well where were we before the bio-medical model came into being anyway?' Births were done on Country, on Missions and in homes.
>
> (Dea Delaney-Thiele is a Dunghutti, Kamilaroi, Yuin woman)

About the authors

Donna Hartz identifies as a descendent of her grandmother's people, the Kamilaroi nation. She is midwife and nurse with 34 years' experience as a clinician, educator, lecturer, manager, consultant and researcher. She is an Associate Professor and has worked at a variety of tertiary and metropolitan health services and universities within NSW Australia.

Aunty[1] Sue-anne Cutmore identifies as a Wandi Wandi woman from Kamilaroi country. Sue-anne is committed to working with communities, families and individuals around equity in all areas of life. She has a mediation background and is moving into Family Group Conferencing. She is currently completing a Bachelor of Social Work after working in the field for 30 plus years.

Dea Delaney-Thiele is a proud Dunghutti, Kamilaroi and Yuin Aboriginal woman birthed on Country at Burnt Bridge Mission, Kempsey, NSW. Dea is an Associate Professor and has over 26 years' experience working within the Aboriginal Community Controlled Health Sector at all levels of the system. She is now the National Executive Director of the Dhiiyaan Mirri Bridging Cultures Unit at OzChild.

Cherisse Buzzacott is an Arrernte woman from Alice Springs, Northern Territory and a midwife. She was the first woman to graduate from the Australian Catholic University (ACU) Bachelor of Midwifery Indigenous course, an Away-from-Base delivery mode. She is the Co-director of the National Strategic Birthing on Country Committee, the Australian College of Midwives Birthing on Country project officer and works and lives on her Country in Alice Springs.

Melanie Briggs is an Aboriginal woman and descendant of the Dharawal and Gumbangirr peoples and lives on Wandandian country in the Yuin nation. She is a midwife with 10 years' experience working with Aboriginal families in the community. She is the Co-Chair of the National Strategic Birthing on Country Committee and works as the Project Officer at Waminda in Nowra for the Executive Shoalhaven Birthing on Country Strategic Committee.

Introduction

There is an irony behind collating a chapter about birthing 'outside the system' for Aboriginal and Torres Strait Islander women. As the oldest surviving culture on earth, our culture, customs and law (lore) – Aboriginal and Torres Strait Islander Dreamtime – has always been and will always be the system for our people (Walking Together Reconciliation Committee, 2017). The irony lies in having to justify our need, in this chapter, to birth within the system – *our system.*

Since British colonisation, the health and welfare of Aboriginal and Torres Strait Islander people has been decimated, resulting in huge health disparities compared to other Australians. There has been a loss of traditional knowledge and practice of Women's Business (Daylight, 1986) throughout the country, including birthing knowledge and practices (Adams, Faulkhead, Standfield, & Atkinson, 2018; Carter, Abbott, Liddle, & Hussen, 1987). British colonisation of Australia meant dispossession of Aboriginal and Torres Strait Islander's Countries and the forced relocation of Aboriginal people onto missions and settlements, where they became disconnected from cultural ways and food sources. This contributed to poor health as well as the introduction of disease. This was further compounded by Aboriginal genocides (Ryan et al., 2017), the fracturing of traditional family structures (kinship) (Boulton, 2016), incarceration (Australian Law Reform Commission (ALRC), 2017) and the removal of children (Human Rights and Equal Opportunity Commission, 1997). 'The fertility and childbirth rate declined and infant mortality rose dramatically' (Carter et al., 1987, p. 6). Those fortunate to return to Country[2] had to deal with added issues: inadequate access to water, housing, food, transport and communication. In essence, the social determinants of health were removed and basic human rights denied. For childbearing, the risks of birth in the bush increased. Modern obstetrics, with structured antenatal care and in hospital birth, despite best intentions has not redressed these risks (Carter et al., 1987; Australian Institute of Health and Welfare, 2018a, 2018c, 2019).

The colonised system of the past few hundred years has resulted in intergenerational trauma tor Aboriginal and Torres Strait Islander people, with the effects well documented. When compared to the non-indigenous population, there is currently, to list a few: (a) a higher mortality rate of 1.6, reflected in a 10.8 year gap in life expectancy (Australian Institute of Health and Welfare, 2018b); (b) higher rates of maternal (Australian Institute of Health and Welfare, 2018c) and infant mortality; (c) higher preterm; and (d) low birth weight babies (Australian Institute of Health and Welfare, 2018a). The last two outcomes predispose people to chronic disease. There are also record numbers of children being removed to out-of-home care, residential services or other care arrangements (Australian Institute of Health and Welfare, 2019).

The traditional Aboriginal and Torres Strait Islander knowledge of childbirth or 'borning'[3] was sacred, passed on by the grandmother and kept secret. For many communities and families, disenfranchisement or forced removal meant the loss of such knowledge. Today, there is a recognition that 'borning' is a two-way process (Carter et al., 1987) involving both traditional ways and modern institutional maternity care practices. The inclusion of traditional knowledge and birthing practices is paramount for Cultural safety and community self-determination (Adams et al., 2018) and essential for improving maternal and infant health, and saving lives (Kildea, Magick Dennis, & Stapleton, 2013).

Stories of resilience

This chapter shares our stories of resilience. The stories of four Aboriginal women sharing their experience of birth, either individually or on behalf of their Community, and how they move between the two worlds. Aunty Sue-anne Cutmore is a Kamilaroi and Yuin woman, and Dea Delaney-Thiele is a Dunghutti, Kamilaroi, Yuin woman. They are mothers and grandmothers who talk of successfully navigating the system and taking control of their births and memories. They also express a sense of loss when it comes to the knowledge of Women's Business. In Aboriginal culture, certain customs and practices are performed by men and women separately. For women, this is referred to as Women's Business. These practices are sacred and, until recently, remained secretive, as with traditional birthing practices or Grandmothers law (Carter et al., 1987; Wall, 2017). Aunty Sue-anne's, and Dea's, resilience is evident, their traditional knowledge embedded in their actions and consciousness, and they have a yearning for the next generation to embrace this. Cherisse Buzzacott is an Arrernte woman and midwife from Alice Springs, and she shares her story of having no control in a system that she trusted to look after her. Cherisse shares an insider's perspective of feeling culturally unsafe and discriminated against. The actions of the staff who were meant to care for her amplified her sorrow over the loss of her baby girl, Senna. Finally, Melanie Briggs, a senior midwife at Waminda, the South Coast Women's Health and Welfare Aboriginal Corporation in Nowra, NSW, shares the story of her Yuin Community's remembering and reclaiming the health system for their childbearing families – implementing Birth on Country model of care and a birth centre (Kildea et al., 2013) that is Aboriginal Community Controlled and governed.

Taking Control

Aunty Sue-anne Cutmore

My name is Sue-anne Cutmore. I was born in Moree and moved to Sydney with my parents and siblings when I was about five or six. My Mum and

Dad always said they moved to the city for employment and a better life for us, their kids. We lived in Balmain and attended Balmain Public School. So, my formative years were spent in a multicultural community that was mostly made up of factory and dock workers. As the eldest child, I went to Riverside Girls High School in Gladesville which, at the time, was the only publicly funded high school in the vicinity. I left school in 1974 to attend business college in the city.

I had my first pregnancy in 1978 at just 18 years of age. At the time, I was working in a solicitor's office as the receptionist. This proved challenging as I suffered severe morning sickness. My bosses and colleagues were very understanding and supplied me with a bucket (in case), lots of tea and toast. My partner and I had a small flat in Kings Cross, conveniently located close to our respective workplaces and Crown Street Women's Hospital. I had my antenatal care at Crown Street. I was very curious about pregnancy and childbirth, so the nurses gave me some information, and I sourced literature to read in preparation for birth. After reading about Leboyer, I decided I was going to have a Leboyer birth. Not a lot of people knew what that was beyond the maternity ward nurses. My family said, 'What is Leboyer birth?' My family thought I was a little bit crazy after I explained what it meant. My Mother and Aunties couldn't believe when I said, 'It's going to be a natural birth, using the Leboyer technique and I'm not using drugs'. Shortly before I was due to give birth, my partner was posted to Darwin, which meant I was going to birth alone.

When I eventually went into labour, I attended hospital with my younger sister who stayed with me for a short time before being encouraged to leave. My labour was a really long one, 26 hours in total. The nurses encouraged me to stay in bed and rest, even though it was uncomfortable, and I wanted to move around. I was told I had to be shaved and be on my back, my legs were placed in stirrups. Further along in the labour, the doctor on duty broke my water. I was embarrassed as I had previously worked for him as a medical receptionist and he remembered me. I felt weird, like, 'Oh, I know you, I used to work with you'. Hours passed and they put me on drugs, I think it was oxytocin and pethidine, and when I hadn't progressed, I was given more drugs. I was then told that because of the duration of my labour, I needed an epidural block. Then, as a consequence of the epidural, I was given an episiotomy, and my daughter delivered with forceps. Because I felt intimidated by the setting, I allowed all these interventions which I would come to question in subsequent pregnancies. I have suffered a weak back ever since. My lasting memory of that time is one of dependence and reliance on nurses and doctors. I felt stupid and inadequate and not confident or in control.

One good thing about the whole experience was moving to the Crown Street maternity annex located in Rose Bay. It was a lovely setting, overlooking the bay and very peaceful, with mothercraft nurses who basically coached new mothers. A friend I attended business college with had a change of career and trained as a mothercraft nurse. I didn't feel so alone, knowing she was practising there. I felt supported, unlike my time at Crown Street Hospital. Three days after giving birth, I began to cry and continued to cry for a few more days. My only visitor was a school friend and, because it was a long way from home, my mother wasn't able to visit. I felt so alone. I went home after seven days to my Mum's place in Mount Druitt.

That experience was enough to put me off hospitals. I didn't like the interventions, or people telling me what to do. Two years later, I was in western Sydney and I had health insurance, so when I became pregnant with my daughter I could choose my doctor. That turned out very differently to what I expected! During the antenatal visits, I shared my thoughts about the type of birth I wanted. He agreed that, as long as there were no complications, we could have a natural birth (no interventions). When the time came to birth, he wasn't available. Once again, my younger sister accompanied me to the hospital but it turned out to be a false alarm. I went home and two days later, I went into labour. I didn't attend hospital immediately until I was certain I was having regular contractions that were intensifying and gaining in frequency. At hospital, I relaxed and walked around, and as soon as I felt the urge to push, I spoke to the nurse. She rushed at me with a wheelchair and off we went to the delivery ward for an examination! She said, 'Right! I think this is it'. Twenty minutes later, after having an episiotomy, which is not a very pleasant experience second time around – it feels like you're cutting through a piece of chicken – I had my baby. No, didn't like that at all. I thought there had to be a better way.

Fifteen years later, I was pregnant again. This time, I was older and wiser, and I knew women who homebirthed, although not Aboriginal women. Just knowing that Aboriginal women years ago had homebirths, or were birthing under trees, near rivers and in special places, I knew I didn't want the hospital experience again. This time, I had enough resources to engage a midwife, and my partner, the father of my youngest three kids, said, 'Look, you've had experience giving birth, I'll trust you to know what to do'.

It was a bit scary the third time around because it was 15 years on, and my body was a lot older. I actually remembered the fear of all the previous interventions, that all came crowding in. My midwife helped me by talking through it. I was still kind of hanging onto this little baby once I went into labour. My membranes had broken and my midwife was concerned that I would get an infection. She said, 'Look Sue, just so that we're safe, let's go to the local hospital. They're expecting you. This is the back-up plan'. I said, 'Yeah, not a problem'. So, me and my army of supporters – it was an army – eight people all carrying various things under their arms, traipsed to the hospital.

Once there, we pulled the mattress off the bed in the family birthing room and placed it on the floor. I was given oxytocin to speed up the contractions and to get things moving. I remember the strength and intensity of the contractions after being given oxytocin and then, I had her, my third daughter on the floor, in maybe half an hour, an hour. I just needed a little bit of help,

I guess. The midwife that I'd had with me all through my pregnancy was there with me. The registrar didn't want me to leave because of risk of infection for our baby. I said, 'Well, what are you going to do that I'm not going to do?' 'We can monitor', the registrar said. 'Well', I say, 'how often are you going to monitor her?' 'Every four hours', was the reply. 'Well, no, that's not good enough', I said. 'I'd be monitoring her every moment of the day. We're going home'. I think, all up, we were there for about two hours – not long at all. I went in, pushed her out, had a shower, got dressed and went home. I still class that as a homebirth for me. I felt in control.

The fourth birth took place here in the Shoalhaven, in the lounge room of our property at Sussex Inlet. I had two local midwives with me, and it was good. I was able to move around, I could lie down if I wanted to, watch TV if I wanted to, cook if I wanted to, and shower as long as I wanted to. I was just in my own home and it was not really a big deal. I was able to put my girl to bed when she needed to go to bed. I laboured by myself for most it anyway, and when it came time, I rang my midwife, I said it's time, she came out, and I gave birth. It all just happened easily, quietly and in the early morning, about four o'clock. When my daughter was born, I was able to say, 'You were born right here'. She says, 'I was born on this Country'.

I became pregnant with my fifth child when we moved to Perth and, once again, I thought 'I want a midwife, I want a homebirth'. I was accepted into the main hospital homebirth programme. It was part of a community health department initiative. The midwives were funded to attend up to a hundred homebirths per year. I was one of them, because I had a good birthing record, no complications. I had my son at home in Fremantle. No complications, with supportive people close by if I needed any help. My midwife was wonderfully affirming and validated my birthing knowledge.

We came back to New South Wales when our baby was seven months old. I dragged his placenta back with me, all packed up in a small esky with lots of frozen bricks. It was important for me to bring his placenta back from Perth because it is Country. I was born in Moree, which makes me Kamilaroi, but my connection, or my spirit connection is here, in this place (Shoalhaven). My kids, because they went to school here, it's their connection. Sadly, they've been told by some Aboriginal people of this community that this is not their Country. I tell my kids, 'If you feel a connection to this Country, this is your Country. Your spirit will forever be tied here until your spirit is called elsewhere!'

I'm the only woman in my entire (and extended) family to homebirth. Moree is a huge community, and I have lots of cousins, lots of aunties. I do not ever remember anyone talking about a homebirth. So as far as I'm aware, I'm the only one, and that's really sad. Even my younger sister wouldn't even consider having a homebirth because in her mind too many things can go wrong.

My Mom said that I was born at the hospital, but in a ward that was for black people only, at McMasters Ward. The hospital segregated Aboriginal women to a separate maternity section. I remember my Mom talking about that ward. She said it was hard, but she never really went into it. For me, it conjured up images of sterile, cold and sparse, with nothing around that was comforting, nothing at all.

Being an Aboriginal woman didn't have any bearing on anything, or any decisions. My parents brought me up to believe: 'You are as good as anyone else'. Honestly, I didn't realise the full implications of being Aboriginal until I was around 30 years old. I had an idea but I didn't fully understand discrimination and racism. The concepts were alien because my parents reinforced that: 'You can do whatever you want, you're just like anyone else'. I developed that mindset but now I'm living with my eyes open. I'm noticing racism and discrimination everywhere. But I didn't notice them as an 18 year old – I suppose thinking about it, there may have been, but it didn't bother me. It's like I said, have the baby, that's it. With the younger three, it didn't even enter the picture.

There's an intuitiveness to birth – I just knew that was what I needed to do for me and my babies. I needed to do it for me as a woman because the first two pregnancies and births were more or less taken out of my hands. I wanted to have my babies my own way, and luckily for me, I had the resources to find the homebirth services and pay for it.

I know, for the women in my family, it's a fairly new thing, even in Moree. My aunties are in their 70s and 80s and even they don't recall any of the Women's Business or practices. A lot of what I know today, I've learned by talking to other women. Remembering my Nana and Auntie who, at times, would speak in language but not tell us what was said between them, because, 'that's our secret language, okay'. As an adult, I realise they were trying to protect us, but at the time, I couldn't understand it, I just thought it was a made-up language.

I'm hoping young women gain confidence in themselves, trust their bodies enough and inform themselves so they can have homebirths in safety and comfort. I'm sure women in the community have birthed at home, but accidentally; they're not planned. I'm hoping, with the support of midwives like Mel Briggs, and others equally passionate about homebirth in Shoalhaven or having access to a birthing centre may be just one step closer to giving our young women control.

Awakening

Dea Delaney-Thiele

My name is Dea Delaney-Thiele. I am a very proud Dunghutti, Kamilaroi, Yuin Aboriginal woman. My Mother, Gwen Delaney (née Campbell), birthed me on Country, at Burn Bridge Mission in Kempsey, NSW. Mum also has cultural connections on the South Coast of NSW as well as the North Coast through the Campbell lineage. A couple of Mum's Great Uncles went from Yuin Country to Dunghutti Country to marry because they knew well and good that you don't marry within the clan. It was usually the men who went outside the clan to find wives and have children.

My Mum and Dad (John Delaney) went from the Mission to Sydney and back again, a couple of times in my early years, to find employment, which was difficult for Aboriginal People in those days for many reasons that were underpinned by racism. My eldest brother, Neville, was born on the Mission, then my parents moved to Sydney for work. My sister, Joanne, was then born at Crown Street Women's Hospital, after which we moved back to Kempsey to be with my mother's family as Dad couldn't find work. I was born on the Mission.

I don't know the exact date of my birth. At the time, from what I understand, the Mission Managers spoke to officials from Births, Deaths and Marriages who would go around to all the missions to count us. Apparently, the officials would say 'Any kids born lately?' My Mum and Elders would say, 'Oh, yeah, well Dea was born three moons ago', or three suns ago, or something like that around the cycles of the moon or the sun because they didn't understand the western ways of the calendar.

I would have loved to know how much I weighed, what length I was and what time I was born – all those little things that you get these days when our kids are born in mainstream hospitals. In 1984, my mother passed into the Dreaming at just 44 years of a massive myocardial infarction so I never had the opportunity to ask those simple but fundamental questions. All but one of Mum's siblings have all passed on too. On the Campbell side, unfortunately, they don't live long lives. We are lucky to have one of our Aunties still living, but she was too young at the time, only 10 years old, so she wasn't around for my birth. Unfortunately, I cannot find my birth record anywhere.

I was really, really angry at the system for many years for not allowing my Mother to birth me in the hospital. Some of our Elders said that it just wasn't the done thing in the Kempsey area at the time. The Aboriginal women gave birth on the veranda of the hospital or just on the Mission itself. But one day, ten years ago, I woke up and thought 'You are such an idiot Dea, you're a complete fool. Because whilst you're angry at the colonising system, the racism and everything that goes with that, you weren't embracing your sacred cultural birthing practices'. That made me think in a more positive light, 'Oh, wow, here's my mother giving birth to me on Country, surrounded by her Aunties and other Elder women, how magical is that!' I am living proof of a sacred, cultural practice on Country that we have used for thousands of years. What an extraordinary practice it was too, as the birthing ritual took place in the natural environment surrounded by the essentials, such as running water and trees for shelter. Our Mob[4] in Kempsey called it a 'crik', for creek. So, I was born on Country under a lovely 'Yerrenin' (Kamilaroi for large gum tree) that gave the shelter my mother needed, next to running water from the Crik, close to the Mission. I don't know how it was done but, I'm here, I survived the cultural birthing experience, and I'm a living example of someone who was birthed on Country. Now, that's a very special moment in time for me – something I celebrate with much pride today!

I realised that it's such a magical part of our culture to continue our future generations. We were birthing on country for millennia and it is not embraced enough, not even by our own Mob these days. Really honouring our cultural practices, especially around birthing, is really important. If my younger daughter has a baby, I'm sure she'll probably want to give birth on Country.

Birthing on Country is a wonderful ceremony. Aboriginal women once birthed in a shady area, near running water, which was really important. And that's probably all I know. It's only a couple of generations, really. Also, many of the birthing areas have been demolished. One area was located near the IMAX centre where the waters are a bit calmer around Cockle Bay, in Darling Harbour (now a busy tourist spot in the Harbour of Sydney). There would have been lots of trees there once. Aunty Muughi (Margret) Campbell knows all the natural waterways around the Sydney area which have been blocked off or rechannelled these days. I live in Western Sydney now, but every time I go back to the bush or even the Blue Mountains and sit around on Country just looking at nature, being among it, is just so spiritually healing and rewarding. Whenever I get into an angry or sad mindset, when the day-to-day hassles of life get in the way, I love to go up the Mountains and watch the trees sway in the wind. That sounds silly, but it's really calming just to sit over a cuppa (cup of tea) and rest and reflect and be absorbed with the nature around you. The Megalong Valley is beautiful as well, or Glenbrook Park, where we used to go swimming a lot when I was younger. I'm still intrigued about the birthing process, but all my Elders on my Mother's side and the people who were around her at the time have passed on now, so I still feel something is missing.

The biomedical model is birthing outside of our cultural ways. For many non-Aboriginal people, they just can't believe we've survived, they can't fathom it. And I'm like, 'Well where were we all before the biomedical model came into existence?' It's only been around since the nineteenth century. I still find it so intriguing that our People actually delivered children the way they did, obviously very well for over 65,000 years. Our cultural ways of knowing and doing obviously kept us in good stead. After all we have survived! And what an absolute privilege it is to belong to the oldest surviving culture on Mother Earth.

Betrayed

Cherisse Buzzacott

This story is about the birth of my daughter Senna Napaltjarri Elsie-Storm. She was born at 20 weeks and four days into my pregnancy, on 11 November 2017. I went to hospital in early labour and my daughter was born two days later, a precious 275 g, but perfect in every way. My experiences as an Aboriginal woman were not unlike many others who have birthed within the system. At no time did I feel safe, supported or like I had a voice. I didn't know my main caregiver, I was not given any information and, at times, I felt hopeless. The health team behaved as though what I was experiencing was not real or as severe as I reported. I kept telling everyone in the room that I was in labour, but at no point was I assured that they could help stop the labour or even stop the pain I was feeling. It felt as if I was going to die.

There were many incidents that occurred, and I believe these incidences and treatment were because I am Aboriginal. A senior health professional came into the room and pushed my stomach as if to feel for contractions. I was feeling severe pain in my abdomen and lower back, and attempted to move and push her hand away. She snapped at me. I told her I was in pain and that she needed to stop touching me. She said 'Well, I can't feel anything, I don't think you're in pain'. Then, she snatched the nitrous out of my mouth and pushed it to the other side of the room. She said I was not cooperating with the exams that the hospital wanted to do. She yelled, 'Put that in her notes: refusal to be examined!' No one had attempted to consult me, console me or explain what was happening to me. They brushed off my pain as if it was nothing.

Another incident took place with someone I discovered later was 'my midwife'. When I asked for some water because I was in pain and had a dry mouth from using the nitrous gas, she replied, 'Say please and thank you'. On at least four separate occasions, she used an assertive, domineering tone of voice when addressing and said, 'Here, we say please and thank you'. Any woman in labour would understand needing support in a time of vulnerability while forgetting manners. I was not being mean and, as midwives, they should understand how to react appropriately. I was in pain, I was helpless, and no one seemed to care.

Medical staff refused me pain relief even though it was blatantly obvious I was in labour. I also have a history of miscarriages, but staff brushed it off saying things like, 'we need to examine you before we can give you something' or 'we need to find out what is happening before we can give you something'. I later found out they were trying to determine the gestation of my pregnancy so that they could determine if my daughter needed resuscitation when born. Afterwards, the birth centre manager told me (at the time of my complaint to the hospital) the team were unsure of how many weeks my daughter was, which is why they delayed pain relief. But I had my morphology (18–20-week) ultrasound scan the day before, I had a dating scan and an early scan at 6 weeks, what further information did they possibly need? Again, it was if they had trouble believing me when I told them how many weeks I was.

My partner suffered immensely and still does now. He was not supported or spoken to at any time, he was pushed to the side of the room. He is seriously scarred from our mistreatment at the hospital. He witnessed every occasion during which I was spoken AT and DOWN TO. He felt scared to speak up for me because he thought he would be branded 'aggressive' and 'troubling'. This was my view also when reflecting on the incidents he witnessed. I was glad he didn't react because I feared him being banned from the maternity ward or the hospital. I have seen this as a midwife, and as an Aboriginal woman; that the stereotyping of our Aboriginal men is so prevalent in the community.

After I received sufficient pain relief, I was left in the room for hours, still with no explanation about what was happening. No one spoke with me, except to let me know that I could eat and that I had an intravenous line for fluid. A midwife told me an ultrasound was booked for 1 p.m. but was only done at 3.30 p.m. By that time, I could feel, by hand, my daughter's head in my vagina, but when I rang the emergency bell, another a midwife just came in and tucked me into bed. At that point, my waters had broken. No one discussed this with me, to either reassure or at least share information as to next steps. Late in the afternoon, a senior consultant came into the room to tell me the inevitable, what I already knew.

The lack of privacy is concerning for any woman, but for someone with a strong voice and who speaks up, it was so distressing to be disregarded. I was dressed in only a t-shirt, with blueys to catch my leaking waters. The curtain was constantly left open and the door left wide open throughout the time I was going to the bathroom and throughout the time I was in pain. I remarked that the door should be closed with several people standing around at the midwives' station.

After the registrar snatched the nitrous gas from my mouth, I made my partner call a friend who I work with to support me. My friend was the one changing my blueys and assisting me to the bathroom. She was my improvised midwife that day and I am forever grateful!

When the evening shift started, yet another midwife transferred my partner and me to a family room at the end of the birth suite hallway. From then, our experience was great. We were supported and had the same midwives over the next few days. We felt like they were listening, and they gave us a lot of choice and opportunities for decision-making in regard to my care. We did not again cross paths with the midwives or doctors who saw us when we arrived. I am grateful that my friend was present as I believe our mistreatment would have gotten worse. My friend advocated for me, asked me if I was okay with staff touching me, which didn't happen before.

I am a midwife. I have attended over 100 births and supported twice that number of women in labour. I have never treated a woman in such a despicable manner, and that goes for the other caregivers, not just the midwives, but all the health professionals present during my birth experience. I understand the frustration that midwives have with women in labour when they are perceived as 'non-compliant' or 'difficult', but I would never mistreat her or make her feel as useless, voiceless and as small as how I felt that morning.

My partner and I both feel we received that treatment because we are both obviously Aboriginal. I told my friend, who supported me, about our experiences before she arrived. She at first assumed we have just experienced substandard care – but once we both explained what happened in detail, and compared that treatment with how a white couple would have been received in the same circumstance, she agreed.

Community culture, resilience and power

Mel Briggs

The South Coast Women's Health and Welfare Aboriginal Corporation, known as Waminda, is governed by a Board consisting of seven strong Aboriginal women from the Yuin nation. Waminda was auspiced as Jilimi, the Shoalhaven Women's Health and Resource Corporation in 1984, and renamed Waminda in 1990. Prior to this, the local Aboriginal community were concerned with the limited cultural understanding and care they were receiving within mainstream services which led to poor health and isolation problems. In response to the meagre service delivery and cultural insensitivity, Jilimi was formed in 1984 and funded by the NSW Department of Health to care for Aboriginal families residing on Yuin country. In 1990, Jilimi was officially changed to the South Coast Women's Health and Welfare Aboriginal Corporation, and is now known as Waminda.

The history of traditional birthing practices in Shoalhaven is not written. It is shared through storytelling, song and dance. The matriarch female elders within the Yuin nation tell stories of racism, isolation and poverty growing up in the area which some elders have said led to the poor health outcomes they suffer as older women. Women tell stories of birthing outside the hospital because they were not 'allowed' in hospital by reason of the colour of their skin. Women travelled by foot and boat across the Shoalhaven River to have their baby at Berry hospital, but birthed in tin shacks out the back. They also tell stories of the women and unborn babies who died making the journey across the river to attend hospital. Some share stories of birth in hospital being traumatic and scary because they were not given any information about what to expect during labour and birth. One elder said, 'It was my first baby, I didn't know what to do, I had no one with me, my mother never told me anything, I was all alone, in a room, in pain, then they put my legs in stirrups and I was told to push' –tears were rolling down her face as she told me this story! At birth, children were whisked away to the nursery where they were placed in rows which one Aunty described as a 'production line'. She did not see her baby except at feeding time, and she stayed in a hospital bed for up to ten days.

The history of mistreatment in birthing has embedded a culture of distrust towards mainstream maternity services by Aboriginal women. The distrust comes from an extensive history of death and child removal which, for Aboriginal families, seriously impacts women's desire to access maternity care today. Aboriginal women fear their child will be taken if they do not 'comply' with mainstream health system demands and therefore resist engagement with health services. The disengagement, in turn, leads to increased intervention by mainstream services and an increased risk of child removal. Women also experience racism, which acts as a major barrier to accessing care within mainstream services. One woman said, 'They called security on my family to ask them all to leave, if they had just asked us first, we would have done it, but they called a man into my birthing room, I was disgusted and disgraced'. A birthing room is meant to be a space for women to feel safe, shared only with family and professionals who are there to care and nurture them through labour and birth – not to create stress and anxiety by removing your voice, your choice or your support systems, such as family.

Hospital maternity services are provided to women experiencing illness requiring medical intervention and treatment. Hospital-based maternity care is fundamentally a biomedical model of health which considers pregnancy an illness and therefore responds to pregnancy in that way. It follows that the biomedical model of health does not factor in the social and emotional well-being of the woman and her family. For many Aboriginal women, family, community and culture will influence her health in one way or another, and this is not even considered, let alone taken into account, within the biomedical model. Waminda has developed a social model of health that centres the woman and her family, culture and community as one. We tailor our care and focus on the woman and her strengths using a strengths-based model. The Waminda team are profoundly aware of the social impacts of health, and our model of care highlights this.

Minga Goodjaga (Mother and Child) maternity services – cultural continuity

Waminda delivers the Minga Goodjaga maternity programme, which provides cultural continuity by ensuring women remain connected to culture through the care we deliver. Non-Aboriginal midwives are mentored by Aboriginal staff to ensure they are practising within a culturally safe way. The Minga Goodjaga midwives listen and validate women's voice in a respectful way to make women feel safe and form positive and professional relationships. These relationships are vital to ensuring women engage and receive care with a known midwife. The Minga Goodjaga maternity team are supported by crucial wrap-around services such as case management, family preservation and restoration, the Dead or Deadly programme, healing counsellors, Balaang Gunyah and tackling indigenous smoking. The Dead or Deadly Programme is a holistic health programme encompassing but not limited to these components: Lifestyle Medicine; Smoking Cessation; Weight Wellness; Yarning groups; and Holistic Health and Physical Activity/Exercise.

Minga Goodjaga utilises the Birthing on Country Model of Care. 'Birthing on Country is a Metaphor for the best start in life for Aboriginal and Torres Strait Islander babies and their families because it provides an integrated, holistic and culturally appropriate model of care' (Kildea et al., 2013, p. 11). In 2019, plans are in place to expand the model to a Midwifery Group Practice at the local hospital. The Waminda Community also plan to build a purpose-built Community-integrated care hub that will house their own Birth Centre – Goodjaga Gunyalamia (Child and Fig birthing tree).

Reflection

This chapter reflects on both the loss of knowledge in traditional birthing practices and the racial discrimination that continues to impact Aboriginal and Torres Strait Islander women. Our deep sense of loss and pain is evident. That said, the stories of the Aboriginal women we shared are also about deep remembering, strength and resilience. These stories resonate with many other Aboriginal and Torres Strait Islander women. The stories we tell are another step along the path to reclaiming traditional Women's Business and Birthing practices, healing and health, and awakening the minds of those who have the power and position to make a difference. Colonisation, and ultimately the domination of the Western biomedical model in childbirth, has led to poorer outcomes in health and birth for Aboriginal and Torres Strait Islander women. As Dea put so simply and eloquently, the '*bio-medical model is birthing outside of our system*'.

The development and implementation of Birthing on Country initiatives in Australia is building on the global movement for Indigenous peoples to reclaim birthing in their own communities (Kildea et al., 2018). Australia's *Birthing on Country* is our 'metaphor for the best start in life for Aboriginal and Torres Strait Islander babies and their families' (Kildea et al., 2013, p. 10). These initiatives are being championed by Communities as described in Melanie's story of the Waminda Community. Not only have improvements in health outcomes for Aboriginal and Torres Strait Islander mothers and babies been demonstrated, workforces are being developed which, in turn, foster other improvements in social determinants of social and emotional wellbeing for the whole community (Zubrick et al., 2014). Hopefully, this will lead to Aboriginal and Torres Strait Islander women being able to birth in their system – one that is both physically and culturally safe.

A way forward

To ensure continued improvement in maternal and infant health outcomes, a way forward is to walk in two worlds: embrace the best that modern medicine can offer and develop maternity services designed and delivered for Indigenous women, such as the Birthing on Country model.

These services need to:

- Be community-based and -governed
- Incorporate Women's Business and traditional practices
- Involve a connection with land and country
- Incorporate a holistic definition of health that will promote health and welfare integrity and redress the impact of integrational trauma
- Increase the Aboriginal and Torres Strait Islander maternity workforce
- Understand that cultural safety is paramount

Notes

1 Aunty is a term of respect and recognition given to a female elder in the Aboriginal community.
2 Country is sacred to Aboriginal and Torres Strait Islander people and denotes the traditional cultural land the 'owns' a group of people.
3 'Borning is used to refer to a much wider and more symbolic process. Where one is "found" refers to the rebirth of a "spirit child" from the Dreamtime ancestors who belong to a particular area of Country which may be the grandmother's or grandfather's Country. The child has strong traditional affiliations to the Country where he or she was found and will later assume rights and responsibilities for Law, the land and its people …

Women with particular familial and traditional affiliations, usually the grandmothers and aunts, are in attendance during birthing in an alukura apmere alaltyeke (a single women's camp in the country)' (Carter et al., 1987, p. 6).
4 'Mob' is a term identifying a group of *Aboriginal* people associated with a particular place or Country. It is a term that is extremely important to *Aboriginal* people because it is used to identify who they are and where they are from.

References

Adams, K., Faulkhead, S., Standfield, R., & Atkinson, P. (2018). Challenging the colonisation of birth: Koori women's birthing knowledge and practice. *Women & Birth,* 31(2), 81–88. doi:10.1016/j.wombi.2017.07.014

Australian Institute of Health and Welfare. (2018a). *Australia's mothers and babies 2016 – in brief.* Perinatal statistics series no. 34. Cat. no. PER 97. Canberra: AIHW.

Australian Institute of Health and Welfare. (2018b). *Deaths in Australia.* Retrieved from: www.aihw.gov.au/reports/life-expectancy-death/deaths/contents/life-expectancy [accesed 18 June 2019].

Australian Institute of Health and Welfare. (2018c). *Maternal deaths in Australia 2016.* Retrieved from: www.aihw.gov.au/getmedia/558ae883-a888-406a-b48f-71f562db3918/aihw-per-99-printable-PDF-of-web-report.pdf.aspx [accessed 18 June 2019].

Australian Institute of Health and Welfare. (2019). *Child protection Australia: 2017–18.* Child welfare series no. 70. Cat. no. CWS 65. Canberra: AIHW. Retrieved from: www.aihw.gov.au/getmedia/e551a2bc-9149-4625-83c0-7bf1523c3793/aihw-cws-65.pdf.aspx?inline=true [accessed 18 June 2019].

Australian Law Reform Commission (ALRC). (2017). *Pathways to justice – Inquiry into the incarceration rate of Aboriginal and Torres Strait Islander Peoples (ALRC Report 133).* Australian Government. Retrieved from: www.alrc.gov.au/publications/history-contact-criminal-justice-system [accessed 18 June 2019].

Boulton, J. (Ed.) (2016). *Aboriginal children, history and health.* New York, NY: Routledge.

Carter, B., Abbott, L., Liddle, H., & Hussen, E. (1987). The Congress Alukura by the Grandmother's Law. *Aboriginal and Islander Health Worker Journal, 11*(3), 7–14.

Daylight, P. (1986). *Women's Business: report of the Aboriginal Women's Task Force.* Canberra: Australian Government Publishing Service.

Human Rights and Equal Opportunity Commission. (1997). Bringing them home: Report of the national inquiry into the separation of Aboriginal and Torres

Strait Islander children from their families. Retrieved from: www.humanrights.gov.au/sites/default/files/content/pdf/social_justice/bringing_them_home_report.pdf [accessed 1 August 2016].

Kildea, S., Magick Dennis, F., & Stapleton, H. (2013). *Birthing on Country workshop report, Alice Springs, 4th July*. Brisbane: Australian Catholic University and Mater Medical Research Institute on behalf of the Maternity Services Inter-Jurisdictional Committee for the Australian Health Minister's Advisory Council.

Kildea, S., Hickey, S., Nelson, C., Currie, J., Carson, A., Reynolds, M., … Tracy, S. (2018). Birthing on Country (in Our Community): A case study of engaging stakeholders and developing a best-practice Indigenous maternity service in an urban setting. *Australian Health Review, 42*, 230–238. doi:10.1071/ah16218

Ryan, L., Richards, J., Pascoe, W., Debenham, J., Anders, R. J., Brown M, … Newley, J. (2017). Colonial Frontier Massacres in Eastern Australia 1788–1872, v2.0. Newcastle: University of Newcastle. Retrieved from: http://hdl.handle.net/1959.13/1340762 [accessed 1 June 2019].

Walking Together Reconciliation Committee. (2017). *Working with Indigenous Australia; Culture*. Muswellbrook Shire Council. Retrieved from: www.workingwithindigenousaustralians.info/content/Culture_1_Culture.html [accessed 6 June 2019].

Wall, C. (2017). *Aboriginal Grandmother's Law*. Australian Insitute of Aborignal and Torres Strait Islander Studies. Retrieved from: https://aiatsis.gov.au/publications/presentations/aboriginal-grandmothers-law [accessed 5 July 2019].

Zubrick, S. R., Carrington, C. J., Dudgeon, P., Gee, G., Paradies, Y., Scrine, C., & Walker, R. (2014). Working together: Aboriginal and Torres Strait Islander mental health and wellbeing principles and practice. Retrieved from: www.telethonkids.org.au/globalassets/media/documents/aboriginal-health/working-together-second-edition/working-together-aboriginal-and-wellbeing-2014.pdf [accessed 11 December 2019].

17 Midwifing women who make 'off-menu' choices

Kathryn Gutteridge and Hannah Dahlen

> Where women choose 'off menu' ways to receive care I have learnt that they have felt disrespected, unheard and by and large dismissed.
>
> (Kathryn Gutteridge)

> I do not believe we need to sell out women's rights to meet our professional responsibilities. I do not believe we need to sell out our professional responsibilities to support women's rights. Supporting women's rights is our professional responsibility.
>
> (Hannah Dahlen)

About the authors

I (Kathryn) am a midwife of many years. I have worked in every setting, including home and free-standing midwifery centres. I undertook (further) academic studies as part of an MSc programme and I later qualified as a psychotherapist; this learning and additional skills enhanced my midwifery practice in many ways. I then began a new era in my career as a Consultant Midwife in a tertiary obstetric unit where I was tasked with developing and creating facilities for normal birth. After a few years and success in this role, I was invited to apply for a second consultant midwifery post, where I was asked to effect the greatest change, not just in terms of facilities, but also in cultural and clinical outcomes. I co-developed alongside and freestanding midwifery units, and influenced a new wave of midwifery freedom in delivery of care. As my role consolidated and awards were won, I was encouraged to put myself forward for the President of the Royal College of Midwives. I was successful in that election and am serving as I write.

As a younger community midwife (Kathryn) in a semi-rural area, I was called early one summer evening to a young couple's home. I was their known midwife; I had delivered their antenatal care and provided their education programme. The labouring woman was in their long, very traditional English garden. It was secluded, with a swing she invited me to use. Her husband was busy in the kitchen. He brought tea and juice with snacks that he had made for us. I could see that the woman was in established labour. I asked if she wanted me to assess her progress and listen to her baby's heartbeat. She declined. She was more comfortable walking around. She was singing and rocking to a rhythm.

As dusk approached, she asked me to assess her. She lay on the swing with a towel for protection. She raised her pelvis up and spontaneously ruptured her membranes. Within two minutes, I could see the presenting part (vertex) at the introitus. I sat with her on the swing as she breathed her baby into the world. She was a primiparous woman. I had only been with her for 1 hour and 15 minutes. Her husband knelt by the swing and encouraged her, magnificently. He then quickly went into the kitchen, switched on the garden fairy lights, and put on that glorious music: the 'Arrival of the Queen of Sheba'. I was enthralled. The woman stood up in her garden and with the baby at her breast, squatted and produced her placenta. She later buried it under a rose bush in the garden.

I remember that birth in so much detail. I was the only midwife (that was how we did it then) but I realised that I was a guest at a very private, spectacular event. A birth that was planned and a labour choreographed almost to perfection. Now, I have been mocked for romanticising this story and reminded that 'birth is not always a fairytale event', but I will still maintain that birth like this is within the grasp of women and midwives.

What I learnt from women has taken me on a journey of trust, faith and belief in women's bodies. No doubt nature can teach us some hard lessons, but women are not stupid – they do not take risks and they trust midwives when presented with the truth.

You have already read my story (Hannah) at the start of this book. I work as a private midwife in a group practice in Sydney alongside my role as Professor of Midwifery at Western Sydney.

The birth of Serenity Birth Centre

Kathryn Gutteridge

My (Kathryn's) journey as a midwife is supported by the generosity of women who tell me their stories. I do not take this lightly; they tell me why they want to choose for themselves and I listen. My work in diverse settings means that I am aware of the risks that birth can present. With age and wisdom, however, I have learnt that women do not put themselves or their babies unnecessarily at risk. Where women choose 'off-menu' ways to receive care, I have learnt that they felt disrespected, unheard and, by and large, dismissed.

While engaged as a consultant midwife in a large urban UK hospital, I developed services that support and respect women. The population was ethnically diverse and had a lower socio-economic profile. More than 100 languages were spoken in the antenatal clinic on any day. This presented its own challenges as the women did not always understand how to navigate the health system. Relationship-based care is the predominant way to ensure that all women understand how to access, and avail themselves of, health services.

I was also involved in designing and setting up the Halcyon Freestanding Birth Centre, 3.5 miles away from the hospital.

Innovation is vital to, and expected of, the consultant midwife. I was delighted to be part of developing three birthing facilities and assisting in advising other services more times than I can remember. My template is simple: base the environment on one that protects women's dignity and respects their choices. I used the *End of Life* model of care to educate and inform facility developers, with a great deal of emphasis on care for the family and not just the individual. Priority is given to comfort and the availability of refreshments and non-medical care options, such as holistic therapies.

The plan for Serenity was simple: self-contained rooms with ensuite facilities, access to a pool, Entonox that was accessible in every corner of the room (including the toilet/shower), double beds hidden away and access to the outdoor space for everyone (see Figures 17.1, 17.2 and 17.3). The model was implemented as an 'opt-out' one: all women without medical/obstetric complications had access to this service. Following birth, they could be home within two hours if they wished. Serenity was designed as a birthing centre – not for postnatal stay – as I knew that women recovered more completely in their own homes. Serenity was situated some way from the traditional delivery suite, giving midwives and support workers control over the environment. The women only attended Serenity for assessment or in established labour.

Within the first year, the outcomes were favourable, with more than 600 women successfully giving birth at Serenity. Use of pethidine was less than 2%, with no major morbidities for women or babies, and waterbirth rates of

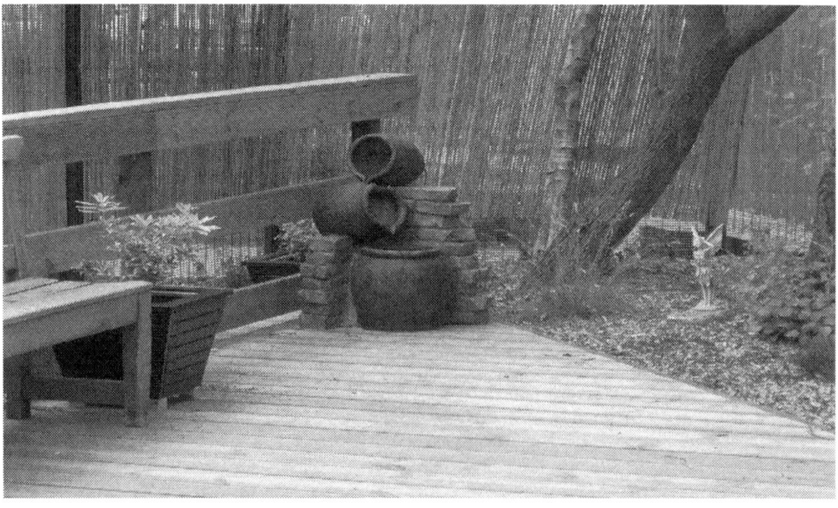

Figure 17.1 Serenity garden

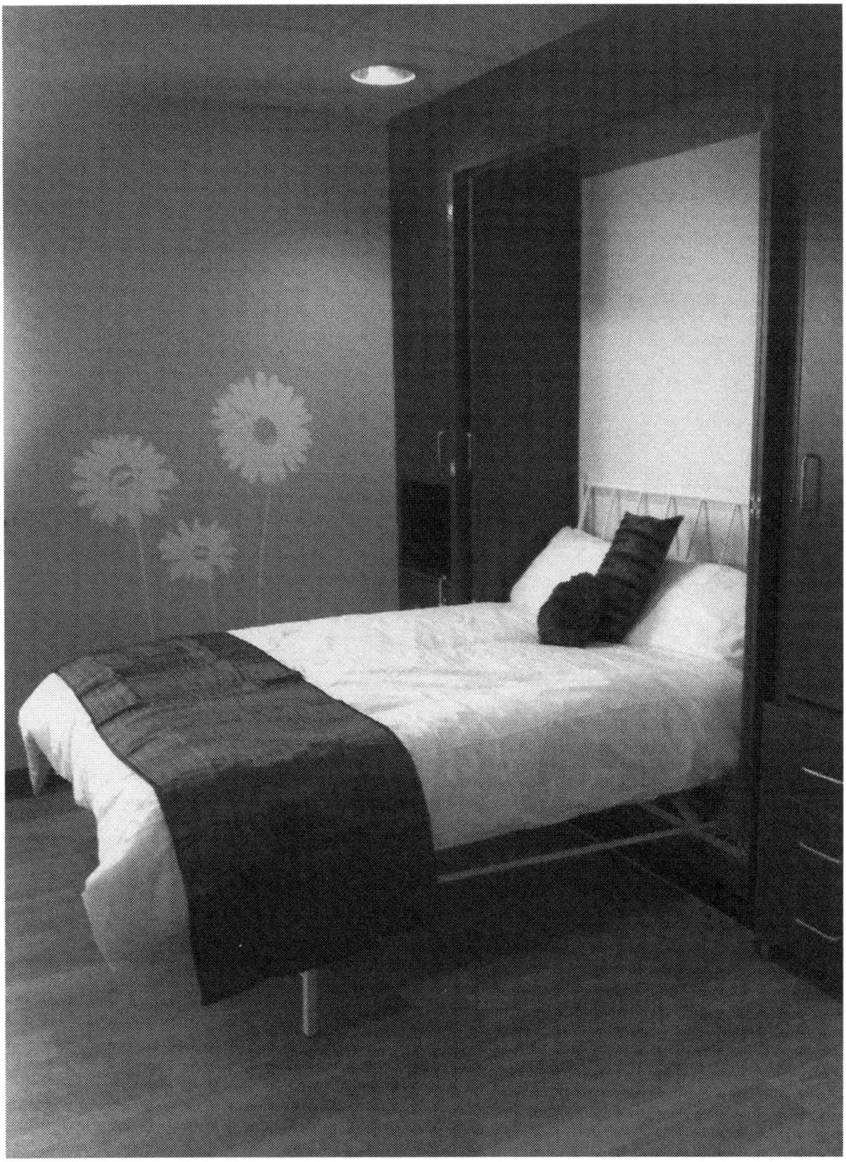

Figure 17.2 Halcyon BC bed in wall

more than 65% (Gutteridge, 2011). It can be very tempting to become overly confident with such positive data, but caution is applied whenever a new service is developed. I kept detailed data on every birth for the first three years to demonstrate the positive morbidity outcomes for all mothers and babies

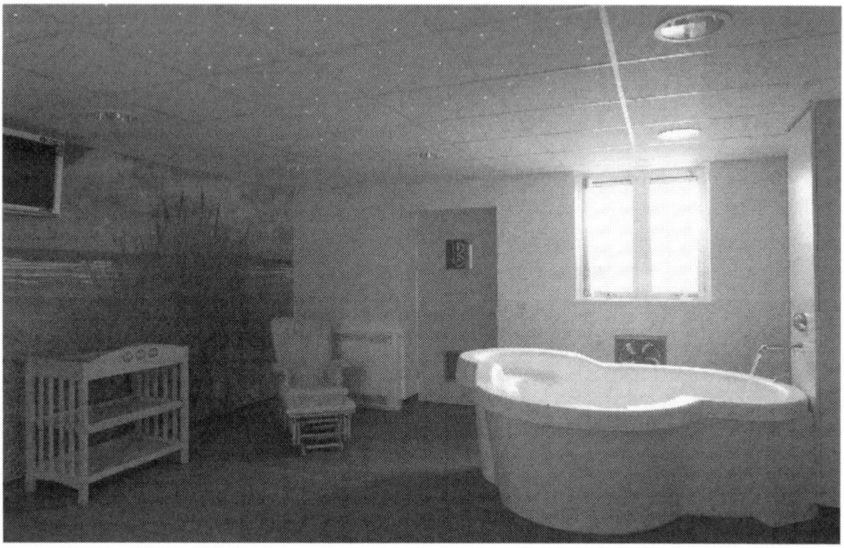

Figure 17.3 Serenity birth room

(Gutteridge, 2013). Scrutiny can be excessively applied where midwifery only services are introduced. I was determined that my team and I would take ownership of our work and clinical outcomes, be they good or bad.

Women are also brilliant at spreading the news about a great birthing facility and that is what happened with Serenity. Phrases like 'my sister gave birth here, can I?' were common. Although in the first instance midwives were clear about offering intrapartum care only for non-complicated women, it soon became apparent that women with moderate risk factors also wanted to access this service.

Vaginal birth after caesarean section (VBAC) in a birth centre

One of the first groups of women to make themselves known to Serenity were women who had a previous caesarean section (CS). While there has been little research into the impact of the birth environment on mode of delivery, we know that if we optimise the first birth for a woman, her risks in future pregnancies are reduced.

I was tasked with setting up a VBAC counselling service for women using the National Health Service (NHS) Trust. My brief was to develop a counselling service for VBAC unless the woman had a preference for a CS. To achieve this, I needed to determine the women who posed a lower risk during labour to women with more complex obstetric histories. On reviewing the numbers, I realised there were potentially at least 20 women per week requiring VBAC counselling. Women choosing repeat CS are referred to the clinic midwife, consented and prepared so that they can enjoy a pregnancy with straightforward antenatal care.

Women who requested VBAC were offered a further appointment with the consultant midwife and Serenity Team Midwife. This appointment is focused on understanding the previous birth from the woman's perspective and how she wants to manage her labour this time. This individualised discussion is important for the preparation for labour and a personalised risk assessment. During the discussion, I make clear to all women that, whether at home or in the birth centre, there will be no continuous foetal monitoring, no doctors and any transfers, in the event of an emergency, can take a minimum of 12 minutes – possibly longer from home – to the nearest hospital. A care plan is put into the woman's facility records and her hand-held notes. A card with details of the agreed plan is held at Serenity so staff are aware of upcoming planned VBAC births.

After each VBAC, data were collected so that we could present women with updated information on current success rates in the midwife-led facilities (96%). This information was also presented to the Maternal and Perinatal multidisciplinary meeting.

Table 17.1 shows an example of a care plan.

It is important to consider midwives' feelings about working with women with risk factors in midwife-only facilities, in order to understand what they need in terms of support, education and senior management. As a confident and competent midwife, I felt that I could easily manage women's wishes, but some of the midwives were early in their career and needed additional support.

Flora's VBAC at the Serenity Birth Centre

Flora suffered terribly after the birth of her first baby. She had an extended recovery and a long hospital stay. Her second pregnancy was unplanned. Flora was initially undecided about keeping the pregnancy but, after much heartfelt discussion, she decided to proceed with caveats. These were to VBAC at home, decline ultrasound scanning and engage a doula.

Her husband (a doctor) was worried; Flora needed a blood transfusion and extended antibiotic treatment for suspected sepsis following her first birth. Flora agreed to meet with me so I could understand what happened with her previous birth and how she had made decisions in pregnancy. She gave me permission to share her story.

> I presented at the hospital after I thought my waters had broken, I was 39+4 days and although I had no pain at the time I felt as if my labour was not that far in starting. I was excited and anticipated that I would be listened to and asked what my needs were for my labour. That was not the case, when I arrived, I had a painful and undignified examination

Table 17.1 Sample care plan for VBAC in the Serenity Birth Centre

Plan	*Frequency*	*Rationale*
Women accept that their request for a VBAC in Serenity has some restrictions but they feel that the benefits for them outweigh any risk. Therefore, this birth plan takes into account the facilities available at Serenity Birth Centre and advice for care. It is important that staff do not cross-examine and question the woman's choices on arrival at Serenity BC. Midwifery constant support and maintaining upright positions throughout labour are more likely to result in a positive VBAC outcome.		
Assess the pregnancy is without complication on arrival in labour	On arrival and continuously through labour episode	The normal pregnancy parameters should be met and within the expected range.
Intermittent auscultation using Pinnard stethoscope and or Doppler	15 minutes 1st stage 5 minutes 2nd stage	Deviations in foetal heart rate may be an indication of foetal compromise particularly if an upward trend in the baseline –inform the woman and transfer to delivery suite.
Observe maternal pulse and BP	Pulse 15 min BP 2-hourly	A rising pulse rate over a period of time (1 hour) and falling blood pressure is an indication of physiological compensation and not normal. Transfer to delivery suite.
Abdominal palpation	2-hourly or prior to vaginal examination	Fundus should be equal to term, abdomen soft and no areas of tension. Presentation should be noted and level of descent documented. This should be repeated 2-hourly and prior to each vaginal examination. A rising fundus, rising foetal presenting part is a sign of scar dehiscence. Transfer to delivery suite.
Vaginal examination	2-hourly minimum	It is advised that vaginal examination is performed routinely on admission and 2-hourly thereafter. Increasing cervical dilatation is a positive sign of progress – if after 4 hours of established labour with no distinct cervical change consider ARM. Wait for 2 hours re-examine if no change – transfer to delivery suite.
Observe for signs of fresh vaginal bleeding	On arrival and continuously through labour episode	May be a sign of scar dehiscence – may also be an indication of full dilatation. Observe amount, mucousy, associated pain, other vital signs. If concerned transfer to delivery suite.

Table 17.1 (Cont.)

Plan	*Frequency*	*Rationale*
Observe for blood-stained liquor	On arrival and continuously through labour episode	May be a sign of scar dehiscence – take into account while observing other signs of labour (fresh blood loss of 20 ml is acceptable, greater than this transfer). Presence of meconium should be observed as usual and appropriate action taken if grade 2–3.
Observe for blood-stained urine using Labstix	On arrival and tested at every void Encourage woman to pass urine at least 2-hourly	Heavily blood-stained urine is a late sign of scar rupture. Fluids and light diet to be offered and maintained throughout labour.
Observe for pain or scar tenderness that is not consistent with contractions	On arrival and continuously through labour episode when contractions subside	Pain can be right- or left-sided not necessarily across the scar. The pain is likely to be there despite contractions and is not relieved with usual measures. If the pain is referred to the scapula (shoulder tip) this is significant and must not be ignored. Transfer to delivery suite.
2nd stage labour management	Should last no longer than 60–90 minutes	May be preceded by a small PV fresh blood loss, SRoM, expulsive contractions change in maternal behaviour and breathing, anal dilatation and visible signs of presenting part at the introitus.
3rd stage labour management	Within 60 minutes if physiological	Discuss on arrival and confirm the preferred method. If waterbirth and active management chosen may remain in the pool until complete.

in a busy triage area where other women were being assessed. I had opted for a waterbirth and the midwife stated: 'you can forget that now my love'. I was shocked at her comment and asked her why she made that judgement; she shrugged her shoulders and said 'you are a primip, SROM and not in labour so I would put money on you needing an epidural and drip'.

I was advised to go home and come back in the morning if I had not come back before in labour. When I asked what would happen I was told that I would be put on a drip and my contractions would be managed to get me into labour. I was told my waters breaking and no labour yet meant that my baby was at risk of being exposed to infection and being ill. All I could think about then was my body not being able to protect my baby and being scared to go to the toilet in case any urine contaminated my waters. I couldn't sleep, eat or forget those words. Next morning, I was relieved to be going back into the hospital and for labour to be managed.

I arrived to be told that I would be sent to the ward and would wait for a slot to be induced. I wasn't sure what that meant and tried to ask what that was but the doctor said they would explain when they were ready for me. My husband was told he had to go home because there were no facilities for him on the ward, I was terrified that he was leaving me as he had been with me for all of our appointments.

Once I was on the ward I was put into a cubicle and left there. Four hours later someone came and saw me saying that I would not be induced today because they were really busy with emergencies and I would be on the list for tomorrow. I rang my husband nearly hysterical now and he came in to see what was happening. We asked if I could go home but they said that was not a good idea as I was at risk of infection. We stated that I was able to assess if I had any signs of sepsis but they were not happy for me to go home. I stayed alone, frightened, upset and worried about me and my baby.

The next morning I was told that I would be going to the labour ward for induction and or augmentation as soon as the round was completed. I waited and waited until 3 p.m. and still I was informed that the labour ward was too busy to accept me. By this time I was frantic and my husband insisted on speaking with the labour ward consultant. Eventually I was accepted on labour ward at 11 p.m. that evening where I was assessed and a syntocinon drip was commenced.

At about 3 a.m. I was starting to have some contractions and because I had not slept for almost 2 days I agreed to have an epidural – the words of that midwife were coming back to me now. I stayed on the drip for a further 12 hours and got to fully dilated but there were no signs of my baby descending into the birth canal. It was noted that I had a temperature and my baby's heartbeat was going up, so I was consented for an emergency CS. The epidural wasn't effective by then and I ended up with a general anaesthetic, I didn't see my baby until he was about 6 hours old as I was bleeding and needed quite a bit of care. I felt as if I woke up in a war zone; the noise, bright lights and cold air was all I could remember but I knew something else had happened but couldn't for the life of me think what.

Later when I woke from a drug-induced sleep I was met by the midwife saying 'you have had a lovely baby boy' and I then felt an immediate sense of panic. Where was he, who was looking after him? I needed to know why he wasn't where I could see him or hold him; in fact he was with my husband behind the curtain who was waiting to be told he could come in to me. I will never forget that feeling of terror and panic.

We went home after 5 days once mine and my baby's care was completed, I was frightened and tearful and although I didn't want to be in hospital I was more scared to be on my way home to care for him. It took me a long time to feel contented with my baby and to master being a mother.

Flora brought this written transcript to our first meeting to convince me that she was eligible for a VBAC. She didn't know that I would not require the narrative, but I still thanked her for allowing me to read about what had caused her so much distress and ongoing pain. We moved to talk about the normal issues that I discuss with all women considering a VBAC.

The most obvious risk for VBAC women is scar dehiscence (scar rupture); this may occur in 1:200 women. There is also the risk of a repeat CS, but this equates to 25% (1 in 4) of all women attempting a VBAC. It is only slightly higher than the risk of a caesarean, which is 20% (1 in 5) for women labouring for the first time. The reasons cited for recommending repeat CS are usually slow progress in labour and/or the baby is distressed. So, the predicted VBAC success in this pregnancy is 80% or 8 in 10 women, although, as you can see, our rate is much higher at Serenity (96%) (see Chapter 7 for more on VBAC). Flora and I discussed the care that is traditionally offered to women, such as a cannula in the hand, continuous foetal monitoring and birth in the delivery suite, with access to a theatre if required. While this information is stark advice, I go on to say that women do not always have to have this prescribed plan and, to get the best from her labour, she should consider what she would find helpful this time. Flora was tearful and, while holding her husband's hand, she said just coming to meet me in the hospital had increased her anxiety, but she was keen to look at what we could offer her.

Flora knew the risks about VBAC in hospital but, after researching VBAC at home, she knew she would feel more able to face labour and all the fears it held for her in that environment. I invited her to walk with me to Serenity, which was not too far from the clinic but away from delivery suite. As we walked through the door, I could see her breathing visibly slow down and her shoulders relax. I introduced her to the Serenity team midwife, who gave Flora and her husband a tour of the facilities. We agreed to meet again when she was 32 weeks to discuss how she was feeling and to start a birthing plan. When we met again, Flora looked a different woman; she was calm, focused and excited. Two days before she was due, Flora arrived in established labour. She had been supported by her doula at home. She declined a vaginal examination on arrival. Her midwife used other measures that I had devised to assess Flora. This consisted of 15-minute pulse rate, intermittent foetal heart rate auscultation, urinalysis, strength of contractions and behaviour signs (see care plan above –Table 17.1; Gutteridge, 2013).

Flora focused on the hypnobirthing techniques she had practised through her pregnancy. We offered the use of a pool for comfort when she found the contractions moving closer and stronger together. As she got into the pool, her membranes ruptured (clear) and she was encouraged to continue the techniques that had got her this far. As she relaxed into the warm water in the darkened room, her breathing became quicker. Her eyes were wide open as she told her midwife, ‘I can feel something in my vagina’. Her midwife encouraged her to relax and wait until her body gave her the next message that her baby was ready to come. This did not take long. Approximately 15 minutes later, Flora was involuntarily pushing. She lost her nerve a bit at this point, as it was clear that her baby would be here soon. With the support of her husband and doula, and her midwife’s guidance, Flora breathed her baby into the water and she reached down to catch her daughter.

Flora was ecstatic; she could not believe that she had achieved this most precious of human events and given birth to her daughter. She stayed in the pool where her placenta made its presence felt; no excessive bleeding, no perineal trauma, no cannula and a well mother and baby.

I was there when Flora arrived in labour. I wanted to support the midwifery staff but also be around if she needed to move to delivery suite. I wasn’t needed, but I was elated for her human fulfilment and her new journey as a mother. I informed the team that we had done much more than enable this woman to birth her baby, we had made midwifery care available to other VBAC women in our service.

There have since been more than 300 VBAC births at Serenity and 11 of those were following two previous CS. The model of care is supported by an Enhanced Maternal and Foetal Monitoring Pathway that closely observes the physiological and psychological elements of labour. Five of the 326 women who started labour in Serenity decided to go to delivery suite and were transferred before admission. Another 21 transferred to the delivery suite, 17 of whom achieved a vaginal birth and four had repeat CS – all with live babies. I believe this offers women another option when they are considering their birth choices. Other maternity units have expressed interest in this pathway and I feel that we should be promoting choice for all women about their care. It is better to try and be flexible in our care than drive women to give birth outside the system. The canary in the coal mine of my organisation continues to sing happily.

Taking on breech birth

When midwives become confident and competent in their skills, they question other norms in the delivery suite. Why are women planning breech birth in the delivery suit if the pregnancy and onset of labour is normal? The answer is usually, ‘just in case there is a problem’. The next question our midwives asked is, ‘If we are in the same building where we are observing carefully and caring for VBAC women anyway, can we not apply the same rule?’

Fair question. I have always been fascinated by breech presentation in birth, mostly because my daughter made her way into this world feet first and I achieved an assisted delivery, not entirely as it would happen today. Furthermore, breech is familial on my husband's side; my daughter's first son was breech at term and three of my nieces have had breech presentations. I too felt drawn to understand breech birth.

At the NHS Trust I worked for previously, we offered as standard ECV (external cephalic version). I trained and maintained my skills in achieving this technique. Only 3–4% of babies will be breech at term, but it is vital for all midwives to competently support a breech birth. With this in mind, I started training and raising interest in breech with Serenity midwives. If the woman was labouring without any sign of abnormality, she stayed on the normal Serenity pathway of: water and pool for pain relief; freedom to move comfortably; and any other usual ways of coping with labour. There are no beds in the birth centre (they are all tucked in the wall) so, in all likelihood, the woman remains mobile and active.

On diagnosing a breech, I encourage the midwives to support women in upright and active positions so that there are no barriers to delaying the labour. The usual clues of an impending breech, however, may not be present, such as fresh meconium, foetal position and auscultation. It is entirely possible for the midwife to discover a breech at full dilatation. The optimum outcome has to be a healthy mother and baby, but if we practise midwifery to its full potential, this is likely to follow. To transfer a woman along a corridor at this point may be distressing, traumatic and does not take into consideration her dignity. Informing the delivery suite and the senior team to be on standby was seen to be more pragmatic. So, this was the approach that we practised for breech presentation at full dilatation at Serenity.

Planning a breech birth, however, is different. This is Asma's story.

Asma's breech birth at Serenity Birth Centre

I met Asma when she requested an appointment to see me in Serenity to discuss her plans for her first birth. Asma has also given permission to share her story. She was 29 years old, 37 weeks pregnant and a lawyer with a special interest in human rights. When I met Asma and her husband, she told me that she knew her baby was in a breech position as she had always been comfortable that way, despite Asma having moxibustion and reflexology, and performing various exercises every day. She was against having ECV as she believed her baby was comfortable and she felt strongly that her baby should not be physically handled.

I listened to her and asked her what I could do for her. Asma said she wanted a vaginal birth. She was convinced that she would cope better if her needs were listened to and she had the freedom to move around. She knew our facilities would enable that, but she also knew the negative aspects of breech vaginal deliveries. She read all of the literature she could access, reviewed the Term Breech Trial (2004) data and made her own judgement about its applicability to her. Asma was slight in build (her BMI was 21) and low-risk.

We discussed what she thought might happen on the delivery suite if she were to labour there. She felt her labour would not respond as it should because the control she needed may not be forthcoming. I asked if she would consider a transfer if any abnormal features arose in labour and she replied that she would. I agreed to support Asma's desire to birth with Serenity as she was already at term and, in my experience, many breech labours start before 40 weeks. I wanted Asma to be confident and relaxed when she went away with a plan that worked for her.

I knew that this was the first time that the Serenity team were planning to receive a woman with breech presentation. I wanted to help them appreciate the normality of this presentation. In discussions, I focused on Asma's history, noting she was not at higher risk of developing a problem if her labour started spontaneously. She had a fully grown, appropriately sized baby and she was informed about the risks and benefits of her planned breech birth. I used the time to remind the team of how breech births usually progress and the benefits of the 'all fours position' at both full dilatation and second stage. We discussed the foetal response in second stage of labour and we spoke about foetal 'cycling' and 'praying hands' as the foetus delivered its own body. As the head is the last part to deliver in breech (the main worry for some midwives), I reassured them that if the body is left hanging and untouched, the physiological manoeuvres would be set in motion for the head to descend. We watched videos of breech birth and we used a pelvis and foetus to rehearse these movements. I reminded the midwives not to panic when the baby is finally born and to be patient when stimulating them as the baby is usually shocked by the rapid descent through the birth canal. I also agreed to be available to them when Asma arrived. Finally, after all that, I said, 'A breech birth is just a variation of cephalic birth, and you all do that without batting an eyelid'.

At 37+3 days, Asma arrived at Serenity in strong labour. She consented to a vaginal examination and her cervix was dilated to 8 cm with intact membranes. The midwives quickly started to run water in the pool. Asma did not plan to birth her baby in the water, but she wanted to at least relax in the pool. It was obvious that this labour would be fast as Asma was soon showing signs of reaching transition with strong and powerful contractions. As she stood up, her membranes ruptured and of course meconium was noted; the midwives did not panic as they knew this would be the case from our previous discussions. They prepared for the birth and were reassured that the foetal heart was both regular and normal. Asma was semi-standing, holding on to her husband who was standing in front of her supporting her arms.

Within five minutes Asma was involuntarily pushing at the end of each contraction and her midwives were kneeling in front of her. As she continued to push gently, the left sacrum appeared and was quickly followed by the whole of the breech making its way through to be visible. As with most breech births, the legs, abdomen and arms quickly revealed themselves, with the foetal nape of the head now visible. Asma lifted her right leg to widen the space available and her midwife caught the baby as she was born. We had prepared Asma for the way her baby may be at birth, so we patiently dried and stimulated her baby daughter who then cried loudly to let us know she was fine.

I arrived as the baby cried, and just about caught the placenta as it plopped onto the floor 12 minutes later. Asma was calm and contented as she sat with her baby across her breast and said she felt as if she had just achieved something magical. In all, Asma's labour totalled 5 hours 15 minutes. She lost a small amount of blood acceptable for her labour and had only a couple of grazes which did not require suturing. Asma said goodbye to the team four hours after the birth and went home.

This was a great success for Asma and a brilliant success for the Serenity midwives who had extended their skills and were once again pushing the boundaries for other women.

Alexa's birth with twins at the Serenity Birth Centre

Many women are helped and fulfilled in childbearing by midwifery skills, but there are times when my role is to help a woman be with a doctor so she can have the best of all of us. Occasionally, women who have suffered at the hands of a clinician during birth will put themselves at risk because of the fear that is now deeply embedded in their psyche. My job, as a midwife, is to try to restore faith and trust in our profession and to enable a woman to receive the best care. If that is not possible, I need to find a compromise that will give her a better chance of a good outcome. One of those times was when I met Alexa.

Alexa had been to four other maternity units in the region before she came to me. She is English but had lived in Greece with her husband, a policeman, where she birthed her now four-year-old son. Alexa was now expecting non-identical twins. She was 32 weeks pregnant and her mental well-being was not good. Alexa wanted a midwifery-supported birth, ideally at home or, at the very least, in a midwifery unit. She came back to the UK for the birth because she wanted to avoid birthing in a Greek maternity clinic. She told me that, when she was fully dilated, she was put into lithotomy and remained there for 2.5 hours in total. She had an episiotomy (cut to her perineum) without consent. She remembers blood everywhere, followed by a forceps delivery which badly bruised her son. She did not want this again.

Alexa told me that, in addition to being turned away from four hospitals, she was reported to social services and even received an appointment for a mental health assessment to determine if she had full mental capacity; something she knew nothing about. I listened to what Alexa said and asked her what we could do that might help her.

She said she wanted to labour in a peaceful and quiet environment with midwives who cared for and respected her wishes. She did not want machines around her as she felt they were distracting. I knew that this was a long way from what Serenity would normally accept, but I could not turn this woman away. I asked my Clinical Director and Serenity team midwife to meet Alexa and me so we could decide the best way forward. Alexa told them she knew that midwives could care for her in labour; she also knew that if her pregnancy was showing signs of problems, she would change her plans. We shared our concerns about listening to foetal hearts in labour as we had no way of determining the presence of each foetal heart separately, unless two midwives listened at the same time for each foetus. Alexa said she knew that, but did not want any monitoring of her babies during labour, as she knew this would disturb her labour.

We agreed a plan for Alexa which included the offer of two weekly appointments with myself and the obstetrician to assess foetal growth and maternal well-being. Alexa agreed to this and was happy to attend. She also agreed to have at least one ultrasound to ensure that the information we had about the pregnancy was accurate and that the babies were growing normally. The scan showed that one twin was slightly bigger than the other, but growth, amniotic fluid and placental blood flow was within the expected parameters.

When I took the plan to the Serenity midwifery team, they were anxious about this woman's expectations and potential risk factors. I agreed to work with their concerns. We conducted several sessions to rehearse Alexa's labour and birth. I also agreed to be there when she laboured.

At 37 weeks exactly, Alexa contacted Serenity to advise them she would be arriving soon. She brought her husband and son, who was half asleep. The midwives tucked him in a blanket in the corner of the room. Alexa was quiet and swaying as her labour gathered pace. We arranged for two midwives to attend her and support each other. The delivery suite gave us extra midwives so other women would be supported.

I arrived at midnight, just as the first baby was being born. This little girl was born quickly while Alexa was in 'all fours position' on the floor. She held her baby across her breast as she relaxed back into her husband for support. I had helped the midwives to prepare physically and mentally for the next part of labour, which would be probably against everything they had ever seen before at a twin birth. No stimulating the fundus, no separating of the cord and no loud noises or disturbances while we waited for labour to resume. It is common practice in obstetrics, following the birth of the first twin, to stabilise the body of the next baby, start a syntocinon infusion and scan the presenting part.

I could feel the midwives' anxiety, but I smiled and waited by Alexa's side as she started to breastfeed her baby. I knew that within about 30 minutes, the uterus would regain its tone and the second twin begin its journey. Just as I predicted, I saw a bag of bulging membranes. Alexa asked her husband to hold her baby as she now felt her contractions re-establishing. In a few minutes, I saw the foetal head crowning and with the rupture of membranes her second baby was quickly delivered into her hands. This baby was shocked and again, I reminded the midwives that this baby had had a rapid descent with limited exposure to extrauterine life, so we should gently stimulate but keep the cord intact. The baby cried after about 90 seconds. Both babies were in Alexa's arms, where she held them with tears in her eyes. Her little boy slept through the whole event.

Alexa birthed her placentas after 20 minutes with only 300 ml of estimated blood loss. Her perineum remained intact this time. After six hours rest and recovery, mother, father, brother and even their dog, which had been housed in our garden at the birth centre, went home (see Figure 17.1). Alexa called her daughters Ophelia and Catherine. They weighted 3.150 and 2.985 kg, respectively, and she breastfed them exclusively for 18 months. She is now in Greece with her family complete.

We reflected on the case in a convened meeting later that week with all staff who wanted to attend. The clinical director (senior obstetrician) and many of his colleagues, midwives from the delivery suite and, of course, the midwives present at the birth gathered to discuss how we all felt about this case. I presented an outline of the case and an overview of the outcome. Some of the midwives, and almost all of the doctors, felt that Alexa had placed her life, and that of her babies, at risk. They felt that she had been 'selfish and thoughtless'. I said, in response, that I could see why they might feel that way, but that was because they had accepted the medical paradigm: that it is normal, in modern society, for women to sacrifice their feelings and let us manage their labours. But I said, as a midwife of many years and one that had supported women to birth twins in their own homes at a time when it was normal to do so, I had a different view. I made the case for Alexa, stating that:

- She was, arguably, mismanaged in her first labour
- She had received poor advice in early pregnancy from other hospital units who refused to help her
- She was probably (and perhaps unfairly) labelled an 'unfit' mother and referred to child protection services by another nearby unit
- She accepted the need to compromise if her babies were not well and she agreed to change course if needed – this does not suggest a woman who is mentally incapacitated
- She attended all the appointments we offered in pregnancy, which showed she had her health and that of her babies at heart
- She knew that, if her labour was abnormal in any way, we would ask her to attend the delivery suite and she agreed to do that

Once all of the above was made clear, the discussion that followed was much more supportive of Alexa's wishes and birth. A junior doctor asked me how I knew not to stimulate the fundus between deliveries and what evidence I had to support that. I replied that I read the work of Ina May Gaskin (2012) and Mary Cronk (1998), a UK midwife, and learnt from my own observations with labouring women that touching and stimulating the fundus was only done in emergencies. Between the birth of one baby to the next, the cervix needs to reform and the uterus to regain tone and strength. Stimulating the fundus will interrupt the natural behaviour of hormones and physiology.

We had a great learning opportunity with the birth of Alexa's babies and we certainly felt as if we added to the confidence of our midwives in supporting the magnificence of the female birthing body.

Reflecting on women who choose care 'off the menu'

I have encountered thousands of women through my career lifetime. Many of them enjoyed the pregnancy and birth that they wanted. Flora, Asma and Alexa, who each knew they were placing themselves at risk of harm if they followed the standard pathway for their birth, took courageous steps off the path and asked for a plan of care that protected them from their fears of the past and respected their hopes for the future. They risk the wrath of midwives and obstetricians, the vitriol of family and that their requests will be dismissed and disrespected. I am so glad to meet and accompany women like them. They make me a better midwife. I can teach others that humanity is more than being alive at the end of labour and birth. Having a live mother and baby is just not good enough when we can offer so much more.

Personalised care is the ideal for every woman and the standard we must achieve. Waiting for women to ask for a choice that is 'off the menu' is simply not what a modern maternity system should look like. For too long, we provided care that babysits the foetus and does nothing for the woman. We see her as a vessel with a precious load. Women are so much more than that; they are not stupid, they are not selfish and they are not putting their own needs before their baby. They are asking to be heard and respected; after all, it is her body we are speaking about. If we do this, we should be able to provide the very best care in any setting, whether midwifery-led or obstetric led units – both should aim high. Once you have lost the trust of women, it is almost impossible to earn it back; let us not lose it in the first place.

Dancing in the grey zone

Hannah Dahlen

Several years ago, I (Hannah) wrote a paper based on a 2011 conference presentation I gave in China called 'Dancing in the grey zone between normality and risk' (Dahlen, 2016). In this paper, I argued that childbirth is mainly grey. At times, the most straightforward of births leads to heart-stopping and unexpected moments. At other times, the highest-risk woman, despite all our fears, birth without any of the imagined horrors eventuating. Midwives and doctors have the choice: be paralysed with fear over birth, or be responsive and respecting of it. Kathryn has illustrated so well how, with some flexibility and careful planning, we learn to 'dance in the grey zone', while meeting our professional responsibilities and obligations, as well as meeting human rights obligations. Sometimes, when it comes to birth we dance the 'waltz', as birth unfolds smoothly and without ripples, but more often than not, there are some ripples in the fabric of birth that call on us to be responsive and change our pace and actions somewhat, if not entirely. We move into a 'tango' at times, intense and dramatic and, at other times, what we do may feel more akin to 'hip hop'. Indeed, I feel I'm doing 'hip hop' when I transfer a woman from a planned homebirth to hospital, when I negotiate the system and the woman's needs.

Childbirth is mostly grey. It is rarely completely 'white' and without any problem at any time, and rarely completely 'black' and problematic all the time. So how can we be more flexible in the shades of grey that are our reality as midwives, so women do not feel they have no other option but to avoid our care?

I have previously written about getting the balance right in birth and that this is

> not about setting a steady course and never deviating from it until we reach our destination, neither is it being so focused on the destination that we don't enjoy the journey. It is like sailing a yacht from the harbour into the open sea – we constantly need to tack to stay on course; we feel the wind, respond to the billow of the sails and the lean of the boat, the messages coming from the depth sounder, the shape of the coast, the signalling of the lighthouse and the direction of the compass. To watch an expert sail a yacht is to see order being made from disorder, and disorder being made from order, until that boat is anchored and still again. Birth is much the same way, and we need to learn to dance through the uncertainty, enjoy each step along the way and not become so focused on the destination that we forget to live life. I do worry that we are losing the joy that comes with being a midwife [and obstetrician], not to mention how our care and fear is impacting on women. It has all become too serious, too stressful and too complicated. It is time for midwives to dance!
>
> (Dahlen, 2016, p. 18)

This is exactly the process Kathryn has demonstrated in her case studies. She showed the consultation, the back and forth, the negotiation, the learning and debriefing, and the personal and professional growth that came from Serenity's midwives being flexible around catering for women's needs. Indeed, this is a messy and, at times, disorganised process that functions best when the care is relationship-based and woman-centred rather than system-centred. It takes time and causes some sleepless nights (which I am sure Kathryn would attest to), so it is completely understandable that busy, complex organisations take an absolute black and white policy-driven, one-size-fits-all approach to this. It seems efficient and easy – but is it?

Two stories where 'off the menu' choices were dismissed

I want to tell two stories of events that happened in 2018 in Australia to illustrate what happens when we are inflexible around women's choices and our assessment of risk. I want you to think about how something that looks like a simple 'black' and 'white' decision aimed at reducing risk in fact causes other risks. Both these stories were written by journalist Cindy Lever and published in *Kidspot* (Lever, 2018b) and *Essential Baby* (Lever, 2018a)

Case one: Katherine's story

Katherine planned a homebirth through a publicly funded homebirth programme in Adelaide for her second baby, after suffering from PTSD from her first birth. When she reached 42 weeks, the hospital managing the programme removed her option of the homebirth due to guidelines that precluded birth after 42 weeks. Here is her story as written by Cindy Lever and published in *Kidspot* (Lever, 2018b):

> 'I got to 41 weeks and it was very stressful. They wanted to induce me and do stretch and sweeps. Being induced wasn't an option. I really wanted this birth to happen how it was going to happen. I was afraid, and I already had PTSD from the first birth', Katherine said.
>
> She was given until 8 a.m. on the day she became 42 weeks to go into active labour. 'My midwife texted at exactly 8 a.m. on the dot and said she couldn't come anymore. I felt very angry, frustrated and exasperated by all the hoops I had already had to jump through. I couldn't believe I was being punished for wanting to trust my body and allow it to do its own thing', she said.
>
> Just over five hours later Katherine went into labour. She texted her midwife begging her to come but the midwife refused. 'I just wanted someone to come so I would feel safe and know when to transfer to hospital.'
>
> Katherine even called one of the two private midwives in Adelaide asking for help but because she hadn't seen her from the start the midwife said she couldn't attend. Labour slowed, and Katherine was able to sleep through the night. Her first birth had taken three days, so she was prepared for the long haul. When she woke at 6 a.m. it had started again and although the contractions were coming thick and fast, she said she was still in denial. 'My husband and friend packed the car, but I got into the birth pool because I thought it would still be a while. Then I couldn't get out of the pool and kept vomiting every time I tried and felt nauseous', Katherine recalled.
>
> Unable to move his wife, John called an ambulance. 'The ambulance arrived as the head was crowing. I yelled out to John to ask the ambulance to wait outside because I didn't want to be disturbed. I was afraid if they came in things could go pear-shaped. They were angry and said they would leave but John asked them to stay and give me five minutes.'
>
> While John went in to ask Katherine again if the paramedics could come in, they called the police, suspecting there could be an unregistered midwife attending. John went back to the door to tell them Katherine

agreed to have them come in, but she didn't want to be disturbed. It was at this point that the first policeman arrived and walked straight in to stand over Katherine as she birthed her baby in the pool. Two more police then joined him. 'The baby came out as soon as they walked in and they wanted me to hand him straight over to the paramedics. I said, "no, everything is fine. I want skin to skin and delayed cord clamping". They wanted to clamp the cord straight away', Katherine said.

The police and paramedics convinced Katherine to get out of the pool and it was at this point that she started to bleed. While lying on the bed bleeding with the placenta still intact police asked her name. 'I remember saying, "have I done something wrong" and he said, "no we just need to make sure everyone is safe. Because there is a baby involved it's a social services issue".'

Katherine said by this stage the bleeding was very heavy and she begged the paramedics to give her the syntocinon she was keeping in the fridge for her planned homebirth, but they refused. 'It became a massive medical emergency because my third stage had been so disturbed and because of my rising cortisol levels. I lost 2.6 litres of blood, most of which was in the ambulance. I was half a pint of blood loss from death. I needed two blood transfusions and an iron transfusion', she said.

Even while Katherine was being rushed off in the ambulance her husband, John, wasn't able to be by her side because police wanted to search the house. Once at the hospital he and a friend were kept outside the room, hearing the screams of Katherine as doctors had to physically remove the placenta, while police continued to question them. Katherine said it has taken her over a year to recover physically, and emotionally she is still struggling 19 months on. 'The implications in terms of my mental and physical health are enormous. I have PTSD. My body has really struggled, and it has impacted my ability to go back to work as a doula. I am so furious because it was unnecessary trauma'.

Katherine said for about three seconds she was ecstatic because she didn't know her body could birth the baby and it took a few days to realise the enormity of the situation. 'My friend had to get legal advice and couldn't even talk to me. She feared she could be charged if police thought she was an unregistered midwife. I feel like they took advantage of the situation. My body knew what was happening (with the police standing over her) and that was why I bled. This is what happens when third stage is disturbed'.

Katherine said midwifery group practice is considered the gold standard in care but unless you tick all the boxes, including mandatory testing you will not be allowed to access it. 'It is basically bribery. I didn't want to freebirth. I would have been better to not call the ambulance. I would have been to freebirth and if that is the case there is something wrong', she said.

(Lever, 2018b)

Asked to comment on this story for the article I (Hannah) said:

> Guidelines are just that – guidance – to enable health providers to provide evidence-based care, but they must never be used to brow-beat a woman or remove a woman's right to make an informed choice. It is quite clear that the safest thing in this situation would have been the presence of a registered midwife who would have given the syntocinon that was in the fridge (placed there for this exact scenario) and could have prevented the massive blood loss experienced. There appears to have been inflexibility about a woman going over due and her choice to have a homebirth and complete ignorance of an even greater risk. This is not a logical, safe or human response.

Case two: Steffanie's story

Steffanie was pregnant with her fourth baby and planned to give birth with a publicly funded homebirth programme in Victoria, as she had done with her third baby. Below is her story as written by Cindy Lever and published in *Essential Baby* (Lever, 2018a).

> When Steffanie Schiavon fell pregnant with her fourth child, she looked forward to giving birth at home – just like she did with her third baby less than two years ago. But a change in the navigation method used by her local hospital in Victoria meant her family home now falls outside the homebirth system and that dream was denied. Ms Schiavon, 28, had her third baby with [a publicly funded homebirth programme] a midwifery group practice in 2016. When she found out she was pregnant again she returned to the programme and at 16 weeks was again assigned a midwife. The hospital at the time advised her that they were now using a different navigation system to calculate distances and, according to the new system she was now one minute outside their 30-minute requirement for a homebirth. Ms Schiavon said this [hospital], and the closer hospital, had both told her she couldn't have her other three children in the birthing room, which meant her husband would be forced to stay at home and look after them. 'At 32 weeks I started to appeal the decision based on the fact I don't have family around to help with my children while I give birth. They declined my appeal despite me giving them my reasons and history of birthing with them', she said.
>
> Ms Schiavon took her complaint to the Health Complaints Commissioner and after a six-week wait received a final rejection letter from the hospital telling her she was one minute outside their 30-minute midwifery group practice. The hospital did agree to let her have her children in the delivery room, however, as she was unable to birth at home, Ms Schiavon chose to give birth at the [nearer hospital] as it would involve less travel once she was in labour. 'They have changed the system in how

> they calculate the distance using a different navigation system since my last birth. I can find it at 29 minutes using Google maps and emailed this to the management but because it is not the system they use they wouldn't accept it. They need to deal with cases in a human way and a case-by-case basis. I am low-risk, and this is my fourth baby'.
>
> Ms Schiavon gave birth to her fourth child, a baby boy she named Saleh, on 10 August. Her neighbour drove her to the hospital at 3 a.m., while her husband stayed home with the couple's other children. The baby was born at 8 a.m. and Ms Schiavon's husband arrived 30 minutes later. 'It wasn't ideal because I didn't have my husband, but he was there within 30 minutes. He kept messaging me while I was in hospital', she said. 'I am upset I didn't get the home birth I wanted, but I can't complain, the midwives all knew what I wanted. Everyone at the hospital knew the story so they knew what I wanted and my birth history. Everyone was beyond supportive of my wishes and what I wanted out of the birth'.

When I (Hannah) was interviewed for the story, I made the following comments:

> The concept of 30-minutes from medical care being a safe distance was arbitrary and unnecessary in every woman's case. There are multiple factors that need to be taken into consideration. It is about risk factors, whether you can get an ambulance into your place, which hospital you are transferring to. Most women give birth between 1 a.m. and 5 a.m., so at those times there would be no traffic. I find it really distressing that people are still using (the 30 minute rule). It is cases such as Steffanie's which are forcing women to freebirth in Australia. It is never about the woman as a whole complex and individual human being with her own unique needs.

These two cases are such a contrast to the stories Kathryn Gutteridge shared earlier in this chapter. In Katherine's case (case one), she ended up with added physical risk because of the inflexibility of the service she was booked into. The irony of having syntocinon in the fridge, just steps away, and no one being willing or able to give it while she nearly bled to death is simply disturbing. This situation was made less safe – physically and emotionally for Katherine. She has a history of PTSD, hence her choice of homebirth this time. The result of this decision by the health service means Katherine has now been retraumatised through her second birth. In Steffanie's case (case two), a one-minute change in a new navigation system, despite living in the same house and being the same distance from the hospital she was for her last birth, meant her husband was not able to be at her birth and she wasted so much time in her pregnancy fighting for her rights and feeling stressed. An even greater irony with this case lies in the fact that, according to the research, as a low-risk multiparous woman, Steffanie had a lower risk birthing at home than in hospital (Birthplace in England Collaborative Group, 2011).

In both these cases, there would have been exasperated midwives (and probably some doctors too) who wished to provide care without repercussions to these women. Guidelines are just that – guidelines, and were never meant to make us abandon our common sense or brow-beat or abandon women when they make 'off the menu' choices.

Legal note from lawyer Bashi Kumar-Hazard: In my view, Katherine's case indicates that South Australia is no longer a safe place for pregnant women.

In Chapters 13 and 14, we discussed how laws are created for the convenience of medical practitioners, at the expense of womens' lives and reproductive rights. In Chapter 11, we discussed how midwives, and women who homebirth, are subjected to discrimination and treated with suspicion and animosity by enforcement and mainstream health services. In Chapter 5, we discussed the recently implemented criminal prohibitions on *engaging* an unregistered birthworker in the State of South Australia.

Katherine's case (case one) is a real-life example of just how those laws and discriminatory attitudes can endanger a woman's life and violate her human right to life and the highest attainable level of physical and mental health. Katherine was abandoned by the health service she chose because of an aggressively mandated and unnecessary guideline. Her husband called an ambulance for help. Instead of expressing concern for Katherine, ambulance personnel became suspicious and, without cause, called the police. Through that same suspicious and discriminatory lens that we see directed at midwives and women, they refused to administer medication which could have helped deliver the placenta and prevent blood loss. If the husband had said he was diabetic and needed an insulin shot, we wonder if the ambulance service would have denied him assistance in the way they denied Kathrine – which almost cost her her life.

The police invaded her home without cause or a warrant because they were more concerned to determine if Katherine had broken the law than with Katherine's safety. They also issued a veiled threat of calling child protection services, again without cause. Aside from an inappropriate exercise of police powers, they contributed to her stress, which led to an excessive and near-fatal postpartum bleed. Katherine was then 'punished' in hospital when she was isolated from her family and her placenta removed without pain relief. The police continued to, again without cause, inappropriately question Katherine's husband while this took place.

Practise within your scope as midwives and continue to advocate for women regardless of scope

As we criticise the many things wrong with mainstream care, we also have to question ourselves as midwives when we get it wrong. Normal birth at all cost is a huge price to pay. I get nervous when we become polarised into positions of always wrong and always right. I am always looking to improve the care I give, reflecting on the evidence and advice I give women based on the best available evidence, without using coercion. I think there is some worrying information given by midwives at times that is dangerous and that really worries me. I have heard and seen the heartbreak of women who feel misled or misinformed. Just because the other side has major fault does not mean midwives have none!

In the paper 'Dancing in the grey zone between normality and risk' I wrote the following:

> Midwives need to practise within their scope and to consult and refer when this is appropriate. If we don't do this, no matter how well meaning it may be, such as seeking to protect women from unnecessary intervention, then we are failing in our professional responsibilities and we will be held accountable. Where midwives get it wrong though is when they abrogate all responsibility to continue to advocate for the woman when consultation or referral is required. Practise within your scope but continue to advocate for women outside of it. Don't be silent and hang your head and purse your lips when you see wrong being done to women. Don't whisper in conspiratorial tones at the midwives' station with your colleagues about 'how unnecessary that was' and how distressing it was for you to watch the woman being coerced. If you say nothing you are complicit in the abuse. If you say nothing you have made as big, if not bigger, a mistake than practising outside your scope. Of course, the best way to reduce the need for conflict with colleagues is to have a shared philosophy around birth, to work in teams where relationships are built and to respect each other. However, above all we need to recognize that the woman's word is final and your job is not to coerce but to inform. I do not believe we need to sell out women's rights to meet our professional responsibilities. I do not believe we need to sell out our professional responsibilities to support women's rights. Supporting women's rights is our professional responsibility.
>
> (Dahlen, 2016, p. 22)

Scaling up the advice

I have been an expert witness in coronial cases and legal cases where midwives have frankly come unstuck. I have found, in most of these cases, that midwives get into hot water when advice to women is not appropriately scaled up to reflect the more serious implications of the decisions being made. Below are some examples of what I mean by this from 'Dancing in the grey zone' (Dahlen, 2016, p. 22).

You could do either or as the evidence is equivocal …

Best use: circumstances where the evidence is undecided, such as discussions on Group B screening, and whether this is routine or based on risk.

There is evidence that this increases the risk for you and/or your baby and so we would recommend …

Best use: when a slightly more direct position is needed, such as advising a woman with raised blood pressure to have a consultation with a medical professional.

The risk for the baby is significantly increased and so I would strongly recommend …

Best use: when clear and unequivocal discussion is needed for, say, a woman with a breech baby or twins who wants a homebirth.

There is a middle ground between 'shroud waving' and always framing everything positively. We can give frank and fearless advice without bullying and harassing the woman, or coercing her into a choice she does not make (see Chapters 19 and 20 for a medical perspective on this). As Kathryn has shown so eloquently, we have a responsibility to try and deliver the elements of care that a woman wants and get as close as possible to her ideal birth. When she does not want continuous monitoring, for example, we need to be able to compromise when this is required. Blatant refusal to consider options makes women feel they have no other choice than avoid our systems of care altogether and this is the worst possible scenario (Dahlen, Jackson, & Stevens, 2011).

When it goes terribly wrong, we are all scarred

We invited women who lost babies during freebirths or high-risk homebirths to tell their stories in this book, and they declined. In discussions before and following our invitation, I (Hannah) came to understand that the refusal is based on these reasons: (1) they don't trust us to truly represent the devastation and betrayal they feel they experienced; (2) they don't want to be attacked by homebirth and freebirth communities who sideline women with negative birth experiences/outcomes; (3) they are considering legal action and don't want to jeopardise their claims; and (4) they are hurting so much, they are not able to rake open the wound again. I have also come to realise a more profound aspect underpinning their reactions, which is based on my own experiences of loss. When women give birth outside the system and something goes wrong, they have no one to share the responsibility, grief and guilt they feel about their choices. Women who birth within the system have either their providers or the system to blame. Their choices are not disparaged as they are for women who birth outside of system. They are not unfairly accused of being bad or selfish mothers. The burden of bearing social approbation and unfair accusations leads some down the path of litigation, and yet others to hunker down with their families and disengage. My own heartfelt experiences, as I recall that dreaded year of believing my choices were the cause of my son Luke's death (see my story in the Introduction), were a burden that almost sent me crazy. But it also set me on a path, to change a system that forces women into corners and to face the heartbreak they would not have chosen in the first place if the hospitals learnt to listen to and respect women.

As reported in Chapter 5, the three women interviewed in the unregulated birthworker survey who had lost babies said they wished they had not chosen the path they did. They said that the problem with 1:100 or 1:1000

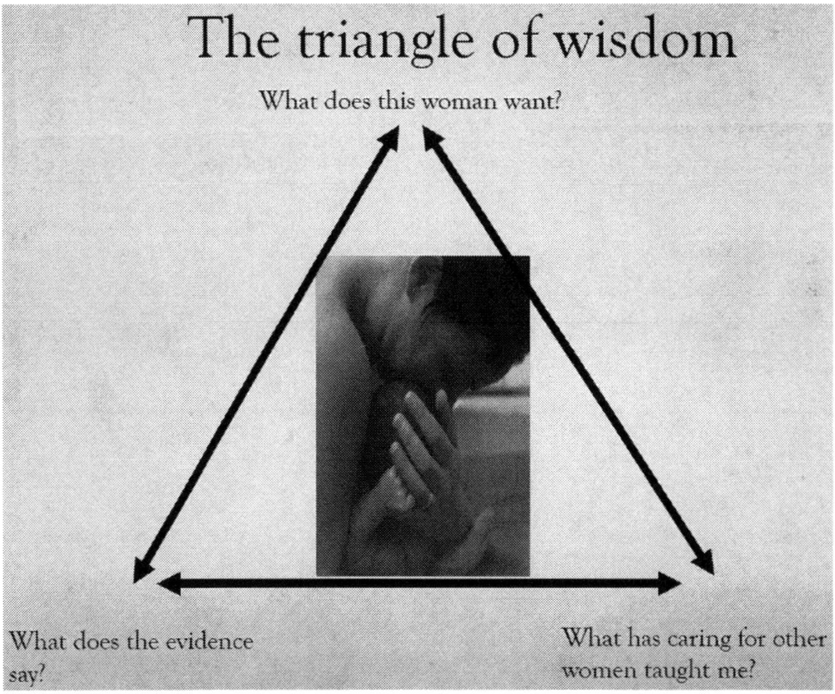

Figure 17.4 The triangle of wisdom
Source: Dahlen (2016).

risk projections is that you never think you will be 'the one'. When social media groups promote only positive stories and sideline or avoid the less positive and medical professionals only emphasise the negative, polarisation in discourse is inevitable. As health workers, we have placed dead babies in women's arms and desperately wished we could have changed it. In this very human response, we can let our scars get the better of us. The answer here is to find that balance. I use the triangle of wisdom to demonstrate safe practice (Figure 17.4). What does *this* woman want? What does the best-available evidence say? What has caring for other women taught me? At all times, the woman's needs and choices remain central to our advice and decision-making, and we safely dance in the grey zone when we consider and respond to these three questions. As Nietzshe said, 'We should consider every day lost in which we do not dance at least once'.

The way forward

- Women do not put themselves or their babies at risk intentionally. If they leave our care because of feeling disrespected, unheard and by and large dismissed, then we must draw them back to us with respect, listening and adapting ourselves to them and not always expecting them to adapt to us
- We need to develop services so that women would feel supported and respected
- We are clever as humans, so be innovative. If you want to say 'no' to a request think what makes you say this and if there is another possible response
- Learn to dance in the grey zone by not manufacturing fear, but also not ignoring the evidence that you need to act
- Midwives need to learn how to say the tough things as well as the lovely reassuring things to women
- Practise within the triangle of safety: what does *this* woman want? What does the best-available evidence say? What has caring for other women taught me? At all times the woman's needs and choices remain central to our advice and decision-making

References

Birthplace In England Collaborative Group. (2011) Perinatal and maternal outcomes by planned place of birth for healthy women with low risk pregnancies: The Birthplace in England national prospective cohort study. *BMJ, 343*. doi: 10.1136/bmj.d7400.

Cronk, M. (1998). Keep your hands off the breech. *AIMS Journal, 10*(3).

Dahlen, H. G. (2016). Dancing in the grey zone between normality and risk. *Practising Midwife, 19*, 18–20.

Dahlen, H., Jackson, M., & Stevens, J. (2011). Homebirth, freebirth and doulas: Casualty and consequences of a broken maternity system. *Women and Birth, 24*, 47–50.

Gaskin, I. M. (2012). *Ina May's guide to childbirth.* New York, NY: Bantam Books.

Gutteridge, K. (2011). Annual Report of Clinical Outcomes 2010–2011 Serenity Midwifery Led Co-Located Birth Centre. Sandwell and West Birmingham Hospitals NHS Trust. Unpublished report.

Gutteridge, K. (2013). Serenity and Halcyon Birth Centres Progress and Clinical Outcomes Report 2011–2013. Sandwell and West Birmingham Hospitals NHS Trust. Unpublished report.

Lever, C. (2018a). Change in hospital 'navigation system' denied mum her homebirth dream. *Essential Baby*. Retrieved from: www.essentialbaby.com.au/birth/birth-stories/change-in-hospital-navigation-system-denied-mum-her-homebirth-dream-20180920-h15mh1#ixzz5mN8gChjk.

Lever, C. (2018b). I went into labour at home and paramedics called the police. *Kidspot*. Retrieved from: www.kidspot.com.au/parenting/real-life/reader-stories/i-went-into-labour-at-home-and-paramedics-called-the-police/news-story/efe1be3e35e580e5b911534027b04edf.

18 Anthropologist, midwife, researcher

A perspective on birth outside the system

Melissa Cheyney

> Women are looking for far more out of their birth experience than not dying or having their baby not die, and we haven't been able to really provide that for them. To bring them back in, what I see women really wanting is to be treated like individuals, with respect and dignity. We need to see and act accordingly in response to their sense that their birth is far more than just a clinical event. How we treat women in birth matters deeply.
>
> (Melissa Cheyney)

About the author

I started my career as a medical anthropologist studying the evolution of human health and disease at an archaeological site in Jordan. I specialised in human skeletal remains from a Byzantine cemetery, and spent four years working in a beautiful little Bedouin village that grew up around the ruins of the ancient town. During my work there, I built many deep and loving relationships, one of which was with the local midwife or *daya*. As our relationship grew, she eventually shared with me that, while I was welcome to study the long-dead occupants of the site, what really mattered to her were the living people in her village who were losing the option of giving birth in their own community as the government encouraged women to go to the closest hospital, some 30 minutes away if you could catch that highly unpredictable bus, to give birth. I am embarrassed to admit that I remember telling her that we didn't have midwives in my country anymore. She assured me that my claim was probably not true and predicted that I would be a midwife someday. The full story is written up in the book *Ways of knowing about birth: Mothers, midwives, medicine, and birth activism* (Davis-Floyd, 2017). This *daya's* patience and wisdom opened my eyes to what can be lost when birth is moved outside of communities, and she planted a seed that eventually grew into my own calling to community midwifery. I am now an Associate Professor of Clinical Medical Anthropology at Oregon State University, with additional appointments in Global Health and Women Gender and Sexuality Studies. I am also a Licensed Midwife in active homebirth practice, and the Chair of the Division of Research for the Midwives Alliance of North America.

Introduction

Recently, I helped someone have an unassisted birth (also known as freebirth). We had begun our care with each other several years ago. In our first birth together, she had cholestasis, so she was risked out of homebirth care and attended hospital where I supported her as her doula. She was traumatised by that birth experience. She did end up with a vaginal birth, so everyone kept saying, 'It's a miracle – with how sick you were that you ended up with a vaginal birth'. In reality, she was thoroughly traumatised and actually struggled with depression and attachment issues with her first child. She's been on quite a journey since then. Her second birth was a beautiful homebirth, with no recurrence of cholestasis. Then, in this last birth, she had the birth that she really needed to heal. She built a little cottage close to a river that runs through her property over the course of her pregnancy and had regular prenatal care with me. She was actually quite intense about having every test she could have to ensure she was healthy and well in every respect. When she felt safe and ready to take full responsibility for her birth, I didn't hear from her again until after her baby was born. She told me that her water broke early one morning a few days after her due date, she walked to her little cottage with her partner and two friends, and in a few hours, had a completely undisturbed birth in the space of her choosing. She experienced birth on her own terms, connected only to what her body was telling her. She felt this birth heal her from her first birth experience, and I can see that she is a different person. She regained something that she has been missing since her first birth experience – a spark, a confidence, a fierceness that is truly beautiful to behold. I would not normally advocate for freebirth, but now I have seen what can happen for women when they tell us what they need to be whole again, and we believe them.

Why women birth outside the system

There is something in women that we don't spend enough time thinking about. We are so concerned about making sure that, at the end of the process, mother and baby are not dead and that they're not infected. I think this is actually a very low bar. Not being injured is also important, but I don't think we really worry about the mom being injured. We may worry about the baby being injured, and that is really not sufficient. Women are looking for far more out of their birth experience than not dying or having their baby not die, and we haven't been able to really provide that for them. To bring them back into the system, what I see women really wanting is to be treated like individuals, with respect and dignity. We need to see and act accordingly in response to their sense that their birth is far more than just a clinical event. How we treat women in birth matters deeply.

I have worked with women who choose homebirth midwifery care even with known risk factors, and I wish people could understand that they are not pursuing homebirth at all costs and they are not cavalier about losing their infant. What they understand (and we often ignore) is that their choice of birth setting is not a one-time thing. Those choices are made throughout the pregnancy and as the pregnancy unfolds. What they're looking for is a chance – for someone to believe in them, and to really give them a chance to birth on their own terms. I don't hear them saying, 'I'm staying home no matter what'. They're saying, 'We believe you need to give us a chance'. Now, we know, statistically, that most of them will go on to have a safe labour. That said, there is a proportionately higher risk of transfer for women with certain risk factors, so we build strong, collaborative back-up relationships and go into hospital if needed. We labour at home only as long as it makes sense. So, I think it is not about women shutting the door, but about them leaving open the space – the possibility – that they could have a physiological birth in the care of a midwife they trust. It's about giving themselves the chance to have the birth experience that they believe will give them the best possible start as a mother. I really understand that desire because I felt it too.

It's so hard for me to hear people reframing a woman's self-protective instincts as a claim of selfishness. It isn't about putting her own needs above the child; mother and baby are inseparable and her feelings about herself, as a woman and a parent, affect how she responds to her child. She knows that parenting from a position of empowerment and strength is different to parenting from a position of trauma. So many women tell me, 'I just want to avoid a traumatic birth because I know, once I have this baby, I'm won't be able to just go to therapy for the next six months to get my mindset back. I will have to care for my baby, and I want to be able to do that from a place of power, not a place of suffering or a place of victimisation'. That is not selfishness. That's understanding that her well-being is tied to her infant's well-being, and what she's asking for is an opportunity to be respected and supported through birth, to protect her well-being.

The other issue is trust. We have to regain women's trust and we have to do it through relationship-building. We've said a lot about person-centred care – woman-centred care – but what I really hear from my clients and our study participants is that it's not just about putting the woman first. Often, women are thinking about a whole array of people in their lives, including their relationships with their other children or their partner. That's why I like to think about it as relationship-centred care. It's about our relationship and it's about what they need to fulfil the relationships in their own lives. If we can't build that level of trust with them, I think what they do is go through their pregnancy very sceptical about the care they receive. Even where the care provider really has the woman's best intentions in mind, she won't always hear or feel that coming from us if we haven't built that trust.

I see that it is not that women reject caesarean (section) altogether. It's that they don't want a caesarean that they know or suspect is unnecessary. The women I care for embrace caesarean when they come to realise it is probably the only way they are going to have a healthy infant. They just don't want one before that time or one that has been precipitated by earlier and possibly unnecessary interventions. When you perform caesareans every day or every week, you can start to think they are not that big of a deal. The women who seek out community birth, that I care for, do not see it that way at all. How we are born very much matters to them, and surgical birth is not a small thing.

We need to create a system of care that women can put their trust in. We can't, in good conscience, advise them to put their trust in the systems we've created now. We understand why they want to go outside of the system to get access to care, and yet, the stark divisions between home and hospital in the United States doesn't serve women. We need an integrated system of care that respects women and trusts them to make choices about where and with whom they give birth. Ideally, the literature teaches us that to provide community birth settings, midwives need to be able to manage first-line complications and, when there's a more severe complication, we need to be able to transfer seamlessly to a higher-level care. That process needs to be respectful, at every step, of the woman. It is just not enough to say her baby hasn't died. We need to strive for something more – that she is not harmed in any way during that process. Until we get that right, people have a very complicated job ahead of them when they get pregnant, having to navigate our very complex maternity health system. Sadly, in the USA, so few people have access to true choice or to continuity of care with a community midwife.

It's a shame that we've constructed this story of women not wanting to give up their birth experience for their baby. I had a birth where there was a cord prolapse, and we caught it immediately, got the woman on her knees and chest, and came into hospital quickly. We explained beforehand that, when we got to the hospital, we would go straight to the operating theatre, they would give her a general, she would be flipped over at the last minute and they would do the caesarean as quickly as possible. She was, as we were coming in, saying, 'I won't move, you can cut me right now, I promise I won't move, just get my baby out'. We were all in tears hearing her say that and thinking she loves her baby so much, she's offering her body as a sacrifice. We explained, 'You don't have to do that, we have time'. It was a lovely outcome, with a very quick transfer and everything going according to plan. That was a home-birthing woman who absolutely embraced the caesarean when she knew it was needed. I think women can do that, but they have to be able to trust their providers.

Working towards harmonious solutions

Where I work in Oregon, we have midwife-to-midwife transfers, and this has evolved over many years of trying to build relationships between home and hospital. Following my very first transfer to the hospital, the ER doctor called the police and accused me of child abuse. Ten years later, we have midwife-to-midwife transfers. Gradually, over time, we've built relationships, so we can consult in the antenatal period if we get laboratory tests back or there is something that we're not sure about in the intrapartum period. Our clients go in to see the nurse midwives in the third trimester, after which they're on call for us. We have these lovely midwife-to-midwife transfers, and if we need them, we come in, we meet the midwife, we work together, and collaborate on the care. The only time we ever see an obstetrician is if we need forceps, vacuum extraction or a caesarean, which is only about 5% of the time, so we don't see them very often. When we do, they're there to do the things they are skilled at doing. Everyone's practising at the top of their skillset, and we all really love that kind of collaborative relationship. This is relatively uncommon in the USA where the interprofessional interactions are actually very stressful relationships generally. When interprofessional relationships are hostile, and women know they are going to have a punitive caesarean when we go into hospital, everyone is more reluctant to transfer and you cannot have that. It encourages midwives to spend more time at home and push that window of safety. Making it work like we do is such a welcoming and positive experience. What it has really done is helped our community midwives transfer for complications, not crisis. Now, the decisions are more about going in when there's still time to do something else. This arrangement has led to very high vaginal birth rates after transfer. Most of the time, people are coming in for an epidural, to rest. They fall asleep; sometimes they don't even have Pitocin (synthetic oxytocin), but when they do, they have just a small amount of it. They rest and then wake up to push their baby out. This has been so triumphant for women. It's a really, really positive experience.

Gentle caesarean sections as part of the solution

We also have 'gentle caesarean' at some of the hospitals we transfer to in our state, which is so wonderful. In a gentle caesarean, the screen comes down and everyone in the operating theatre is told to treat the birth as though it were a vaginal birth. The rationale is that the incision is just a few inches away from the vagina, so let's just behave as though she's having a birth because she is! This is a momentous occasion, and we're going to give her all of this loving attention, so the baby comes out very slowly out of the incision and she reaches down and lifts baby up to her. At first, everyone thought women wouldn't want that because they can see the incision, but they really can't because they only kind of sit up a little bit – just enough to see the baby. They wait for the cord to stop pulsing, and it's a really beautiful experience for women. This is about humanising the whole of birth rather than feeling like you've got this one option for community-based humanisation, which can lead women to make choices that sacrifice the benefits of hospital in order to get the benefits of care at home.

Collaboration is key

Some communities have successfully established collaborative models because there's mutual respect between community midwives and hospital providers. Through mutually respectful working relationships, we share our knowledge bases when we need to, which makes care safer both physically and emotionally for women. Receiving providers develop an understanding of what our clients want, and they offer this incredible medical expertise that we sometimes need. When communications and mutual expertise flow smoothly between providers, that's much, much better for the client. Of course, the inverse is also true in the USA where a transfer to the hospital means that the midwife is likely to be reported, the woman subjected to some sort of punitive intervention or caesarean, and the family shamed and blamed for their choice. That is very difficult because now the woman is processing not just the loss of the birth she hoped for, but also the disrespect she felt. I will say that, even when practitioners are kind to the woman but rude to the midwife, the client who is very connected to the midwife still sees the disrespect and abuse towards her midwife as a negative strike towards her. She feels the receiving provider is indirectly judging her choice, which, of course, they are. That needs to be addressed. We see outcomes are generally worse in the states in which those kinds of relationships prevail, and it's usually because of delayed transfer and punitive treatment.

Homebirth after caesarean (HBAC)

In regions of the USA where VBAC is readily available, mainly the Southwest and West Coast (especially the Pacific Northwest) of the United States, homebirth VBAC (HBAC) represents a smaller percentage of overall births. HBAC is happening more in regions where women can't get VBAC support in hospital – the Southeast and in the Midwest of the United States. There's not only more HBAC happening, there's also higher-risk HBACs in these regions. Women with multiple caesareans and then additional risk factors on top of that find that no one will support their VBAC in the hospital, so they seek out a homebirth provider. How can we change that? I don't think VBAC bans are ethical. Women cannot be forced to have another caesarean against their will, and homebirth or freebirth should not be their only options when they choose to labour after a caesarean.

Unlicensed birth providers

The other issue is that, in the USA, there are unlicensed midwives or midwives who identify as traditional midwives. Their practice is not constrained by guidelines or protocols, like licensed midwives. So you have this curious situation where the most experienced, skilled, licenced midwives, who are best equipped to manage complications, are doing the lowest-risk births at home. By contrast, unlicensed midwives without the skills or equipment (like carrying Pitocin to manage haemorrhage) are doing the highest-risk births because they don't have a licence to worry about. So, the least-experienced midwives who are doing infrequent births and are least able to manage a complication are taking on the highest-risk births in some areas. Again, we need to think about ways to remedy this situation that acknowledge a pregnant person's right to make choices about their own body.

How midwives get labelled as good or bad

One of the most challenging things we face in our communities in the USA is the phenomenon of the 'good midwife' and the 'bad midwife'. Some of it is luck of the draw. If your first transfer, the first time hospital staff interact with you happens to be one which didn't go smoothly, you get labelled the 'bad midwife'. After that, it becomes very hard to figure out who's initiating the hostile relationship. Is it the referring or receiving provider?

I actually think that our hospitals bear the majority responsibility for making people feel welcome when they attend, and where a midwife who is treated very poorly becomes defensive, the hospital needs to extend an olive branch to make it a safer place for her to come in. That's not to say that we can't hold midwives to a professional standard in terms of interprofessional communication. I've certainly seen rude, disrespectful, obstructionist attitudes coming from midwives too, but because we're coming into your home (i.e. the hospital), it would be really nice to see hospitals extending some courtesy to midwives, especially in the moment when the client is most in need of interprofessional collaboration and communication. Once a midwife has had that kind of very negative experience, it really shapes her future interactions. The midwives in our state and across the US have done so much to build those relationships. When they (hospital staff) find out that we carry the same neonatal resuscitation certification and antihaemorrhagics as their staff and can start an IV, it becomes very difficult (except for the ones that really have an axe to grind), to hold the line on 'no homebirth ever, no community birth ever'. We have to remind them that they have seen the times when women come in, just have their baby really quickly and don't really need them. I think they have to eventually come around to the idea that homebirth can be okay for certain subsets of the population. Of course, it's made more complex by the fact that they only see the ones that don't work out at home, the ones that require transfer.

Interprofessional training is key

We've got to build interprofessional relationships. I would love to see some kind of interprofessional training. When we've taken neonatal resuscitation training at the hospital and actually go through those classes together, that has been really, really lovely. I have always wanted to bring hospital providers to some homebirths, and I would also love to see community midwives be able to see physiological births in the hospital. It would also be wonderful for community midwives to be able to have more opportunities to keep up their skillset because it can be very, very challenging, for example, with breech birth. We did a survey of midwives who are attending births in the community setting and we found that they have breech births once every three to five years. You can't keep up your skillset if that's how often you're seeing a breech birth. Many of the women in our care also don't tear, so it's very hard to keep suturing skills well-honed. There could be this really beautiful collaboration where hospital providers see unmedicated, undisturbed births at home but also see midwives manage first-line complications. I think that would make them feel much better, and then, we can attend some hospital births to see that physiological birth can in fact happen there, and that there are many hospital providers working to promote vaginal birth and undisturbed birth. The relationships that could emerge out of these shared experiences would transform our system.

I knew a doctor who asked to bring students whenever there was a home to hospital transfer of someone still wanting an unmedicated birth – like this woman I was caring for who needed to be induced at 37 weeks. The doctor invited three medical students to sit in the corner and watch the birth. Once her labour got going, she had this really beautiful birth. He was kind of narrating through the experience, 'Watch how the midwife uses personal connection to manage the mother's stress level. Notice how she touches to comfort rather than just to hurt like when you're starting an IV'. He then says, 'She likes hot towels right now. Get some hot towels'. He really got it and the students knew they had just experienced a really unique learning opportunity. There was really no way for providers see a homebirth in the USA, but he was trying to emulate it in hospital for those who were wanting those kinds of experiences, and I think that was helpful. Certainly, the students expressed a greater willingness to work with midwives and a respect for their skillset and approach.

Culturally and socially matched

It is really important for women to feel like the person caring for them is part of their community. It is partially about where they've come from, what they have faced in their life, what they struggle with. Can my provider relate to me and what I am experiencing now? Is there a cultural or social divide that we have to traverse to develop a relationship of trust and mutual respect? I think about this when I provide care across different social race categories. I know we can build a strong relationship, but it seems to me, and I've had clients tell me, they would love to have a black midwife or a midwife who speaks Spanish as their first language or an indigenous midwife whose face looks like a face they know. They say, 'That's someone who comes from my community, that's someone who knows what is important to me'. It can be very difficult to perform in a way that you think you have to perform in order to fit in with a midwife or doctor who either does not speak your language or share some part of your heritage. I think that's a lot to ask of someone who is in the middle of labour and how wonderful to have a known and respected sister from your own community actually caring for you. Regardless if people want to birth at home or birth centres or hospitals – whatever it is – the first person you meet in your care should be someone you know from your community, who feels like a member of your community. I think it would help to facilitate trust. I'm not positive it has to be culturally or socially matched to see some of the positive outcomes we've seen in community doula programmes and community midwifery programmes in the USA, but I think it would be my ideal. You would meet that person in your community and then, the vast majority of women would be attended by a midwife. Instead, we have a system that's really kind of upside down, where the vast majority (89% of women in the United States) are being cared for by a surgical specialist – an obstetrician in a hospital in a for-profit system where it's just astronomically expensive. We have to flip that around and understand that, while some people will be attended by an obstetrician or by a maternal–foetal specialist, all women should have a midwife and ideally, a socially or culturally matched one.

Continuity of midwifery care is key

We should be aiming for relationship-based care so the woman knows there's some continuity of care that's going to span the entire course of her pregnancy and then maybe future pregnancies as well. I think that would actually save the US system quite a bit of money, and you would have obstetricians operating at the top of their licence. I actually think the obstetricians would like it better. From what I can tell, they don't love being on call all the time and coming in for long labours and sleeping in the on-call room or running back and forth between the hospital and clinic.

Increasing the midwifery workforce and looking at funding systems

We need many more midwives. I don't even know where the US would start. We have such a small number of midwives. We would have to train those midwives, and restructure our systems to gain improved access to higher education. How can you afford to pay for higher education when you're from a poor, black community? Basically, the whole system has to be torn down and built up from scratch. The rampant inequality that we have in the USA, which ironically is supposedly a classless society (and we all know that that isn't even close to being true) – that is what keeps midwives from all communities from being trained. That said, I can't imagine it would be any more expensive than what we're doing right now because the USA is spending half of all the world's healthcare dollars on a system which produces some of the worst outcomes, so there really isn't any point in continuing down the path that we're on or tinkering with the present system. The entire system is broken and putting a Band-Aid on it is not going to fix it at this point.

For-profit medicine is really problematic, and it actually gives you the outcomes that we see. It seems to me that there has to be a system where, financially, we incentivise physiological birth rather than medical interventions. Of course, that's the exact opposite of what we do now in the USA. To make money, you have to create disease and then treat it – at an astronomical cost. The whole system needs to be overturned so as to incentivise healthy outcomes, physiological birth and low intervention rates. We try, we tinker with that through quality metrics, but that too has now become a whole separate and lucrative industry. Every time someone tries to introduce a systems-level intervention or systems-level change, a whole new bureaucracy quickly builds up around developing that system and its associated metrics. We now spend hundreds of thousands of dollars a year trying to develop patient-led metrics and public health safety nets, and still, very little of that money goes to the person who actually needs the medical care or social supports that are so hard to access and so expensive to fund. We've got to find a way to cut out the massive bureaucracy and the huge sums of money that go into the wrong pockets.

Midwives need to take responsibility

Community midwives also need a more nuanced identity that isn't just defined by opposition to the mainstream. Some US midwives don't want to give Vitamin K because it is given in hospital and hospitals do things that are often unnecessary. There's got to be another reason for not giving it, so we don't just define ourselves in opposition to hospital. Birth *is* natural, but so is death, and sometimes we don't want a natural outcome. We want a culturally mediated outcome. Here's another thing that I hear midwives saying, 'Listen to your body, listen to your body'. Unless of course your body is telling you something that you don't want to hear and then we'll pretend that's not happening. It's head in the sand and looking the other direction. I understand why that sometimes happens. We love our clients, and we know they may not get the birth they are hoping for because of certain risk factors, but ultimately, there's no real empowerment if you're not holding a healthy baby in your arms. Sometimes, we have to say the hard things and be realistic with clients about what it is they're facing as they go into a medically complex birth, and I do think we should take full responsibility for that. Andrew Kotaska (see Chapter 20) takes a radical autonomy approach. I think it really resonates with the way I practise, but I also love the work of Paul Burcher, who emphasises professional responsibility. We need some kind of balance between those two things. We understand when we say birth is normal, trust birth, but we also know that when you go to a birth, there's always a little bit of death sitting on your shoulder saying, 'Look out for me. Watch out for me'. I actually think that's okay. It can promote safety and shows that we really value the life of this mother and baby. We know she wants to hold that baby in her arms and that there are worse things than a hospital birth. I don't like the idea that a transfer to hospital is thought of as a morbidity. It's a successful outcome, it's a perfectly predictable, expected outcome of a decently triaged system. We can't think of transfer as failure. Absolutely not.

We have to change that. It's a success. We had a case in our state recently where there was a threat to sue the midwife for transferring care because the woman wanted to stay in homebirth care, but she was outside our protocols. I don't think we have to support those kinds of choices. Professional responsibility has a role to play and when you are at the end of your skillset, a transfer might be the appropriate thing to do. It's different for a physician who is the end of the line for referrals. They have to do the best they can for the person, while respecting the patient's right to choose – even if they don't respect the choice that person is making. It is more complicated for us because we have the option of referring to someone else who is likely more experienced with whatever complication we are grappling with. We need some balance between autonomy and professional duty or responsibility. This is what we really need to be reflecting on as midwives and part of that is not working outside of our skillset or beyond our experience level whenever possible.

Physicians need to reflect on what community midwives are really asking of them. If we have someone who's had a long, non-progressive labour, they're stuck at six centimetres and we transfer from home, what's really the problem? Why are hospital providers so upset about that? They actually like mothers to do as much of their early labour at home as possible. They don't really want to admit them until they're four to six centimetres. What are we actually asking you for when we come in the vast majority of times? Pitocin and epidural, and perhaps a caesarean birth if those options do not lead to a timely vaginal birth. You're telling me you have a problem with that? That's what you do all day long, every day. We're coming in asking you to do the thing that you do very well and are very familiar with. Why are you so upset? What are you so worried about? It's about power, control and fear. The care you're actually being asked to provide is perfectly within your everyday scope of practice, and it's much better for women if we all just admit that and work together.

Looking at birth as an anthropologist

In anthropology, we say normal is simply what you're used to. If all you ever see is hospital birth, it might be really hard to envision an alternative. That's your normal. We have to imagine that 100 years ago, people thought very differently about their birth than they do today, so hopefully in the next few decades, the same will happen. I often wonder about the children at homebirths, who see these incredibly triumphant homebirths or they see their mother being strong and giving birth and being elated – what are they going to think about when they have their baby? They're going to have a very different perspective on what it is like to give birth.

There is this fear of birth; this perception that women's bodies are defunct and can't give birth without thousands of dollars of medical interventions. As an evolutionary biologist and medical anthropologist, it makes no sense to me.

It's impossible. Natural selection operates fiercely on reproductive function. Women are not incapable of giving birth. It is mind-blowing when you look at birth intervention rates in the USA and beyond. We have to be reminded that women's bodies can indeed give birth. It is both strange and intriguing to me that we have set up what has always been the way we as humans give birth as this thing that we should study to see if it is safe. Some women are pushing back against this assumption, and if we don't support them, they do look to birth outside the system.

I remember there was a debate in my community about whether baby should go skin-to-skin after the birth and also delay cord clamping. To have to argue for the evolutionary condition of humankind is just so bizarre to me, really. This is the normal human condition. But what's really bizarre is talking with someone who works in the hospital about it and having them not understand what you're talking about. You've got to do studies to support skin-to-skin? Of course, we do and how many thousands and thousands of dollars are spent demonstrating that the normal human condition is advantageous. As an anthropologist, I love it. It's fascinating, but I can also see that it is not that fascinating for many women who have to navigate a highly medicalised system. When the ARRIVE (Grobman et al., 2018) trial was published (a randomised controlled trial of routine induction for low-risk women at 39 weeks), I was so excited to read it and talk about it because I thought only in this country would you spend thousands of dollars to study whether one intervention could prevent another intervention. We often forget that we need to understand the range of normal for humans and that means trying to understand when induction is truly needed.

The way forward

- We need socially and culturally aligned relationship-based care as the standard for maternity care in the USA
- We need to invert the current medicalised structure in the USA, towards 89% midwifery care, rather than 89% physician-led care
- Every pregnant person would have access to a midwife whom they know, and some will also have a physician to care for them
- The USA needs to identify funding arrangements that optimise care to the woman's advantage
- Interprofessional training and collaboration needs to occur across all birth settings and provider types. This means we will transfer women in from homebirths for complications, not a crisis
- Hospitals need to extend some courtesy to midwives, especially in the moment when the client is most in need of interprofessional collaboration and communication
- Birth is far more than just a clinical event. How we treat women in birth matters deeply and we must recognise this and act now

References

Davis-Floyd, R. (2017). *Ways of knowing about birth: Mothers, midwives, medicine, and birth activism*. Long Grove, IL: Waveland Press.

Grobman, W. A., Rice, M. M., Reddy, U. M., Tita, A. T. N., Silver, R. M., Mallett, G., …, Macones, G. A. (2018). Labor induction versus expectant management in low-risk nulliparous women. *The New England Journal of Medicine, 379*, 513–523.

19 A conversation with the 'breech whisperer'

Andrew Bisits (interviewed by Hannah Dahlen)

> The solution to this [breech birth] is not simply to do more caesareans. You've got to look at understanding processes. What makes something safe? What makes it unsafe? And it's more than just numbers, it's a whole social fabric and approach to birthing that constructs safety.
>
> (Andrew Bisits)

About the author

I (Hannah Dahlen) interviewed Sydney obstetrician and Associate Professor Andrew Bisits to understand how he presents risk and choice to women who have a baby with a breech presentation (i.e. presenting bottom down), where they are making the choice between a vaginal breech birth and a caesarean section. Andrew has now supported over 500 breech births in his career and is known around Australia and internationally for his unique and very woman-centred approach. As you will see in this interview, while Andrew prefers the birth stool for vaginal breech birth as he sees it making the most physiological sense, he is also very clear about being guided by what women want too. Andrew has been coined the 'baby whisperer' by our Australian media, but I like to call him the 'breech whisperer'. I have had the pleasure of knowing and working with Andrew for many years. Whenever I have a client with a breech presentation, we have talked with Andrew. Once one of my clients filmed the external cephalic version (ECV) he did on her and posted it online, it went viral. After a successful ECV, I love sending Andrew pictures (with the woman's permission) of the woman holding her baby following the birth (mostly at home). He texts back lovely comments like 'Woohaa Hannah! Delighted for her, pass on my congrats'. His hands have a gentle knowledge that is hypnotic to watch. Perhaps this also comes from a responsiveness he gained playing the violin. Yes, Andrew is an obstetrician who plays the violin, loves a good red wine and tends to get very loud when watching rugby matches (especially if Australia wins). What you read in the following interview is what makes Andrew the way he is and how he presents risk to women when they are deciding what to do with a breech pregnancy at term. If we had more Andrews in the world, we would probably have fewer women seeking to birth outside the system. Andrew not only keeps the proverbial *canary in the coal mine* singing, he accompanies their song with his violin!

The very first question I (Hannah) asked Andrew is what led to his interest in vaginal breech birth? What sparked it?

Andrew: Look, it was in the mid '90s (around '94) that I noticed an increasing frequency in caesareans and I noticed there was this almost facile reasoning around it, which I've mentioned many times; it's where, essentially a woman says, 'I'm scared' and the obstetrician replies, 'Well, I'm scared too. Let's just do a caesarean'. That seemed to me to be the sum total of the discussion and, yes, it might be cloaked in various risks, but that was the sum total of it. That sort of reasoning clearly struck me as a bit facile. I could just see this 'unthinking' drift towards more caesarean sections. This happened for women with a breech presentation at term prior to the Term Breech Trial (Hannah et al., 2000). The thinking seemed to be, 'Oh, it's clearly more dangerous and we should just do a caesarean' and then, I kept hearing, 'Well, you never get in trouble for doing a caesarean' and so, with my questioning approach I asked, 'Well, are breeches really that unsafe and do women really just have to be railroaded into decisions like that?' Then, in 1994 and 1995, there was this talk about doing an international term breech trial and I thought to myself, why do you need to do a trial? This looks safe. Then I saw the way the trial was designed and I had worries. Mary Hannah (trial lead) came and spoke to us, but I didn't want to be part of the study because I could see that the trial recruitment was gravitating towards smaller institutions that weren't doing many vaginal breech births at all. I was very worried then that it was going to be biased, unintentionally, towards a better outcome for caesarean sections.

Then, of course, the Term Breech Trial study was published in 2000. On seeing the results, I thought to myself, is this game over? Is this the final word on the subject and we have to stop any consideration of vaginal breeches? Of course, the answer was no, but there followed considerable professional pressure to abandon planned vaginal breeches, and in fact, any vaginal breech! There were clearly many problems with the trial design. First, there were the statistical problems. It's statistically very difficult to analyse a study involving multiple centres and a limited number of outcomes, and where the treatment arms are unbalanced in each centre. So that already leads, from a strictly statistical point of view, to requiring much bigger numbers to make firm conclusions, particularly about subgroups.

There is no denial, however, of the overall result. The message appeared to be that there are no circumstances in which a vaginal breech is safe and that, to me, appeared overstated, because they were treating the findings as though it concerned one population. In fact, it's not; it's a series of mini trials at various centres, and as soon as you adjust for that, your confidence intervals change. I'm sounding like a statistical nerd here, but I did think about this for a long time. There was the reality that practices varied between the centres, despite the rigorous prescription for both trial arms. There were significant doubts about the skill level of the practitioners involved in the trial; breech birth skills had already declined among obstetricians and midwives were mostly not allowed to support breech birth because, in many institutions, it was deemed outside their scope of practice. In some countries, healthcare providers like Ontario midwife Betty-Anne Daviss helped maintain and reclaim this lost skill.

I had a lot of contacts in Norway at the time and they didn't want to be involved in the trial. I thought to myself this couldn't be the last word on it; more importantly, there will still be women who want a vaginal breech birth despite the trial conclusions. Women are not going to accept the dictum, 'There's this trial that shows this and therefore we can't support it'.

So, it was a conglomeration of factors that led me down the road of developing skill and interest in this area.

The Term Breech Trial's conclusion – that no set of circumstances could reassure us that vaginal breech birth can be as safe or safer than Caesarean section – bothered me. I thought that it prohibited any further thinking and research about breech birth (and it almost did). The Term Breech Trial was done in a climate when randomised trials were really becoming a sort of dogma; it was labelled as a new paradigm of research into clinical outcomes. In one sense, obstetrics led the charge on randomised trials because of Archie Cochrane's accusation that obstetrics was the least evidence-based of the professions – and gave it the wooden spoon along with psychiatry (Cochrane, 1979). A substantial number of obstetricians and obstetric academics were particularly enthusiastic about this challenge. In response, a strident, righteous mindset developed about this paradigm, and they really wanted to find areas where such a mindset would be justified. The issue about mode of birth for term breech was clearly ripe for such investigation and mindset. And, of course, the actual clear result of the trial was a real trophy for the evidence-based medicine paradigm. However, a single trial cannot give us an absolute answer to a clinical question and this one had significant limitations. It gave us valuable information, there is no question it did, but it did not mean that you had to stop thinking about or stop doing [breech birth].

In my early days of increasing interest in vaginal breech birth, I found myself thinking about normal birth a lot. I was thinking about normal birth – in ways I took for granted in a cephalic birth – I thought this is good because I am gaining new insights about the panorama of normal birth. Among the many discussions about vaginal breech in and around 2000 (the year of publication of the Term Breech Trial), I became aware of how much a particular paralysing and anxious fear dominated such discussions. There was continuous mention of being sued, being traumatised – what if this goes wrong and that goes wrong. It also dominated every other area in obstetrics. I then became aware that this was a broader social phenomenon summarised in a book by Frank Furedi, a UK sociologist, *The culture of fear* (Furedi, 1997). The insights in this book made me understand why obstetricians just jumped in and responded in a knee-jerk way to the Term Breech Trial; it was part of an ambient fearful environment, where we are constantly looking for excuses to jump out of anything that looked risky. This was fuelled by the anxiety about the Millennium bug in computers and a fear that Western countries would shut down amid a reign of chaos. At the same time, we were also very close to the HIH collapse[1] and that dragged out for a few years, and left a huge impact. You have to acknowledge these things are influential, but the solution is not to simply do more caesareans. You've got to look at understanding processes. What makes something safe? What makes it unsafe? And it's more than just numbers; it's a whole social fabric and approach to birthing that constructs safety.

The whole area of risk fascinated me as well. Yes, there are these risks, but how do people process those risks? What does it mean when I say that something occurs 1:200? How do you communicate these things? How do people process that? I will always remember one woman who had a history of breast cancer – she survived that, apparently against the odds – and they saw me about a breech birth because someone had said, 'you can't do this'. We talked and they expressed it very nicely. They said, 'We're sick of hearing about averages because I was told that about my breast cancer'. They appreciated the discussion with me because I was trying to individualise it. They said, 'Thank you for not just treating us as though we're condemned to averages'. That's probably a really important point, we have all these figures and information about risk – wonderful – but as I say to women, there are averages and, in the end, we should make some sort of statement as to which side of the average an individual falls. Short of that, it just becomes a very sterile, bland and near meaningless exercise.

I (Hannah) asked Andrew about how he communicates with women about breech. I asked him to take a scenario where a first-time mother has found out her baby is breech at 36 weeks, she attempted an ECV which was not successful, and now you've come to the discussion about whether she has a caesarean section or a vaginal breech birth. What sort of things do you say and how do you present that risk to the woman?

Andrew: I don't launch straightaway into the numbers. I first describe how the baby 'does it' (the mechanisms) because if you don't do that, then the numbers that you present are interpreted in this sort of vacuum, which tends to be purely negative; whereas when you talk about it in the context of this mechanism, that works pretty well, that's pretty clever, the women then, almost universally, take on the subsequent information in a different way. What I then say is, 'if you look at one thousand women having a vaginal breech birth, mostly where the conditions for vaginal breech have been met (baby < 4 kg, pregnancy normal, frank or complete breech), the consensus about the frequency of severe outcomes (baby dies or there is a damaging shortage of oxygen) is about two to three in a thousand. That's a fairly agreed consensus from large observational studies and some randomised trials. If you look at the same situation for a thousand women having a cephalic birth, where the criteria for a normal birth have been met, the same risks are about one to two in a thousand. For a planned elective caesarean section, it's more like a half in a thousand or one in two thousand. Then I make reference to a slightly increased frequency of, say, more minor, short-term events and then I make reference to the frequency of caesarean section in labour (30–40%). I emphasise that a caesarean section in labour is not a wasted effort, mainly because the baby does get exposed to the whole process of labour, which has its own benefits, and it is also good for future births. I have rarely seen any of the women, who have been motivated to have a vaginal breech birth, be disappointed about attempting the vaginal birth. None of them have ever said to me that was a waste of time. In one sense, this says so much. It has been many women now, who have said that to me.

After presenting the numbers, I say in the discussion, 'Look, the numbers that I've presented to you are an average'. I then say to women which side of these averages they sit. Recently I saw a woman who was about five foot eight, she's had a baby before, the baby's bottom is in the pelvis, we couldn't turn the baby, the baby's already comfortable there. I said to her, 'To me, you are on the better side of that average'. Every now and again I have to say that 'I'd be slightly more concerned about your situation compared to the average', but most of the time, because of our population [South Eastern Sydney, where Andrew works, is quite advantaged], I would say, 'I think you're on the better side of the average'.

I also talk about the implications for the future with the caesarean; yes, it's straightforward to do, it is safe for the baby, and we do them very well. The reality is, most of the time, once you've had a caesarean, for a range of reasons, you will have another caesarean and, of course, you can have a vaginal birth but it imposes a risk on future births. So now generally, the women have heard enough information and it's a fairly difficult area to process. I get them to read the executive summary of the Royal College of Obstetricians and Gynaecologists Breech Guidelines from 2017 (Royal College of Obstetricians and Gynaecologists, 2017). I then get them to ring me back and I say, 'Well, I'll go with whatever you feel comfortable with (once you have processed all the information)'. I answer any other questions that arise after this.

Part of the discussion, of course, is very much the whole process of having a caesarean, the whole process of having a vaginal breech and, around both of these, the fundamental safeguards. When I mention risks, I always talk about the safeguards that minimise those risks. This is about the sum total of what I say. Usually the discussion takes a minimum of 30 to 45 minutes.

Of course, the discussion about vaginal breech birth is very much about a normal birth. There is all this information out there that you have to have this done for a breech and that done for a breech. I say to them, really, mostly our hands are off and we're very concerned about positioning and doing all those things that encourage a normal birth.

I went on to ask Andrew about his preference for women being upright on a birth stool for a breech birth. I wanted to know why he liked this birth position.

Andrew: I first saw the birth stool used by Monika Boenigk (an Australian midwife). I watched her look after a woman using a birth stool and I became more interested in her approach. It just immediately made sense to me. Since that time, it's just been reinforced that, with the birth stool, the babies descend by themselves, with minimal manoeuvres required, and the women seem to exercise a 'rewarding' sense of control. Even if there is a problem, the babies are so low down that the access to the baby is straightforward. So I have never seen a very difficult mechanical problem using a birth stool. However, I am constantly open to other insights. In Denmark, where I visited recently, there was emphasis on the hands and knees position for birth, but I think the main approach should be whatever the woman feels will help get her baby out; therefore, there needs to be flexibility around the choice of birthing position. In Germany they advocated this hands and knees position as well. My one concern about this is the frequency with which they have to do fairly invasive manoeuvres to free awkward arms. It's just raising the question whether, as a primary position, it is the optimal position. Betty-Anne Daviss (a Canadian midwife who attends breech birth) concurs with me about this. The birth stool just offers a flexible starting point. If problems arise, women can easily adopt the hands and knees position. My other observation has been that once the baby's trunk and arms have birthed the head follows more easily without assistance when the woman adopts a hands and knees position. The birth of the head occurs spontaneously because the weight of the body facilitates this. So, I keep thinking about these things and sometimes women just say, 'Look, I feel better pushing on hands and knees', which is fine. It's really an issue of flexibility but, yes, I do favour the birth stool as a primary position.

I then asked Andrew about how important it was to understand the physiology behind a breech birth.

Andrew: Understanding the physiology behind breech birth is so important. Being present at a breech birth is a great opportunity to intensely think, 'what is happening here?' If I leave things alone, how is this happening? Exactly where is this arm? What angle is this? With vaginal breech birth we are forced to engage in quite an intense observation and hence are led into an increased understanding of normality. Further, we can observe how women pick normality. There is a discernment going on at the time. Again, we work with this rather than trying to control it, and that is what makes all of this so interesting. Normal is never boring!

I asked Andrew about what he felt when he watched women give birth and did he admire them. I have observed that really woman-centred obstetricians like Andrew have a deep respect and admiration for women.

Andrew: Yes, yes, yes. Now, how can I just quickly elaborate on that? I am constantly amazed by just what goes on at the time of a birth and how these adaptations happen which are not just a physiological, primal thing, they are better seen as quite a determination in women. The normal birth process evokes a real determination and will that is unique. I feel it as an overwhelming energy in the room. So, yes, I'm just quite amazed and full of admiration.

Talking about these matters with some obstetricians can be difficult. Too often there is a lack of understanding that birthing women (a) really appreciate the many issues that affect them; and (b) understand the many issues around the birth and, at the time of the birth, they will make decisions.

I remember this woman who was pushing on the birth stool as a student midwife came in and introduced herself. The woman (sitting on the birth stool) says, 'Hi, my name's Mary and this is my vagina'. Of course, everyone started laughing and then she's pushing and she feels something's not quite happening. So she says, 'Look, I think I really need to be on hands and knees'. And I said, 'All right. Let's do it'. And she just pushed the baby down. And again, that sticks in my mind. Really her whole comment about 'Hi. My name's Mary and this is my vagina' was her saying 'I know what's going on here' and then she demonstrated that. She was in control of that situation. She claimed her power. When she said, 'Look, I need to get over on hands and knees', I believed her. There have been many other occasions where, in the course of a normal birth, women have made statements that reflect the fact that they are in control of the situation and they know what is going on. We simply have to listen and work with these insights.

I went on to ask Andrew if he thought that the way doctors and midwives discuss risk can be part of the problem in the rising rates of freebirth and high risk homebirth.

Andrew: Yes, definitely, because it can be couched in that subtly coercive way; it is all in the tone of the voice; it is all in the information that you pick. While it looks subtly coercive to us, to the woman it is obviously coercive. Such coercion is not malicious; it arises from deep fears about birth. And I don't need to tell you, but the women pick up immediately, they hear, 'this person is absolutely petrified of this thing, they do not want to me do it, they're not going to support me' and (a) 'I feel coerced'; and (b) 'actually this is the very thing they're scared about and there's no way I'd feel safe in their hands because of that'. So, it's a very undermining approach. A classic example in the breech scenario is when people say they're counselling someone and they'll say, 'Oh, do you know your baby could die?' That's the extent of the counselling. Or they say, 'Your baby's head could get stuck'. Now that tells you one thing: *I'm scared.* They should be saying, 'I'm scared, I'm very scared of the baby's head getting stuck. You need to know that I'm scared', but instead, they just say, 'The baby's head could get stuck'. Of course, the woman immediately picks up that this person is absolutely petrified. And then, that not-so-subtle coercion is perceived in the woman's eyes as something that will dominate the entire birthing process – that they will be greeted by all this apprehension and fear, and of course this can happen every day in our birthing units. So, yes, I have no doubt we coerce women into the choices they make. At times, it is done in the way we communicate numbers and risk. For example, if you use the relative risks and/or if you communicate a number without any qualification. Whenever I present numbers, I place emphasis on absolute risks, saying to women, 'These numbers for everyone will be different. They will mean different things to different people and you have to decide'. I have found that women do relax when you say that and it is because we are not constraining their understanding. You are treating them as an individual who will have some sort of perspective because of experiences x, y and z, and it will allow them to make sense of it.

I asked Andrew about the worry all health providers deal with when caring for women and how he managed that worry when it came to breech birth.

Andrew: The main task is to take a step back. The conversation I will have in my head is 'you've seen this before, you know it can work'. Again, it's taking a step back from the ambient pressure on you and saying the reason that you're feeling like this is you do have a lot of people breathing down your neck. And the response to that is, you can't be bullied out of things by what other people think. Whenever I'm awaiting a breech birth, I'm always wondering, 'is this going to happen?' And there might be a lack of progress, there might be a few worrying decelerations, but it is about calling on a certain belief, saying, 'you've seen it happen before, you've thought about this a thousand times and you know that as soon as that bum comes out, if it's slipping out, you know it will be okay'. But that's an ongoing work. It really is. You could almost say that you're aiming for a type of enlightenment. It's an ongoing task, even now after many years of experience. But I do have to keep talking to myself and I say things like, 'Why are you so anxious about this situation now? Is it actually about the birth or is it about something that someone's said?' To ease some of this 'worry', one strategy, while waiting for the breech birth, is to talk with the registrar and midwife, 'Let's just go through a breech birth. This is how it will happen, all right?' And then we all know what to do and while that's one way of spreading or sharing the 'worry', it's another way of just saying, 'look this happens by itself'.

The last question I asked Andrew was what is the way forwards? We've got increasing numbers of women traumatised by birth, seeking other options of care or no professional care at the birth at all. So what is the way forward as an obstetrician and how can we re-engage women?

Andrew: Now that is really difficult. The only way I can see it happening at a social level is if there is better financial compensation for a vaginal birth compared to a caesarean. I think a large part of the obstacle we face in this area is due to private practice. There is big machinery there. This was fuelled in Australia by the safety net (a scheme by which private obstetricians had their salaries augmented by a number of government allowances) so that obstetricians made a lot of money from uncomplicated normal births. Obstetricians are trained to deal with the abnormalities surrounding birth. While it is important they are able to appreciate the bounds of normality, normal births are the province of midwives. Obstetricians need to focus on the abnormal and deal with those situations in a competent and confident way. Due to the culture of private obstetric practice, there is an understandable defensive attitude about any threats to it. Private practice administers care to an influential strata of the population. Mostly these are educated, well-resourced women who, in many instances, do not need the services of an obstetrician. This in turn creates a culture of practice where often obstetric-led care is seen as the best and safest, because of the higher cost of the service. And so we have our culture of birth in Australia. This culture will determine 'best practice' rather than best evidence. Therefore, economic incentives have the best chance of changing this. Change can occur if there were less reliance on the adversarial system for compensation of injured babies and mothers; therefore, we need a no-fault compensation system similar to New Zealand or Denmark. Private obstetricians working by themselves can feel very exposed. This, in turn, fuels a particular approach to understanding and talking about risk.

I have just been to a rural hospital in Denmark. This was my second visit. I watched the way they work in this particular department. It's a midwife who leads the handover and they are very much on the same level of power and knowledge with the obstetricians. Their roles and functioning are different but complementary. They are viewing the birthing process and its complexities with different perspectives, all of which are legitimate. We need to adopt such a system. You're both viewing the same phenomenon in different but mutually respectful ways and this approach is strongly embedded in countries like Denmark.

One way forward is to choose one or two birthing institutions in Australia where the staffing will be purely staff specialist obstetricians with no private practice at all. All the primary care will be midwifery and the role of the obstetrician will be very much: if there are problems and its only 'if'. In turn this would create the possibility of better cooperation and cohesion. In Newcastle, where I worked previously, all consultant positions were converted to staff specialists, this in turn led to more cohesive practice and the rates of intervention dropped.

Powerful cultures have been set up around various financial interests and fears, which in turn are a huge obstacle to progressive change and they further a system which subtly leads to coercion and traumatised women who feel let down. They create these, unfortunately, very unwelcoming environments for women. We're just starting homebirth here at the Royal Hospital for Women in Sydney and, for me, it's just highlighting the cultural resistance – and it's very clear to me why women want their baby born at home.

The way forward

- Dedicated clinics and teams for women with breech and twins
- Midwives to play a pivotal role in the care of women with breech and twins
- Midwives do the counselling around breech births
- All institutions should have a goal of creating confidence around breech births and twins as cases of complex normality (Shawn Walker)

Note

1 HIH Insurance Group was a publicly listed primary insurance company – one of, if not the, largest in Australia at the time – which collapsed in 2001, compromising insurance coverage for many industries, in particular medicine.

References

Cochrane, A. L. (1979). 1931–1971: A critical review with particular reference to the medical profession. In G. Teeling Smith & N. Wells (Eds.), *Medicines for the year 2000* (pp. 1–11). London: Office of Health Economics.

Furedi, F. (1997). *Culture of fear: Risk taking and the morality of low expectation*. London: Continuum.

Hannah, M. E., Hannah, W. J., Hewson, S., Hodnett, E. D., Saigal, S., & Willan, A. R. (2000). Planned caesarean section at term versus planned vaginal birth for breech presentation at term: A randomised controlled multicentred trial. Term Breech Trial Collaborative Group. *Lancet, 356*(9239), 1375–1383.

Royal College of Obstetricians and Gynaecologists. (2017). Management of Breech Presentation (Green-top Guideline No. 20b). Retrieved from: www.rcog.org.uk/en/guidelines-research-services/guidelines/gtg20b/.

20 Obstetricians discuss the coal mine and the canary

Alison Barrett and Andrew Kotaska

> There's another special kind of blindness that happens when people refuse to see things that they'd rather not see: willful blindness.
>
> (Alison Barrett)

> Much of the current medical establishment's approach to women birthing in hospital is 'you do it our way or you take the highway.' Women who are birthing at home with risk factors or unattended are saying to us that they choose the highway rather than submit to the coercion implicit in hospital policies and guidelines.
>
> (Andrew Kotaska, 2019)

About the authors

Alison Barrett is a Canadian-trained consultant obstetrician and gynaecologist. She lives in New Zealand, where she continues to practise medicine while finishing a law degree at the University of Waikato. Before she went to medical school, she studied ecology at the University of Toronto. Alison is a member of Ora Taiao, the New Zealand Climate and Health Council, and is also a member of the professional advisory group of La Leche League New Zealand.

Andrew Kotaska is an obstetrician and gynaecologist at Stanton Territorial Hospital in Yellowknife, Canada. He is president of the Northwest Territories Medical Association and has academic appointments as Adjunct Professor with the School of Population and Public Health at the University of British Columbia and Lecturer at the Universities of Manitoba and Toronto.

Iatrogenesis in the coal mine

Alison Barrett

In a blog post, the scientist Meghan Duffy (2019) asked other scientists, 'when did you realize you were studying climate change?' This is a great question in its own right. But this is a book about birth. So in this chapter, I'm going to show you that this question gets at something really important about maternity care too.

Let me explain. My husband has been a climate change scientist since the embryonic stage of his scientific gestation. The first experiment he designed, as an undergraduate in the 1980s, looked at the effects of climate change on biodiversity. I helped him collect samples, because I studied science too, before I was accepted into medical school.

Back then, there were all kinds of scientists: marine and freshwater biologists, microbiologists, plant scientists; a friend of ours studied feral donkeys in the Australian outback. They didn't necessarily begin their careers in climate science, but what seemed to become apparent to the author of the blog was that all were obliged to become climate change scientists over time. The species or the phenomena they studied didn't exist in a parallel non-climate change-affected universe. As they monitored, measured and made observations in their specific branch of science, the natural laboratories they worked in were experiencing climate-induced perturbations. Duffy recognised that most scientists eventually had to become climate scientists, given their observant, scientific minds.

This year, the World Health Organization (WHO) put climate change first in its ranking of the top ten threats to Global Health (WHO, 2019). While the recognition of climate change as a major health hazard was commendable, there was a concerning omission from the list: iatrogenesis. Yet, iatrogenesis, the harm caused by treatment, is now the third leading cause of death in developed parts of the world (Makary & Daniel, 2016).

A charitable view of the omission would be that the WHO knows that, in too many other parts of the world, people are dying due to a lack of medical services. It may seem wrong to worry about the harms of overtreatment when people are dying from undertreatment in less well-off countries. But as we continue to export the medical model elsewhere, we must tackle this problem of medically induced harm. We are already infecting many emerging healthcare environments with the virus of iatrogenesis. We've exported plenty of other harms, communicable diseases and non-communicable (like obesity and type 2 diabetes). We've erased indigenous knowledge about sustainable development practices. So before we compound our mistakes, we must confront the reality of iatrogenesis.

Like the scientist who sees climate change in the science she studies, doctors like me see iatrogenesis everywhere now, no matter what field of medicine we practise in. Iatrogenesis has always been a part of medicine, but it is now a considerable threat to everyone's health (Peer, 2018). Like tobacco companies that simply will not quit, and continue to expand into new markets to maintain profits, medicine has succumbed to the forces of neoliberalism and become an equally unstoppable and equally invasive monster – possibly just as harmful. Drug companies, device manufacturers, insurance agencies and various opportunistic businesses all clamour for their market share in fighting the illnesses they have, in part, created. Doctors become their willing servants, some knowingly complicit, others duped. Some are too overworked or too burned out to care.

For me, I realised early on as a doctor that, even as I tried to help people and wanted to be part of their healing, a lot of my work is about rescuing people from harms caused by treatment. Within the maternity system, I work to keep women and their families from having their pregnancies unnecessarily medicalised in the first place. The problem of the canary in the coal mine is fundamentally a problem of iatrogenic harm. We have literally dug the woman a mine. No canary would really enter it with truly informed choice.

Yet, the charity Birthrights says that the most common call they get is from women who want an elective caesarean section in their current pregnancy and have had that request denied (Birthrights, 2018). According to Birthrights advocates, the women have made an informed choice to have a medically unnecessary procedure. The most common reason for their request, for what is termed a maternal choice caesarean, is a previous traumatic birth (Birthrights, 2018).

It could seem paradoxical that a woman who has been harmed by the medical model of birth might chose to go back to the perpetrators for more. Indeed, some women with previous traumatic experiences in the hospital system do the exact opposite, in the most extreme cases choosing an unattended out-of-hospital birth instead. But the fact remains that women who choose birth by maternal choice caesarean are undeniably assuming a significantly higher risk of severe acute maternal morbidity than if they have a straightforward vaginal birth (Korb et al., 2019). Any harm they might suffer during their unnecessary procedure is a harm caused indirectly by the previous harm. So why would a woman sign up for a highly medicalised form of birth – a surgery with no medical indication?

The women who contact Birthrights have made thoughtful, considered decisions. Knowing the physical and emotional trauma they experienced the first time, many feel their best bet for limiting future damage is to plan surgery within the system. This is quite a sensible decision when examined close up. It's even a sensible decision – given the alternatives – for women who are having their first baby. This is because every attempt at vaginal birth exposes the woman to a risk of an emergency caesarean.

There are only three ways to get a baby out. It's like the game show – with Doors Number One, Two and Three. Door Number One opens to vaginal birth. Door Number Two opens to an emergency caesarean section. Open Door Number Three and you get a planned caesarean section. But the only door with a label on it is Door Number Three.

The certainty of opening Door Number Three is that it removes any chance of a normal vaginal birth – but this may be a price the woman is willing to pay, particularly if vaginal birth in her particular coal mine isn't ever 'normal'. In some places, attempting to birth vaginally means experiencing degrading and disrespectful treatment and lots of interventions (O'Reilly, 2019), and with all that, no guarantee of success. In some clinical settings, for example, a women having her first baby and being induced has a 50/50 chance of succeeding vaginally (Vahratian, Zhang, Troendle, Sciscione, & Hoffman,

2005). Not surprisingly, many women just cut to the chase and opt for Door Number Three.

An elective caesarean offers certain 'advantages', such as choice of surgeon. Private obstetricians can be charming and subtly persuasive. In most publicly funded maternity systems, an emergency caesarean will be done by whoever is on call that day. Sometimes that person is a trainee. Even in hospital systems where most providers are competent, there could be that one doctor everyone avoids. Scheduling surgery means you may avoid leaving your surgeon to chance.

Choosing an elective caesarean is like that canary picking out the loveliest cage they'll be housed in once they've entered the mine, when they can fly free – still trapped inside the walls of the system, of course. It is hardly surprising – if there's a significant chance of ending up with a traumatic emergency caesarean section – that women plan an elective one, with their provider of choice. They are making reasonable calculations about the unpleasant choices on offer in that medicalised menu.

Then there are women who choose not to enter the mine at all. An increasing number of women choose to birth without any care provider, completely outside the system (Dahlen, Jackson, & Stevens, 2011). Some make the choice for the same reasons given for planning a caesarean: a previous traumatic birthing experience within the system and a belief that they will retain autonomy and control in their own environment (Feeley & Thompson, 2016). When women vote with their feet in this way, doctors vilify them without accepting, acknowledging or realising their own role in the woman's decision-making process. Doctors cannot see that the women they hurt aren't so keen to put themselves in iatrogenic harm's way again. The ones that perform caesareans on request are not necessarily facilitating a 'free choice'. Doctors who take advantage of the situation are blinded by their own self-interest, and perhaps some guilt.

Most scientists today see climate change in their work, and almost no scientist is a climate change denier. Unfortunately, it seems the opposite is true of doctors and iatrogenesis. Instead, as Hannah Dahlen (2014) wrote, maternity care has become a 'super trawler of risk'. Dahlen uses the analogy of the super trawlers, now banned off the coasts of environmentally aware countries, to explain: these giant fishing boats cast gigantic nets to catch as many fish as possible, but inadvertently trap dolphins, turtles and other species along the way. Everything that cannot end up on the dinnerplate is called the 'by-catch', and simply tossed back into the ocean, often damaged or dead. In maternity care, the super trawler obstetric net is cast wide. Not all women need to be captured in the net. Most women still have pregnancies that are low-risk. But year on year, fewer pregnant women escape being medicalised through pregnancies and births as the super trawler net of risk gets bigger (Dahlen, 2014). In the fishing industry, super trawlers are valued because they catch large numbers of fish quickly and incredibly efficiently. Similarly, industrialised, medicalised systems of care also pursue efficiency as an end goal. In serving efficiency, and out of fear of risk, women are subjected to interventions they don't need; in other words, it is 'better to be safe than sorry'. There is even a term for these women: *the numbers needed to treat*. The numbers needed to treat are the 'by-catch' – the many inadvertently captured in the net in the pursuit of desired fish. Doctors console themselves for the harm they do to women by telling themselves – repeatedly – that they are only erring on the side of caution.

If you can rationalise the iatrogenic harms experienced by the 'by-catch', you can convince yourself of the benefits of this so-called 'efficient' maternity health system. The alternative – individual, relationship-based care – takes time and seems old-fashioned and unscientific, despite the overwhelming evidence that supports it (Renfrew et al., 2014). Sadly, there are no sales reps or glossy brochures to promote relationship-based care.

There are so many problems with the super-trawler model. For example, the team can be so busy caring for women who don't need care such that, when a mother or baby really do need the urgent treatment hospitals can and should provide, *they don't get it in a timely fashion*. It seems that, every other day, there's another hospital involved in a scandal where the provision of maternity healthcare fell well below standard, and mothers and babies were harmed. Yet, doctors continue to claim that hospital is the safest place for babies to be born (RANZCOG, 2017).

There is a special sort of blindness that develops when you are literally surrounded by something and still unable to see it. Marsden Wagner (2001) described this phenomenon in the maternity system in a paper entitled 'Fish can't see water'. He explained that the medicalisation of birth had become so mainstream, people working within the system could no longer see the damaging side effects of it. This way of birthing had become the norm (Wagner, 2001). The WHO put it like this:

> By 'medicalizing' birth, i.e. separating a woman from her own environment and surrounding her with strange people using strange machines to do strange things to her in an effort to assist her, the woman's state of mind and body is so altered that her way of carrying through this intimate act must also be altered and the state of the baby born must equally be altered … Most health care providers no longer know what 'non-medicalized' birth is. The entire modern obstetric and neonatological literature is essentially based on observations of 'medicalized' birth.
>
> (World Health Organization, 1985)

For an example of how the downstream effects of medicalisation hide in plain view, consider a recent study that found that homebirthing women were twice as likely to establish and maintain breastfeeding as women who delivered in hospital (Quigley, Taut, Zigman, & Gallagher, 2016). The authors were unable to explain the phenomenon – they could not fathom any physiological mechanisms that could account for their findings. They simply concluded that the findings were 'unlikely to be causal' (Quigley et al., 2016, p. 1). This is despite the fact that the difference in breastfeeding rates persisted, even when the study controlled for the increased interventions in the hospitalised group. The authors were unable to see that birthing in the hospital is itself an intervention. Their only explanation for the finding was that women who birthed at home must be different in their desire to breastfeed and their persistence in doing so (Quigley et al., 2016). In other words, they concluded that the difference was due to the personal characteristics of women who birthed at home that carried over to their commitment to breastfeeding: i.e. the women were simply being stubborn. The researchers didn't consider that aspects of the hospital environment itself could alter the woman's state of mind or body, detrimentally affecting the release of oxytocin or other hormones needed for successful breastfeeding. They were unable to code the failure of lactation within the hospital setting as another example of iatrogenic harm. As fish cannot see the water they swim in, maternity researchers cannot see the iatrogenesis that follows on from the normality of medicalised birth.

The inability of doctors to see their role in the harms they cause has a long and continuous history (Best & Neuhauser, 2004). You'd think we learned something from all those previous denials: the germ theory of disease, thalidomide, lobotomy, Essure, vaginal mesh, Vioxx, New Zealand's cervical cancer enquiry AKA 'The Unfortunate Experiment' (Jones, 2017) and the UK's current tainted blood scandal (Walker, 2019). This special kind of blindness, which happens when people refuse to see things that they'd rather not see, is a willful blindness. A doctor's duty is to 'first, do no harm', but it is hard to know that the care you give is hurting people when you aren't collecting (or even looking for) the receipts. In any case, the harm keeps occurring regardless of the truth of who causes it. Whether in malice or through ignorance, when doctors refuse to accept their role in causing harm, the patients bear the cost. And this brings us to another way of framing the issue: as a moral hazard.

A moral hazard refers to the risks people take when they know they are insured against loss. It is a term attributed to the insurance industry and further developed by economists (Rowell & Connelly, 2012). When we examine people's behaviour, we find that they are tempted to take greater risks when someone else is assuming the costs associated with the risk. It is called a moral hazard because the risky action wouldn't occur, but for the insurance. The moral component occurs when the risk-taker knows the scales are tipped in their favour. The same moral hazard applies in medicine. Doctors prescribe medicines or treatments that are known to have risks. They benefit from you taking these medicines or treatments, they are incentivised to encourage you to take them, even as they are incentivised to ignore, disguise or minimise the harms. A patient can be blamed for any negative outcome.

A great example today is how doctors claim that rates of caesarean section are on the rise because mothers are fatter (Berendzen & Howard, 2013), older (Gordon, Milberg, Daling, & Hickok, 1991), and becoming 'too posh to push' (Song, 2004). If the hospitals they work in widely differ in institutional rates of intervention, they maintain that the differences are due to the hospital's 'case mix'. A 'case mix' is the name given to the mixture of women who present to a facility, whether high- or low-risk. Doctors can, and do, claim that their hospital has a high caesarean section rate because their district is full of high-risk, impoverished or non-white women. But the evidence shows otherwise. A Massachusetts study showed that the 'case mix artefact' applied as an excuse for high rates of surgery could not be explained by maternal characteristics (Cáceres et al., 2013). Instead, hospitals actually differ in how readily they intervene based on hospital culture. Hospitals that do lots of surgery simply do lots of surgery, regardless of the 'type' of woman who walks in the door. The likelihood of a woman getting a particular intervention has more to do with the hospital she attends than any other factor. She is usually blamed for the outcome when it has nothing to do with her.

Other forces well beyond a woman's control conspire against her too. For example, the way doctors are paid can influence the way they practise. One study compared funding models for obstetricians with an added twist: it looked at what happens to intervention rates when obstetricians paid under different funding models had patients who were doctors, compared to patients who were ordinary members of the public (Johnson & Rehavi, 2013). They found that obstetricians offered doctor patients different rates of caesarean section based on the way they were paid for their services. If the obstetrician was paid a fee for every procedure they did, thus giving them a financial reason for doing the procedure, these obstetricians were *less* likely to operate on colleagues and *more* likely to operate on non-doctor patients. Perhaps this was because they could pull the wool over the eyes of ordinary people, who aren't as likely to question if monetary motivations are behind recommendations for surgery. The opposite effect was seen for obstetricians paid a salary for their work. These obstetricians are not financially incentivised to perform extra procedures. In those conditions, obstetricians were *more* likely to offer a doctor colleague a caesarean section. Maybe surgery is a kind of perk for club members. While they weren't benefiting directly, the procedure may have been a chance to show off what a great doctor they were, doing that extra work for free. These obstetricians may have been driven by their ego's need to show their colleagues special favours.

Maybe there are other, more charitable reasons for the differences I've been discussing here. There is still a big problem, however, when different surgical strokes are being offered to different folks. When care is unevenly delivered by hospitals influenced by pro-surgery culture, or racism, or by doctors' financial motivations, it becomes more obvious that women's rights are being violated.

Here is a fairly typical story of what we are up against.

A woman was sent for an ultrasound to check placental position late in pregnancy, after her anatomy scan showed the placenta was low-lying. Most times, this situation resolves itself as the uterus grows, and indeed this was the case. Two weeks before her due date, her midwife wondered if the baby was breech and sent her for another scan to check. The baby was head down;

however, the scan apparently showed there had been no growth of the baby at all in the interval between scans. Medical staff advised an urgent induction. The frightened couple were admitted to the ward. Hours passed and finally an induction process was begun with prostaglandin gel. Nothing happened. At the next decision point, where more medication or assessment needed to occur, the ward was busy with other, more pressing issues. A day passed. The couple became irritated. They were sold a sense of urgency that now seemed unwarranted by the treatment they were receiving. If things were not urgent, they wanted to be discharged home. The hospital staff became annoyed. They asked, 'Don't you want what's best for your baby?'

There are two possible endings to this story. The first is that the couple agree to wait for the next stage of treatment. Then, after many different interventions, including rupturing the membranes, IV oxytocin, epidural, fever and antibiotics, the baby becomes distressed, they end up opening Door Number Two and 'elect' to have an emergency caesarean section. There may or may not have been complications after that. The family is encouraged to view their procedure as life-saving and necessary. 'A healthy baby is all that matters', they are told.

But what really happened was the second ending: the couple left the hospital, which made them sign forms to discharge themselves against medical advice.

After they left, the couple decided to book themselves in for another scan, in a different ultrasound clinic. It had only been three days since the previous scan was done, and technically, this is not 'allowed'. They made some excuse to get the scan, and they didn't tell the sonographers about the one they'd just had. Sonographers will tell you that no meaningful data can be obtained by scans done too close together. It is like stepping on the scales to weigh ourselves every day. We cannot really know for sure whether we have gained or lost weight when we take two measurements so close together. For a foetus, we have data to support a gap of two weeks between scans to ensure information collected on weight is reliable. Estimates of foetal weight do not give interpretable data when they are done less than two weeks apart. The margins of error within any measurements mean that there will be overlap between these margins of error of one measurement and the margin of error on the other. The two data sets don't overlap until a reasonable amount of time elapses.

When a foetus really falters in its growth, there are often other warning signs. For example, the amniotic fluid also can decline or the blood flow in the umbilical cord can be abnormal. We should have been suspicious of the second scan, the one that doctors based their decision to recommend an induction, because there were none of these signs. In medicine, we really shouldn't pick the results we like and ignore the ones we don't. We shouldn't pick the best two out of three scans, but that is what this couple did. The new scan had a much different result. If you ignored the one that showed no growth, assuming it was the outlier, the data now showed the baby's growth to be tracking beautifully. The scan that failed to show growth was probably incorrect.

I know all this because this couple was booked into my clinic the day after they discharged themselves against medical advice. I was instructed by the Head of Department to make them stay and persuade them to try induction again. Instead, the couple went home and had their perfectly well-grown baby there a few days later.

Not too long after this event, I found myself at a party, standing beside a stranger. To fill an awkward silence, I asked the safe question 'What do you do for a living?' The man replied, 'I work for an oil company'. 'Oh', I said, trying to seem neutral, 'So, if you don't mind me asking, what do you think about climate change? Do you think the scientists are right?' He replied 'The scientists are 100 percent right. It's for sure a real thing'. He looked genuinely sad as he said, 'I have children and I worry about their future'. He added, 'But I have to feed my family'.

I haven't been able to get that little conversation out of my mind. We all need to eat and support the people we love. Many of us do work that harms other people in the service of that goal. When I think of all the damage done by doctors, I am not sure we are any different from this man. We cannot claim the moral high ground.

In the recent Netflix documentary *One Planet*, David Attenborough said, 'If I were to give one piece of advice to people regarding the preservation of our planet, it would be "Don't waste"'. He went on. 'Don't waste food. Don't waste water. Don't waste power. Don't waste time' (Fothergill, 2019). We have only a small amount of time to act before the harm we do to the climate is irreversible.

What we have done to women and birth is also a waste. Think about all the unnecessary things that were done to the couple who had the scans. The unnecessary scans. The unnecessary worry. The hospital time and resources that could have been used elsewhere. Some may not see the connection between what is happening to the planet and what is happening to women's bodies, but in truth, they are inseparably connected. For the sake of the planet and the women and babies it supports, we need to shut down all the mines.

In the next section, Obstetrician Andrew Kotaska give us his perspective and advice on how to talk to women about risk so we don't alienate them.

We need to stop the 'my way or the highway' approach

Andrew Kotaska

> Much of the current medical establishment's approach to women birthing in hospital is 'you do it our way or you take the highway'. Women who are birthing at home with risk factors or unattended are saying to us that they choose the highway rather than submit to the coercion implicit in hospital policies and guidelines.
>
> (Andrew Kotaska, 2019)

About the author

My interest in obstetrics probably came from my mother, who was a nurse educator. On a deep level, she was convinced of Mother Nature's wisdom, but she also had a scientific mind that sought evidence to prove things. This rubbed off on me. In medical school, I was exposed to obstetrics and saw the magic in the birth process. It is dynamic, intense and carries an intimacy through which you really get the depth of what it is to be human. This intimacy is shared with by those working in palliative care, so it is perhaps not surprising that I was drawn to both birth and death when I was training as a physician.

It was also the late 1980s, when Obstetrics was coming out of a period of overintervention and paternalism. There was a movement well under way to support physiological birth and only deviate from it with good reason. This was the philosophy of a group of family physicians and midwives who were not yet regulated in British Columbia, but would bring clients to hospital if the women wanted to birth in hospital. These women, their midwives and their family physicians shared a belief in the physiology of normal birth. Being exposed to that passion opened my eyes to the magic of birth. I saw that it was a transformative, empowering experience for women. A woman who has had a baby becomes almost a different species: not only in an obstetric sense, but in many aspects of her life.

For me, the beauty of family practice was the ability to witness that transformation longitudinally, through birth, parenting and women's relationships with their partners. This gave me a rich insight into what birth means to women. Having earned the obstetrics prize at medical school, it was assumed that I would go on to become an obstetrician, but I wasn't drawn to a practice that predominantly involved intervention in an industrialised setting. I was already practising in a hospital setting, but with a group of health providers that would turn the lights down, give women privacy and make the environment as home-like as possible. I would also see obstetricians come in, turn the lights on and intervene – often out of necessity, but also according to the old medical obstetrical paradigm.

I didn't initially pursue obstetrics as a specialty, partly because I was averse to the way it was practised in large urban hospitals, but also because I did not want to conform to that culture. I became a family practitioner and modelled myself after my midwife and family physician mentors who valued and protected physiological birth. I ended up having a rich, half-dozen-year career as a family doctor in obstetrics. During that time, I ventured to rural areas where I learned to do caesarean sections from another mentor, Ewart Woolley, who was both a very accomplished obstetrician and very supportive of physiological birth. His skill and keen understanding of the physiological process of birth enabled him to safely attend the majority of vaginal breech births in British Columbia for decades. He provided an exceptional example of how obstetrics should be practised – waiting in the background with well-developed skills, applied only when necessary. Not surprisingly, his hospital had the lowest caesarean section rate in the province for many years. While learning with Dr Woolley, I also attended a presentation by Michel Odent in Vancouver. His book, *Birth reborn*, was full of epiphanies. It eloquently described the physiology of birth as I had observed it and outlined how industrial obstetrics is interfering with the birth process.

I went on to work in rural settings where my skills were challenged to their limit. It was good to realise that high-level interventional skill is essential to modern obstetrics when physiologic birth becomes complicated. Given that I knew I was going to spend much of my career in rural or remote settings, it made sense to return to a tertiary care centre for a four-year residency of high-volume surgical training. And if I wanted to influence the future of the obstetrical profession, it would help to be an obstetrician. Entering residency in Obstetrics meant sacrificing my involvement in the holistic part of the birth process in exchange for a more incisive, interventionist role in the birth process, but also a future in obstetrics. I now live in Yellowknife, Northern Canada, where I work as a generalist obstetrician with a fantastic team of family physicians, midwives and obstetrical nurses to provide a culture of physiology-based obstetrical care that places women's choice at the centre of every management discussion. I also teach residents and students in obstetrics, midwifery and family practice, speak at conferences and write academic papers.

Thinking differently about risk and how to talk to women

A major problem with risk is distinguishing between numerators (the person affected) and denominators (those who aren't). Numerators are flashy and we live in a flashy world addicted to the dramatic. Attention to risk numerators in everyday life is amplified by mass media and instantaneous news feeds, so much so it's easy to forget the denominators. A plane crashes and 70 people are killed. It is broadcast worldwide, yet few will remember that 100 million passengers travelled safely by air that same month. Similarly, many doctors, nurses and midwives aren't trained in epidemiology or numbers in a way that facilitates an understanding of large denominators in a clinical context. A one in a thousand chance of a poor outcome might make a c-section appear worthwhile to avoid that poor outcome, but when you consider the collateral risk of the c-section in the other 999 women, it is not so clear. Balancing those odds is not something that we are well-trained in.

Overall, our tolerance for risk has gone down because life has become much safer. We have antibiotics and seat belts. We are not smoking as much. Air travel is safer than it has ever been. We have high-reliability organisational principles that work for air traffic control and nuclear power plants. In obstetrics, perinatal mortality is very low. So we have expectations of very low levels of risk. But when you start talking about small risks, you really have to understand numbers in a way most people don't, and you have to understand the difference between 'causality' as distinct from 'association'. We need to explain to people that childbirth is not a zero-risk game, it consists of shades of grey – a value judgement as to how much risk you want to take, for what benefit. In the 'I' era, people expect to determine all kinds of details in their lives. It is a natural extension that they get to decide how much risk they want to take in birth.

Health providers are part of the problem

Women who 'freebirth' or homebirth with significant risk factors are telling us that, if we continue the 'my way or the highway' approach, they will choose the highway. Hospitals' and clinicians' unwillingness to accept that women should have the locus of control is a threat of coercion. This threat pushes women to choose high-risk homebirth or unattended birth with much greater risks to baby and mother than birth in a hospital that values guidelines and hospital policies over women's choice. While some women have such a strong aversion to hospitals that they would never choose a hospital birth, many are being driven away because they are not 'allowed' to determine the level of risk they are willing to accept in labour.

Women with a breech presentation, for example, have a perinatal mortality of approximately 1 in 700 with a hospital vaginal birth, which is higher than with a caesarean section (1 in 2000). Most women choose a planned caesarean section because it is safer for the baby. However, some women want to take this extra perinatal risk to avoid the surgical risk to them in this and future pregnancies and to provide the benefits of labour for their babies. Yet when they ask for a planned vaginal breech birth in hospital, a physician or hospital will often only 'offer' a c-section because they feel vaginal breech birth is too risky. This is akin to saying 'our way or the highway'. Faced with this coercion to accept major surgery, some women choose the 'highway', which in this case is home breech birth. The risk of a home breech birth, however, is ten times as high as in hospital-planned vaginal breech birth, approximately 1 in 70. When a woman says, 'I don't want a c-section, so I'll birth at home', the establishment is partly responsible for the extra risk she is taking. It is disingenuous to say, 'Oh, it's the woman's fault. She wasn't willing to come into hospital and accept a caesarean section'. The ultimatum is set by the institution and its practitioners and the woman is not willing to accept that ultimatum. This is coercion. The fact that women are willing to take on significantly more risk to their baby with a home breech birth than submit to coercion should tell us something: not that they are crazy, but rather, that we are not respecting their autonomy. We need to talk to women about the level of risk they are comfortable with, regain skills with supporting vaginal breech birth and respect their informed choice.

Informed consent and refusal: midwives' and obstetricians' approaches to 'recommending' expose their vulnerabilities

When I give a talk on risk and consent, it is interesting to see how it taps into both midwives and obstetrician's vulnerabilities. The vulnerability of many obstetricians is that they are still somewhat paternalistic. I ask them to learn to relinquish the locus of control, be objective about risk and let women decide the level of risk they can accept. This protects the therapeutic alliance, but can be challenging when a bad outcome occurs. When a woman declines advice in favour of a riskier option, I advise clinicians to keep caring for their patient and detach themselves emotionally (as much as they can) from possible bad outcomes that can occur from the woman's decision to decline an intervention. Ethically and legally, the clinician is not responsible for harm that stems from a competent woman's informed refusal. Acceptance of this tenet allows clinicians to maintain their therapeutic alliance with women, which both increases the chances of better decisions (if risk increases further) and aids the process of acceptance should a bad outcome occur.

On the other hand, midwives' vulnerability often stems from a preoccupation with trying to counteract paternalism – so much so, they're afraid to make a 'recommendation' because it might become coercion. Instead, there is a tendency to 'offer' everything, even when there is clearly a path that is the safest. As in, 'Would you like a glass of white wine or a gin and tonic?' That is fine if the two options are equally beneficial or risky, but it is not adequate when there is a clearly safer choice. We would not say 'Would you like cooking wine or a bottle of champagne?' The message should be loud and clear: the champagne is better! Midwives sometimes worry that recommendations might restrict women's choice, so they do not *recommend* the safer option. Provided the midwife objectively presents the risks associated with various options, this worry can be alleviated by recommending the safest option, while letting the woman know that she can decline that option if she chooses.

These vulnerabilities plays a role in the tension between obstetricians and midwives. Obstetricians sometimes feel that midwives have 'no spine' when it comes to giving advice and may perceive their approach as tacit support for risky choices (nudge and wink). When the obstetrician has to 'pick up the mess' afterwards, they may rightly feel that the patient was neither well-informed nor clearly advised to take the less-risky option. Collaboration and collegiality between midwives and obstetricians can be improved by addressing these vulnerabilities openly. Obstetricians can let women and their midwives know that they respect autonomy enough to accept informed refusal without taking it personally or being resentful. Midwives can let women and obstetricians know that they know the difference between 'offering' and 'recommending', can give mild or strong recommendations to women as needed, and can clearly communicate with obstetricians that these recommendations have been given. It is good to involve obstetricians early when a woman's informed refusal increases her risk significantly.

This approach helps everyone. When a midwife says to an obstetrician 'No, really, I told her she should take the safer option and she said "no way"', the obstetrician realises that the midwife did her duty. If possible beforehand, the obstetrician can add his/her weight to the recommendation, but in the end, a woman's choice prevails. If something goes awry, both midwife and obstetrician know they have done their best. They have not accepted the woman's choice; rather, they supported her right to choose. Any bad outcome is secondary to the woman's choice, not to poor counselling or inappropriate support for a risky plan.

A common problem in obstetrics is the dichotomous 'black or white'; 'right or wrong'; 'safe or unsafe' thinking; none of which is usually a good approximation of the actual risk associated with medical and obstetrical conditions. A 1 in 2000 risk is not white and a 1 in 500 risk is not black, but they are often treated that way. Real life and most risk equations involve shades of grey. Women realise this, which is what rouses their suspicions when presented with only one 'safe' option. It is far better to explain levels of risk – the shades of grey – giving mild recommendations for small increases in risk and strong recommendations for higher levels of risk. This approach maintains clinicians' credibility, acknowledges a woman's ability to appreciate varying risk and supports her right to choose her level of risk.

An example of counselling about risk with VBAC

When counselling women about VBAC, I talk about recurring versus non-recurring indication and the likelihood of successful VBAC: approximately 80% with non-recurring indication and 60% where there was a recurring indication for the first CS. A successful VBAC confers a lower risk of maternal infection, bleeding, surgical damage, venous thromboembolism and complications in future pregnancies, including placenta accreta and praevia, and that's better for women and future babies. However, this benefit must be balanced against the 1 in 200 risk of uterine scar rupture with spontaneous labour and the possibility of perinatal death or newborn hypoxic ischemic encephalopathy. If you're in a big hospital, the risk to the foetus is about 1 in 2000, which can seem high or low but is brought somewhat into perspective by the risk of maternal death from complications of caesarean section of approximately 1 in 5000.

I then explain the dynamic nature of that risk/benefit equation: it can change depending on clinical circumstances, before or during labour. For example, if she chooses a vaginal birth after caesarean section and gets to 41 weeks with an unripe cervix and oligohydramnios needing induction, I will recommend a caesarean section because the balance shifts: a lower likelihood of success (< 50%) and a higher likelihood of uterine rupture (1%). On the other hand, if she chooses a repeat caesarean section and presents to hospital a week early in good labour, 7 cm dilated, with a low head, I'm going suggest letting a VBAC happen because the likelihood of success is high – perhaps 90% – and some of the risk of rupture is behind her. Every woman understands this dynamic balance and the shades of grey.

I also talk about the measures we use in labour to maintain safety: placing an intravenous (IV) cannula, foetal monitoring and close monitoring of labour progress. I engage the woman in understanding that failure to progress in labour with good contractions is a very significant risk factor for uterine rupture. Coomb hospital in Dublin has a uniquely coloured partograph for women having a VBAC that acknowledges this fact; their success rates and rupture rates are the best I have seen published. So, if our labour unit is busy and a woman is being neglected in labour, she needs to say, 'Hey, when are you going to check me? Because if I'm not progressing, I need a caesarean section'.

Where I practise in Northern Canada, we don't have full-time in-house caesarean section coverage, so we adjust our risk estimation accordingly. We don't restrict choice as many similarly resourced hospitals in the USA have done. Instead, we inform women about our hospital's limitations. Because our surgical response times are longer in the middle of the night, we double our risk estimate to 1 in 1000 risk of perinatal mortality or brain damage, instead of 1 in 2000. We give women the option of birthing instead in a larger centre, but I have not had a woman say that 1 in 1000 is too high a risk while 1 in 2000 is acceptable.

Some women wanting a trial of labour decline safety measures. When they decline an IV cannula or continuous electronic foetal monitoring (CTG), I discuss why we have those parameters in place. We have an IV in place so that we can react quicker. If you've got big veins it will only take a minute to get the IV in and there is probably not much difference to safety. For a woman with difficult veins, however, the risk of delay might be significantly higher. With foetal monitoring, a drop in fetal heart rate (FHR) is occasionally the only indication we have of uterine rupture. How often is that the only sign in a woman who doesn't have an epidural? That is hard to know, but less often than in women with an epidural. If a woman wants time off the monitor, what is the risk? If the risk is 1 in 200 over a 10-hour labour, then the risk of uterine rupture while she is off the monitor for one hour is perhaps 1 in 2000. If the nurse is listening with the Doppler every 5 minutes, how much riskier is that than continuous monitoring? Again, probably not a large difference. So we inform women of our recommendations for safety, then discuss what is acceptable to them, understanding that the further they move away from the recommendation, the more risk they take. We make it clear that it is their choice, but also that they are responsible for taking the risk.

What if a woman is five hours from the nearest operating theatre and wants a VBAC?

We have had women choose a VBAC in a small rural town that offers midwifery-attended birth but not surgical services – effectively five hours transfer time from an operating theatre. In this scenario, I have a teleconference with the woman, her husband and their midwife. We explain: 'If you have a uterine rupture, you're very likely going to lose the baby. So the risk to the baby isn't 1 in 1000, it's more like 1 in 200. If there is uterine rupture, there is also a chance that you, the mother, would die during the four or five hours it would take to transfer you'. After these discussions, we have had two women say, 'That's still worth it for me – I will have my baby in my home community'. So how do we respond to that? We don't try to coerce or abandon her. We don't say 'our way or the highway'. Instead, we keep the alliance with the woman and mitigate the risk. 'Okay', I say, 'When you're 36 weeks, we're going to get a few extra pints of blood into your community, just in case. When you enter labour, come in right away so we can get an IV in, watch the FHR closely and see how you're progressing. If you're not progressing or there are concerns with FHR, we'll hopefully have time to get you to Yellowknife in time to intervene, if required'. We do not coerce or exaggerate risk, but we make sure their eyes are wide open. These are very stark conversations. I can think of a few women in my career with whom I had such a conversation and who chose paths with risk to their baby of perhaps 1 in 100 or 1 in 200. In all cases, the outcome was good. Had a tragic outcome occurred, however, I believe they would have felt in control and cared for, which was of paramount importance to them.

The law on consent in Canada clearly establishes that a woman is responsible for harm that results from her informed refusal, but it is important to ensure that she is aware of the pertinent risks. For common scenarios that involve varying degrees of risk and choices, we have pre-printed information and consent forms for VBAC, breech birth, term prelabour rupture of membranes, post-dates and induction of labour, each of which incorporate women's choice. If a woman decides a path that involves a significant increase in risk, we often get a second opinion and always suggest to midwives and family physicians that they involve an obstetrician to share the burden of responsibility. Midwives often have the most extreme requests; for them, it is very important to share the burden and document communications very carefully.

Wrapping up with Andrew

I have given presentations on risk, and informed consent and refusal, at various conferences. Perhaps the best compliment I have ever received was at a talk in Ontario, Canada several years ago to a group of about 500 obstetricians. It was a talk about the balance of autonomy, beneficence and non-maleficence, and the need for obstetricians to accept that the locus of control in medical decision-making in modern obstetrics rests with the woman. Afterwards, three senior obstetricians approached me and one of them said, 'We're all at the end of our careers, getting ready to retire, and we have been coming to these conferences for years. It's not very often we hear something new. I wish I'd heard this talk 30 years ago, because it would have changed everything'.

Why did I become an obstetrician? I admire women and I am inspired by the power and resilience they demonstrate in birth. Obstetrics involves an interesting combination: most of the time it requires patient observation of a physiological process that is best left undisturbed. At other times, urgent, sometimes dramatic intervention is life-saving. In a process as varied and dynamic as birth, how do we avoid disturbing normal physiology, maintain adequate vigilance and make the right decisions, under pressure, about when and how much to intervene? It is an amazing challenge and an incredible privilege for an obstetric team to be entrusted with that role and responsibility. I love the dedicated team of nurses, midwives and family physicians I work with, and I share their dedication to finding the balance of just enough intervention to keep birth both safe and as physiologically normal as possible.

Although it involves challenges, one of the most liberating things an obstetrician can hear is a woman who says: 'I know that my choice involves extra risk, but it is worth it to me to take that risk'. Vaginal breech birth is one such example. It involves more perinatal risk than a caesarean section and it is a heavy responsibility to have a woman trust our team's skill and judgement; however, guiding and accompanying her through that process is an incredible experience and a remarkable privilege.

The way forward

Alison Barrett

- It is clear that the problem of iatrogenesis is increasing within every healthcare system, including the maternity system
- As we move away from fossil fuels and realise the impact of our use of the earth's resources, it is time to harness the zero-carbon gifts of human nature
- Relationship-based maternity care is not only effective, it is low- or no-carbon generating
- We must plan for a sustainable future in maternity care, building on women's capacity, trust and hope while centring on kindness and compassion
- All this is possible if we want it enough and we care enough about the future of the planet and our species

The way forward

Andrew Kotaksa

- All care providers need to understand that obstetrical risk is rarely black and white. They need to become conversant in shades of grey and communicating varying levels of risk to women
- When there is a clinical choice that is clearly safer, midwives need to own their duty to recommend, rather than offer. Women can decline any recommendation, but they need to know, clearly, the recommendations regarding the safest option
- When a woman's informed refusal puts her at risk, midwives should call obstetricians to ensure they have a common understanding of the risks, develop an optimal plan to mitigate risk and share responsibility

- Obstetricians must realise that the locus of control for decision-making is not theirs – it belongs to women. They must be careful not to coerce women into following recommendations, even where the recommendation is objectively safer. Amplifying risk, whether intentional or not, is a form of coercion
- When a woman declines a recommendation, the clinician must not take it personally. Ensure that refusal is informed, protect the therapeutic alliance and continue to provide excellent care for the women, mitigating risk as much as she will allow
- When there is a difference of opinion, stating explicitly that a woman can decline your recommendation yet still receive your care can magically remove tension and strengthen the therapeutic alliance
- Midwives and obstetricians need to talk more: about risk, the locus of control, informed consent and refusal, recommending versus offering, the therapeutic alliance and the avoidance of coercion. A better relationship and a common understanding of these themes leads to better counselling, greater choice for women, fewer unattended and high-risk homebirths, and happier obstetricians and midwives who are better able to deal with the emotional burden of obstetrical care

References

Berendzen, J. & Howard, B. (2013). Association between cesarean delivery rate and body mass index. *Tenneseee Medicine*, *106*, 35–37.

Best, M. & Neuhauser, D. (2004). Ignaz Semmelweis and the birth of infection control. *BMJ Quality & Safety*, *13*, 233–234.

Birthrights. (2018). *Maternal request caesarean*. London: Birthrights.

Cáceres, I. A., Arcaya, M., Declercq, E., Belanoff, C. M., Janakiraman, V., Cohen, B., & Subramanian, S. V. (2013). Hospital differences in cesarean deliveries in Massachusetts (US) 2004–2006: The case against case-mix artifact. *PLoS ONE*, *8*(3), e57817. doi:10.1371/journal.pone.0057817.

Dahlen, H. (2014). Managing risk or facilitating safety? *International Journal of Childbirth*, *4*, 66–68.

Dahlen, H. G., Jackson, M., & Stevens, J. (2011). Homebirth, freebirth and doulas; Casualty and consequences of a broken maternity system. *Women and Birth*, *24*, 47–50.

Duffy, M. (2019). When did you realize you work on climate change? *Dynamic Ecology*. 4 February. Retrieved from: https://dynamicecology.wordpress.com/2019/02/04/when-did-you-realize-you-work-on-climate-change/

Feeley, C., & Thomson , G. (2016). Why do some women choose to freebirth in the UK? An interpretative phenomenological study. *BMC Pregnancy & Childbirth*, *16*, 59.

Fothergill, A. (Director). (2019). *Our planet* [Motion Picture].

Gordon, D., Milberg, J., Daling, J., & Hickok, D. (1991). Advanced maternal age as a risk factor for cesarean delivery. *Obstetrics and Gynecology*, *77*, 493–497.

Johnson, E. M. & Rehavi, M. M. (2013). *Physicians treating physicians*. Cambridge: National Bureau of Economic Research.

Jones, R. (2017). *Doctors in denial: The forgotten women in the 'Unfortunate Experiment'.* Otago: Otago University Press.

Korb, D., Goffinet, F., Seco, A., Chevret, S., Catherine, D.-T., Group, E. S., & EPIMOMS Study Group. (2019). Risk of severe maternal morbidity associated with cesarean delivery and the role of maternal age: A population-based propensity score analysis. *Canadian Medical Association Journal*, *191*(13), E352–E360.

Makary, M. & Daniel, M. (2016). Medical error – The third leading cause of death in the US. *BMJ*, *353*, i2139.

O'Reilly, C. (2019, May 22). 'I FELT VIOLATED'. How 'birth rape' affects millions of mums – but why do doctors perform invasive procedures without our consent. *The Sun*. May 22. Retrieved from: https://www.thesun.co.uk/fabulous/8778305/birth-rape-obstetric-violence-mums-doctors-childbirth/

Peer, R. S. (2018). Iatrogenesis: A review on nature, extent and distribution of healthcare hazards. *Journal of Family Medicine and Primary Care*, *7*, 309–314.

Quigley, C., Taut, C., Zigman, T., & Gallagher, L. (2016). Association between home birth and breast feeding outcomes: A cross-sectional study in 28 125 mother–infant pairs from Ireland and the UK. *BMJ Open*, *6*(8), e010551.

RANZCOG. (2017). *Position statement on home births.* East Melbourne: RANZCOG.

Renfrew, M. J., McFadden, A., Helena Bastos, M. H., Campbell, J., Channon, A. A., Cheung, N. F., … Declercq, E. (2014). Midwifery and quality care: Findings from a new evidence-informed framework for maternal and newborn care. *The Lancet*, *384*(9948), 1129–1145.

Rowell, D. & Connelly, L. B. (2012). A history of the term "moral hazard". *Journal of Risk and Insurance*, *79*, 1051–1075.

Song, S. (2004). Too posh to push? As more pregnant women schedule c-sections, doctors warn that the procedure is not risk-free. *Time*, *163*(16), 58, 60.

Vahratian, A., Zhang, J., Troendle, J., Sciscione, A., & Hoffman, M. (2005). Labor progression and risk of cesarean delivery in electively induced nulliparas. *Obstetrics and Gynecology*, *105*, 698–704.

Wagner, M. (2001). Fish can't see water: The need to humanize birth. *International Journal of Gynecology and Obstetrics*, *75*, s25–s37.

Walker, A. (2019). What is the contaminated blood scandal? *The Guardian*. 30 April. Retrieved from: www.theguardian.com/uk-news/2019/apr/30/what-is-the-contaminated-blood-scandal.

World Health Organization. (1985). *Having a baby in Europe.* Marmorvej: Regional Office for Europe.

World Health Organization (2019). Ten threats to global health in 2019. Retrieved from: www.who.int/emergencies/ten-threats-to-global-health-in-2019.

21 Conclusion

Keeping the canary singing into the future

Hannah Dahlen, Bashi Kumar-Hazard and Virginia Schmied

> Until you do right by me everything you even dream about will fail.
>
> (*The Color Purple* by Alice Walker, 1986)

This book has been a long time in the making and has only been possible because of the many who have contributed. That said, we are mindful that it symbolises the suffering of millions of women around the world, caused by their experiences both within the system and, for some, outside out of it. If we are to succeed as a society in the new millennium, we must 'do right by women'. Do we really value women's voices and choices? It seems an odd thing to say, but this book reflects the stark reality which shows that, often, we don't. It is to all of our detriment, particularly the well-being of mothers and babies, to ignore what the 'canary' has been telling us for some time.

Maternal rights are human rights

It may come as a surprise to many that our international human rights instruments are by and large silent on the rights of women as *mothers.* The Universal Declaration of Human Rights (UDHR) makes just one indirect reference to women in their capacity as mothers. Article 25(2) of the UDHR recognises that the condition of 'motherhood' is entitled to special care and assistance. This wording is significant, because it does not recognise a woman's right to directly seek special assistance, on her terms, as a mother. Rather, it recognises the disembodied condition of 'motherhood' as needing special care and assistance. This, by and large, reflects the development of maternity healthcare services today, as Nation States provision services by reference to politically charged (and regularly altered) notions of motherhood.

In 1981, the Convention on the Elimination of All Forms of Discrimination against Women (CEDAW) was introduced to protect women's rights within political, civil, cultural, economic and social life, but made no reference to maternal rights or the specific rights of women as mothers. In 1993, Article 2 of the International Declaration on the Elimination of Violence against

Women recognised the right of women to be free of violence in a number of settings, but makes no mention of violence in medical facilities.

The quest for equality between men and women, as currently enshrined in human rights instruments such as CEDAW, has seemingly erased and, at the same time, diminished the very substance of women that distinguishes us biologically from men. As this book demonstrates, for as long as pregnancy and motherhood are treated as temporary ailments and not a substantive element of being a woman, we will not be able to free ourselves from systematic subordination, vulnerability to violence, socio-economic dependence, poverty and ill health.

The world is speaking up and so must we

The epidemic of mistreatment during childbirth in health facilities has finally attracted the attention of researchers (Renfrew et al., 2014; Bohren et al., 2015; Miller et al., 2016), the WHO (World Health Organisation, 2014) and non-governmental organisations (The White Ribbon Alliance For Safer Motherhood, 2011; Human Rights in Childbirth (HRiC), 2019; Safer Motherhood For All, 2019).

The WHO, in response to alarming reports about mistreatment in facilities, issued a statement which said, 'Every women has the right to the highest attainable standard of health, which includes the right to dignified, respectful health care' (World Health Organisation, 2014). In 2018, the new WHO *Intrapartum Care for a POSITIVE [emphasis added] Childbirth Experience* Guidelines (World Health Organisation, 2018) listed the following top four recommendations for the provision of care: (a) respectful maternity care; (b) effective communication; (c) companionship during labour and birth; and (d) continuity of midwifery care. These simple yet highly effective mechanisms were raised, time and again, as being absent in both the research and stories detailed in this book.

Safe Motherhood For All and the White Ribbon Alliance for Safe Motherhood state that 'motherhood is a social justice and human rights issue' (The White Ribbon Alliance For Safe Motherhood, 2011; Safe Motherhood For All, 2019). In a document entitled '*Tackling disrespect and abuse*', the White Ribbon Alliance identified the seven rights of childbearing women that are being regularly violated in the provision of maternity healthcare: (1) freedom from harm and ill treatment; (2) right to information, informed consent and refusal, respect for choices and preferences, including the right to companionship of choice; (3) right to privacy and confidentiality; (4) right to dignity and respect; (5) freedom from discrimination; (6) right to timely healthcare and to the highest attainable level of health; and (7) right to liberty, autonomy, self-determination and freedom from coercion (The White Ribbon Alliance For Safe Motherhood, 2011).

In the past decade, several surveys have been conducted on women's birth experiences and their satisfaction with care. These include, but are not limited to, the first national survey on obstetric violence in Italy, where 21% of mothers reported experiencing obstetric violence (OVOItalia, 2017); The Safe Motherhood Australia Survey, where 26% of women felt the birth they had was negative and this was more likely if the birth was instrumental or by caesarean section (Safe Motherhood for All Inc., 2017); the Mothers on Respect index (MORi) in Canada (Vedam et al., 2017) found that 1 in 10 mothers felt coerced into accepting options recommended by their care provider and that this was much less likely when women were under the care of midwives or planned to give birth at home.

In 2019, the UNHCR Special Rapporteur on Violence against Women, its Causes and Consequences called for submissions on mistreatment in facility-based childbirth. Many individuals and organisations, including HRiC, submitted reports. This is a significant step forward in the international recognition of this all too often overlooked subset of state-endorsed violence against women, and the outcome is eagerly awaited.

The way forward

We asked every author to recommend 4–5 points at the conclusion of their chapter on what they thought was the best way forward for reconnecting women with maternity health services. We analysed these points using a content analysis and grouped them into five key categories:

(1) Make respectful care a reality, not a mantra
(2) Emancipate and support midwifery to emancipate and support women
(3) Support women's access to their chosen place of birth and model of care
(4) Offer more flexible, acceptable options for women experiencing risk factors during pregnancy and/or birth
(5) Get the framework right and the rest will follow: policy, guidelines, education, research, regulation and professional leadership

The Way Forward, as set out in the table below, is aimed at maternity services, governments, educators, regulators, professional bodies, the legal profession, policy makers and research leaders (Table 21.1). For the more visually oriented, we created a word cloud (Figure 21.1).

Some advice from our leaders on the way forward

In the next section, we hear from three leaders in women's health. They share their recommendations for the way forward, which align with many of the concepts discussed by the authors in this book.

Table 21.1 The way forward

Categories	*Concepts*
Make respectful care a reality, not a mantra	Listen to women and communicate clearly and non-judgementally to gain trust and increase your knowledge of a woman's individual needs Get consent and respect refusal. Don't coerce, punish or give women inflated risk data or ultimatums Uphold maternal autonomy and advocate for women Provide women with judgement-free, evidence-based information so they can make informed decisions and maintain trust in the service and health providers Facilitate respectful communication and collaboration between providers, as they will reflect this respect in interactions with women Provide culturally sensitive information and care, including more midwives of colour. Support and celebrate cultural diversity by being open and curious rather than ignorant and nervous For Indigenous women, remember that connection to country and cultural traditions carry deep significance and must be respected. Cultural safety is paramount to a positive experience Address covert and overt racism in the system and change structures that reinforce racism Ongoing training is required for health providers on respectful care, trauma informed care and PTSD Make sure all staff have education and awareness of women's ethical, legal and human rights Respect the mother–baby dyad and implement care practices that keep them together (i.e. optimal cord clamping, immediate skin-to-skin contact and support with breastfeeding) Humanise maternity care through implementing continuity of midwifery care, support in labour and intervene in birth only when necessary Have a Respectful Maternity Care Advocate to provide on-call, real-time support and mediation
Emancipate and support midwifery to emancipate and support women	Build strong professional bodies/associations to give a voice to midwives and advocate for midwifery at country level and beyond The midwifery profession needs to be regulated, educated and managed by midwives and seen as a separate and independent discipline to nursing Ensure midwifery regulation protects women's rights by not punishing the midwives who support them Enable clear pathways of consultation and referral for midwives working in the community Make continuity of midwifery care a reality with genuine support given to this model and the midwives who work in it at every level of the maternity service

(*continued*)

Table 21.1 (Cont.)

Categories	*Concepts*
	Support the development of private midwifery, including giving these midwives visiting rights access to health Facilitate the education of more midwives of colour and/or from culturally diverse backgrounds through targeted pathways and genuine and ongoing support
Support women's access to their chosen place of birth and model of care	Provide environments that promote, facilitate and respect physiological birth Every woman should be able to have the family/support people of her choice with her and they should be made to feel welcome Enable and facilitate access to homebirth that is equitable and available to women who request this option Make sure transport and transfer from home to hospital is seamless and formalised handover expected and respected. Include what is important to the woman being transferred as part of this and welcome and treat their community or private midwives with respect Expand birth centres that are both standalone and alongside hospitals Create more home-like environments in hospital Provide medical and non-medical options of pain relief, including water immersion/water birth Every woman should have access to a known midwife where trust can be developed across the childbearing continuum, regardless of her obstetric risk Support appropriate training of staff so they have the skills to support women's choices
Offer more flexible, acceptable options for women experiencing risk factors during pregnancy and/or birth	Create flexible guidelines for women seeking a VBAC, vaginal breech birth or vaginal twin birth Support midwives and obstetricians to develop skills, such as with breech and twin birth within the system so confidence is built in 'complex normality' and more options become available When women express their specific needs, be willing to compromise. It is not your body or your baby Multidisciplinary clinics and models are needed for women with risk factors who make 'off-menu' choices Engage allied health workers when caring for women with social, perinatal mental health and special physical requirements (i.e. social workers, mental health teams, disability teams, physiotherapists, etc.) Obstetricians need to understand the locus of control is not theirs, it is women's and don't take it personally when women decline recommendations Midwives and obstetricians need to have more honest conversations about risk and work together to protect the therapeutic alliance with women Engage with traditional birth attendants and unregulated birthworkers so they don't go underground. Consider pathways of education to engage them into the system

Table 21.1 (Cont.)

Categories	*Concepts*
Get the framework right and the rest will follow: policy, guidelines, education, research, regulation and professional leadership	Include women in service and policy development, guidelines and research from inception Guidelines are important, but they are guidance and should never usurp a woman's choice Set research priorities with women and value their involvement Ensure midwifery education programmes meet the ICM standards of education and that contemporary evidence-based midwifery is taught to prepare midwives to work wherever women need them to work When midwives are reported to the regulator, make the investigation timely and the response appropriate to the issue at hand. Interview the woman involved (if they are willing) and don't presume the midwife has misled them Design funding models focused on women and involve women in the design of these models Sustainability and fiscal responsibility need to be considered in the debate on place of birth and model of care Clear documentation processes and living flexible care plans and pathways are needed for women who make 'off-menu' choices Lawyers, courts and coroners need ongoing education about unique issues associated with childbearing women and the international issues being raised in this book when it comes to birth trauma Explicit international human rights treaties and country-based legislation is needed to protect women's reproductive rights including care during pregnancy and childbirth

Fran McConville – Midwifery Expert at the World Health Organisation in Geneva

Fran McConville has been working as the midwifery expert at the headquarters of the World Health Organisation (WHO) in Geneva for nearly seven years. Fran began her studies in Life Sciences under the inspirational David Attenborough, then her head of zoology. She became fascinated by mammalian reproductive behaviour at a time when feminism and women's reproductive rights were high on the political agenda. As you can imagine, it was not a leap to pursue midwifery studies. After working for many years in Africa, Asia and the Middle East with NGOs, UNICEF and the UK's Department for International Development (DFID), the WHO beckoned. Fran has led several key global reports on midwifery including the *Midwives' voices midwives' realities* report (World Health Organisation, 2016) in collaboration with ICM and The White Ribbon Alliance. This report gives visibility to the voices of 2470 midwives in 93 countries, highlighting the socio-cultural,

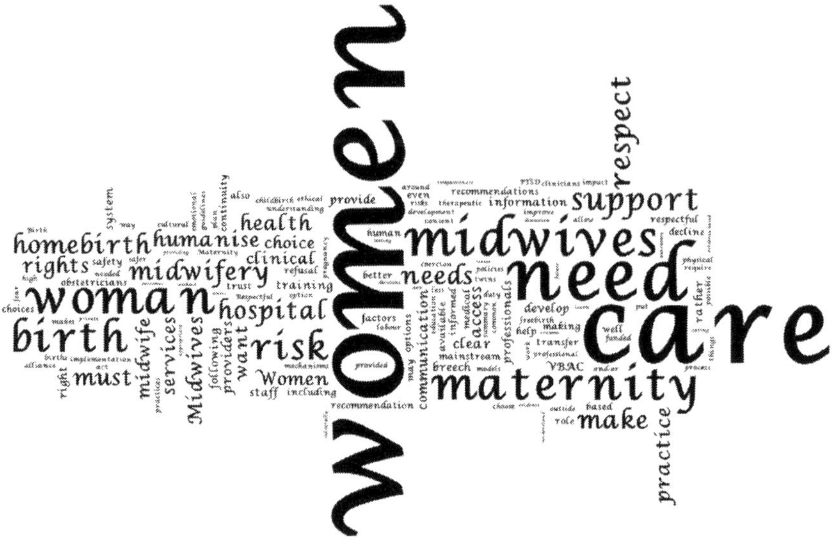

Figure 21.1 A word cloud on the way forward

economic and professional barriers midwives face all around the world, and demonstrating that addressing gender inequality is critical to improving quality of midwifery care. Fran also led the *Strengthening quality midwifery education for Universal Health Coverage 2030: Framework for action* (World Health Organisation, 2019) report, developed in collaboration with ICM, UNFPA and UNICEF and launched by Ministers of Health at the World Health Assembly in May 2019.

With her bird's-eye view of maternal and newborn health care, I (Hannah) interviewed Fran and asked her to share her insights into what she thinks is the way to better engage women in our maternity care systems. We wanted to know, in anticipation of the 2020 *International Year of the Nurse and Midwife*, what we need to do to move maternity care towards a respectful agenda that engages women into care rather than alienates them.

WHO is important

I believe in the WHO. Along with many other UN organisations, the WHO was established, after the devastation of World War II, to improve global health and reach all people. At its best, the WHO is absolutely amazing. The impact from one evidence-based recommendation, from one document, is incredible because of the involvement of the 194 member states (countries) that work together to agree the global health priorities. For example, the recent WHO Framework for Quality of Care includes both the provision and experience of care (including providing respectful care), and this is enabling new language and approaches to maternity care to be embedded globally.

Engage women from the beginning

What we need to do to address the issue of women birthing outside the health/midwifery system is to engage women in the whole process. We need to get better at asking women not only what they want (this is improving gradually), but to be engaged throughout. This includes asking women: what kind of midwifery care do you want? How can we build a midwifery programme in this country that suits your needs? How do we educate our midwives to provide what you want? Getting women, families, and communities engaged – right from the beginning – is critical. We tend to forget that. We also need to ensure that they are proactively informing policy and education programmes.

Women, and their families, should also be encouraged to hold their government to account for what happens in maternity services.

We need to strengthen leadership in midwifery, and we need to respect midwives

Midwifery is not always given its due professional respect and place at the table at high-level government policy and decision-making meetings. Too few Government Chief Nursing and Midwifery Officers (GCNMOs) are afforded the visibility, or equality of opportunity, to make their voices heard and influence decisions made on behalf of women. This must improve to achieve the same impact we see in countries where strong leadership in midwifery has led to improvements in care for women, newborns and their families. We have strong ICM, WHO, UNFPA and UNICEF leadership, and superb midwifery research leadership. The really good news is that we've moved rapidly from almost no midwifery-led research to global recognition of brilliant world-class research programmes. The next step is to improve how we communicate these research findings at the high political level, as well as to midwives and women, so people listen and act with the right information. That is our next great challenge.

Don't ignore reproductive rights issues or the biological impact of kindness

We must keep the focus on reproductive rights, and the positive impact of rights based approaches on accessing quality care, where women feel empowered and trust the health services. We need to show the impact of kindness and humanised care on biology; that this is not only about being respectful and kind, but that compassionate care actually influences the functioning of the all-important endocrine system, for example, to release naturally occurring oxytocin. We need to clearly explain the new science and complex messages around the microbiome, epigenetics and the benefits of normal birth.

We must unite as health workers for women – our time is now

Working in an interprofessional team in a system historically structured on gendered hierarchies of power can be tough. As midwives, we need to acknowledge and address the barriers, lead on excellence in team work and demonstrate the evidence-based impact of continuity of midwife-led care on outcomes. For the sake of women, we must unite with colleagues who make such an important contribution to the care of women and their newborns, especially where complications arise.

At the 2019, World Health Assembly, all WHO Member States endorsed 2020 as the inaugural Year of the Nurse and the Midwife, we have an extraordinary opportunity. We are working together to ensure strong, global, evidence-based advocacy in support of women and midwives, wherever they want to give birth. The future is exciting. After centuries of discrimination and ignorance of the value of midwives caring for women wherever they choose to seek care, our time to support women in the best way possible is now.

Franka Cadée – President of the International Confederation of Midwives

Franka Cadée is the President of the International Confederation of Midwives (ICM). She is a Dutch midwife who has brought a new and refreshing hand to this role, engaging in social media and stepping out to make strong, brave statements on behalf of women and midwives. I (Hannah) interviewed her and, when I pointed this out, she told me she is 'getting braver'.

Franka's first degree was in anthropology, where she became fascinated with the concept of pain and cultural expressions of pain. When she finished her degree, she wanted to do something that was 'hands on', so trained to become a midwife. Franka was bought up abroad and lived in many countries, and this also prepared her for her role as president of ICM. I asked Franka what midwives need to do to re-engage women in our system.

Be brave and be political

We need courage and to dare to stand on our own feet, taking responsibility for ourselves. Midwives worry about repercussions on them. It takes courage to stand up for what you know is right and to fight for women's rights. As ICM president, I like to think I am helping to support midwives to take responsibility and to have the courage to speak out. I think we need to be more political. That's one thing that I really believe. That's something that's grown in me over the last few years – I've realised that midwives are not political enough.

It should always be a woman's choice

Sometimes supporting women who make choices to birth outside the system will lead to poor outcomes. I don't believe that any woman wants anything bad for herself or her child – even a woman who chooses not to have her child, still that woman inside knows this is the best because she and her child are one. We understand more and more that, if that union works well and if there is also support, then this is the best thing for that child and that woman and for our future. It's a woman's choice, and I think it's important politically to say this because it's part of the right of a woman to stand when she wants to give birth or say yes or no to certain interventions and decide on her place of birth. Beginning to mess about with that right is a dangerous thing and will only lead on to altering other rights women have.

Freebirth is also a woman's right

I remember attending such a birth myself as a midwife in the Netherlands. The woman had given birth to her first child at home. Now you would think, 'Oh, she gave birth to her child at home and that it means that she had a good birth'. But, of course, those two do not always go together. She was not happy about her first birth so this time she wanted to give birth alone. She wanted no one with her and we had all kinds of discussions about sitting outside in the car, sitting outside in an ambulance, whatever. We had all kinds of options lined up. But one of the reasons why, in the end, I was able to say, 'Okay, you do that and we'll find our way in being around somewhere', was because other healthcare professionals supported me, understood and respected that I had done everything I could and this was ethically the best thing that we could do for this woman. We have a duty not to coerce, but we also have a duty to make sure choice is informed. She gave birth by herself as she wanted and everything was okay.

We need to build relationships with women and each other

Trust is essential, and building trust happens by building relationships. I think we need to build relationships with each other – women, midwives and doctors.

Don't put so much emphasis on the place

Another thing I find interesting, especially of course in countries where the system does not support safe homebirth, is the emphasis on place of birth. I love it when you don't even have to discuss the place of birth, just let the place of birth be where the birth starts and where the woman happens to remain feeling best. If that happens to be at home, then it's at home. If it happens to be in her garden or a hospital or wherever she wants to be, then that's where she moves and you move with her, trusting her. But we are far from that because, as soon as you say that, you are looked upon as being someone that encourages people to do this or that, and this stops us talking to each other.

Engage midwives in the system just like we need to engage women

Midwives are human beings too and this is something we tend to forget. Rightly, we talk about women's rights, but we also need to talk about midwives' rights. What happens with midwives who support women to give birth in what we perceive to be 'extreme circumstances' presents the same conditions behind why women give birth outside the system. Just like women, midwives are often forced into a situation where they are not 'allowed' to do all kinds of things, and then, they become worried about going into hospital and what might happen when they get there. So midwives start behaving in a covert way to avoid criticism or ridicule. I think it's exactly the same response that women have to the inflexible, judgmental system. We need to ask why, what is the question behind the question? As in, not just how we make sure a midwife realises what her responsibilities are but also how do we engage midwives in our systems with respect and tolerance, just as we need to do with women? As midwives, we also need to have a good look at ourselves and be brave enough to do that.

Hospitals represent power and this affects midwives as it does women

As a midwife, I think I'm quite assertive. I've always been quite assertive but I still know that when I'm with a woman at home and move with her to hospital, my heartrate changes and I change my behaviour. When I'm in a woman's home, I'm different because I'm the guest; my power relationship with her is clear. As soon as I'm in hospital, however, the obstetrician is so often the boss and I do tend to start behaving differently. I start trying to please him or her (i.e. the obstetrician). I know I do it and I don't want to do it, but I know I do it. So why don't we understand that the same thing will happen with women when they enter our institutions and come under our power. When you look less at them and more at us, you start to really see the same dynamics that are at play that lead women to birth outside the system and midwives to work outside the system. In my view, the solutions are the same – respect, choice and communication.

When you hold the power you don't see it

When you are the person holding a position of power, you see this less clearly. It is like being white and privileged, and believing that racism does not exist. You are unaffected and so, from your point of view, it probably does not exist. Others, however, will tell you clearly, when it affects them, that it does exist. I was involved in a debate recently at the Women Deliver conference where I told a story about an interaction between obstetricians and midwives that I felt could damage the woman. The first person to respond in the debate was an obstetrician, who felt it was a really bad thing to tell these kinds of stories because it was 'putting salt in the wounds' and we needed to look forward. She also said she didn't feel that such interactions happened any longer. In my view, that is a problem because when you don't feel it, how can you see it? We know very well that within abusive relationships, the abuser often doesn't see it as abuse. We need to start comparing this dynamic in abusive relationships to how we treat women and how midwives are treated, to show this dynamic for what it is. Some obstetricians don't want to, or can't see it, because they are in a bubble. We are all in a bubble when it comes to women. We need to talk more and listen to each other more. Continuity is great for women because they feel free to talk and they feel heard and we also need continuity principles for health providers so relationships of trust can develop.

Our obsession with risk is a massive problem

We need to talk about our obsession with risk. We are ignoring the full dimension of safety when all we focus on is death – what about suffering? What do our institutions do to women and to midwives when the whole focus is on risk and what can go wrong? There is proportionately less focus on the joy of having a baby and how we can make the birth optimal. I find it deeply painful, because we know what institutions do to people, in circumstances where we as human beings live in institutions. You see it in orphanages; so, what do you think happens to women when they're institutionalised during birth? Why can't we see that? Why are we surprised when some women say no to our institutions and make different choices?

We need a 'Me Too movement' for birth

People today can suffer from what we do to them; for example, more people are dying today from bad-quality care than no access to care. This is huge, but it's not being shouted out. Someone is profiting from this, otherwise we would have changed it a long time ago. And I think I go two ways. One side of me thinks we need to try to join forces more than we do, speak in one voice, kind of carry on the road we're going. And another part of me at times thinks, no! What we really need is a big 'Me Too campaign' for birth. This is definitely not just about obstetricians – midwives too are part of the abuse. It is a systems issue. I'm sure in my career that I've done it as well. I find that deeply painful, but I do know that, in certain circumstances, when I'm tired or stressed, I will have manipulated things in such a way so that it also worked out better for me. And that is where we really need to support each other, look each other in the eye, admit we can do better and that we have at times all done wrong. In order to do this, we need good leadership. Good leadership makes us all want to do better and be better people. I think the way forward is trying to bring people along, see the leadership strength in all of us, speaking to each other about where we do wrong and daring to face this. We must dare to because midwives are some of the worst in carrying out this abuse. We do some really, really awful things, and I can understand it sometimes because midwives also are so often abused.

Michael Klein's birth dystopia – 'The Dissident Doctor'

Michael Klein is an American-born family physician and family medicine professor who spent most of his professional career in Canada and has just written his memoir, *Dissident doctor: Catching babies and challenging the medical status quo*. He has been described as Canada's dissident doctor. He embraced midwifery when it was not yet regulated because he understood that what was important was what women wanted, not what doctors wanted. In 1994, Michael conducted the only randomised controlled trial of episiotomy in North America, which found that routine episiotomy caused the very trauma it was supposed to prevent, and it was the main cause of third-/fourth-degree tears. Despite this significant and substantial finding, he had a difficult time publishing the paper because it challenged deeply held medical beliefs at the time.

I (Hannah) follow Michael on his amazing multidisciplinary *Maternity Care Discussion Group* and regularly experience his wisdom when thoughtful, and at times vigorous, debate ensues on practice matters. On one occasion, he sent around his take on the state of childbirth, which he called 'Michael's birth dystopia', written in the style of novelist Margaret Atwood's *The Handmaid's Tale*. To my delight, he gave permission to publish his piece in our book.

If she is too small, [caesarean] section her
If she is too big, section her
If she is too late, section her
If she is too early, section her
If she is breech, section her
If she has twins, section her
If she is too old, section her
If you think that her baby is too big, section her
If the induction that you did for no good reason fails, section her
If you do not have a nurse or midwife to look after her, section her
If you are too busy, section her
If the unnecessary, or too early epidural stops her labour or creates a malposition due to the deflexed head that you caused, section her
If she is not in labour (but you think she is), section her
If she has a uterine scar, section her
If her risk score is too high, section her
If she is afraid of birth, section her
If she has, or is worried about urinary incontinence, section her
If she is worried about sexual functioning, section her
If her husband is worried about his sexual functioning, section her

For those remaining irresponsible women who insist on a vaginal birth (they are really guilty of child and pelvic floor abuse), but if they insist, they will need a consult to 'attempt' a 'trial' of vaginal birth. Or if they really insist on a vaginal birth, who will look after them? Midwives and a few screwy family doctors both working closely with a few dedicated, but likely very strange, doulas.

Since vaginal birth will become obsolete, the specialty of Obstetrics and Gynaecology will become Gynaecology only, as it was before 1921 when Dr Joseph B. DeLee recommended routine episiotomy combined with outlet forceps in part as a way to sideline midwives and general practitioners from birth and 'birthed' the new specialty of Obstetrics and Gynaecology. Caesareans will now be part of that skill set. But who would want to be an obstetrician if there were no decisions to be made, and he/she would become a caesarean technician. But wait, the US Army has successfully trained medical technicians to do caesareans. If all that is required is to know how to do a caesarean section, why not have technicians for birth? In the future, everyone can have a caesarean and large surgicenters can be established where all women will come for their booked caesarean. Rural maternity care will of course disappear and, shortly after that, so will family doctors doing obstetrics, then midwives, then doulas.

Is it possible that vaginal birth is becoming an extreme sport? Midwives and family physicians will become ecotourist guides who cater to those super athletes (read 'nuts') who insist on subjecting themselves to obsolete and dangerous practices. They will practice their arcane rites in secret, usually in rural and remote settings, with the 'back to the landers', the 'end of the worlders' and some throwbacks from the sixties. All will retreat deep into the wilderness to continue to practice their 'arcane' beliefs. If caught, the caregivers will have licenses removed, be prosecuted or burned at the stake once more, while the birthing women will be charged with child abuse.

Sound absurd? Read and re-read Margaret Atwood's *The Handmaid's Tale* and look around you. What can we do? Education, research, analysis, critique and engage women in the struggle to get childbirth back on the women's health agenda.

Has neoliberal feminist ideology impacted the surveillance and management of pregnancy and childbirth?

Michael Klein's birth dystopia illustrates starkly where we may be headed in childbirth if we do not wake up and act now. This book has shown that women and birthworkers are already 'retreating deep into the wilderness' in many countries. We ask, where are the feminists on this issue? We also simultaneously claim to be part of a new wave of feminism picking up the ball that was dropped in the past.

Early second-wave feminists saw pregnancy, birth and mothering as a natural reason for women's oppression (Friedan, 1963; Snitow, 1992), believing nothing would change for women as long as natural reproduction remained the rule. Mainstream discussions around childbirth – even among self-proclaimed feminists – have been mired in, and confused by, complex and heavily contested discussions about fertility and motherhood (Allen, 2005). There are historical reasons for this myopia around childbirth which suggest that our mainstream understanding of its systemic management (and deficiencies) as part of state policy still has a very long way to go.

Attempts to govern fertility have historically reflected the racial, social and structural fissures (Solinger, 2005) we see exemplified and perpetuated in the polarised childbirth discussions published on social media. Gains were often pursued at the expense of women who are poor, of colour or indigenous, have disabilities or identify as LGBTQI (Ross, 2006).

By the early twenty-first century, antifeminist backlash and white supremacist ideologies appeared to join forces to usher in a new era of white liberal feminism through the reconceptualisation of motherhood. Motherhood (and feminism) were reframed from notions of equality to a series of all-attractive neoliberal 'individual choices', together with the pursuit of a new feminist ideology: 'the cult of true womanhood' (Wolf, 2011). Compliance is relabelled 'sensible choice' and individual responsibility – not structural inequality – blamed if things weren't going according to plan (Hallstein, 2010). The 'good mother' ideology valorises the nuclear family and the absolute dedication of the mother. In this narrative of motherhood, the middle-class mother who professionalises homemaking, runs domestic life like a corporation and is highly sexualised has become the symbol of aspirational femininity (Goodwin & Huppatz, 2010) and is contrasted with single, welfare-dependent mothers or women from culturally and linguistically diverse backgrounds (Schmied et al., 2018).

The reconceptualisation of the neoliberal 'good or ideal' mother created an inescapable moral dimension for all women, in both the construction of identity and the assessment of risk. That moral dimension begins at conception, if not earlier, to construct the pregnant woman's identity in binary terms (good/bad, working/stay at home, helicopter/absent, sensible/silly) by reference to her individual ability to anticipate, assess and manage risk (Fixmer-Oraiz, 2019). This mother strives for perfection and compliance, while simultaneously encoding the trope of the 'bad' mother for all the others who are not members of the wealthy, ethnic majority's heterosexual family group. In as much as 'good mothers' are affirmed by the state for their pregnancy, compliance and self-sufficiency, 'bad mothers' – especially women of colour or working-class women – were disapproved for choosing to *become* mothers (Waggoner, 2017).

It was inevitable that neoliberal feminist ideology impacted the surveillance and management of pregnancy and childbirth as has been shown so clearly in this book. Medical maternity care focuses, not on systemic failings in healthcare, but on the individual's compliance with the system. The 'good mother' will anticipate risks, exercise biological prudence and self-governance

(Roberts, 2009) and undertake responsible decision-making (Piepmeier, 2013), in consultation with medical expertise (Rose, 2007). She will submit, without question, to increased surveillance masquerading as 'choice', such as ultrasounds, drugs, tests and genetic screening. When she does not do this she is recast as a 'bad mother', as was the case for many of the women who were interviewed for the research reported in this book.

By the time of her birth, the combination of aforementioned forces will render her powerless, while holding her and her body responsible for any outcome. Restrictions or mandated hospital policy will be presented as 'choice', surveillance technology used to disembody control, and adverse events couched as individual failings or physical shortcomings. It is not surprising in this context that, by the time of birth, women who resist or challenge systemic control or structural deficiencies, like the many we profile in this book, are subject to verbal or physical abuse, neglect and coercion. They are considered the 'bad mothers' and judged by all.

Most of us are unfortunately schooled on childbirth issues through the polemics of medical professionals, women (popularly named 'the mommy wars') or journalists, most of which stem from singular or anecdotal perspectives which assume the neoliberalist ideology without question. We hope this book, aside from busting a few well-known myths and judgements about the women who were brave enough to challenge the maternity health system, will inspire feminists to take a closer look at all aspects of reproductive rights, including the politics of modern childbirth.

Human rights in childbirth have been neglected

As we have shown in this book, human rights, respectful care and informed decision-making are the fundamental aspects of maternity care we have neglected, sometimes as a result of mainstream institutional cultural conditioning, sometimes because we don't believe it is important, and sometimes because we are too egotistical and patriarchal in our attitudes to women. Whatever the reason, they are not valid excuses, so we need to stop making them. We may appear good at saving lives in the developed world today but, in the process, we have become skilled at destroying minds and souls. This can never be seen as an acceptable trade-off. We can have safe and satisfying births now more than at any time in the history of humanity, and we must strive for this and only this. There is no either/or option here. Human rights in childbirth are the greatest challenge facing us today when it comes to maternity care. If you are not up for this challenge as a maternity healthcare provider, it is time to get out. It really is that simple.

We can't be divided over the politics

As we were finalising this book, a long-running investigation and criminal prosecution of an Australian midwife was brought to a close. On 4 June 2019, a South Australian court found a (voluntarily deregistered) midwife not guilty of manslaughter for the deaths of two infants at homebirths she supported in the period between 2009 and 2011. In 2009, Lisa Barrett surrendered her midwifery practising licence and became a birthworker. She supported several high-risk homebirths as an unregistered birthworker in three separate states, including in circumstances where the mothers were cautioned against homebirth by medical professionals and refused by registered PPMs. Following inquests into the deaths of four infants (see Chapters 5 and 14), manslaughter charges were brought against Barrett for two of the deaths. Barrett was prohibited from being around pregnant women and placed under covert surveillance for several years. The judge did not find sufficient evidence to establish manslaughter convictions. The case was dismissed, but not without strong judicial critique of Barrett's practice as falling well below the standard expected of a midwife.

It begs the obvious question: what standard can we impose on a midwife who surrenders her registration? If the detriment associated with registration is greater than the benefits to a midwife, is the process fair and reflective of the realities of woman-centred midwifery practice? What of the role of women in the transaction? They knew that she was not a registered midwife. In all the cases, the women tried to engage with mainstream healthcare services which, despite being well-funded tertiary medical facilities, offered – as Dr Andrew Kotaska put so eloquently (Chapter 20) – 'their way or the highway'. The women chose the highway. To this day, the hospitals and their providers have not been held to account for their role in facilitating the injuries suffered by these families.

Women who cannot access midwifery care that is respectful and that supports their needs will seek support elsewhere or reject professional support altogether. If it isn't already obvious from this book, women across the globe are pursuing their instincts to have a birth as unhindered as possible, in order to protect themselves and their unborn from facilities that present a known or perceived threat to them and their well-being. If midwives are continually pulled into technocratic paradigms of care, women will continue to seek what they instinctively know, or have learned from past births, is safe (woman-centred holistic care). How do we keep missing this message when it is right before of our eyes? How many inquests and prosecutions must we have before we acknowledge the obvious?

The question that we need to ask is how we make the system more responsive to women's needs, while creating standards of care that are as safe as is possible. We believe the safest system, in terms of physical outcomes for women and babies, involves professional midwives working in collaboration with medical practitioners when consultation and referral is required. However, many women, and the researchers leading chapters in this book, have told us there is more to safety than a live mother and baby – there is also morbidity and psychological, social, cultural and spiritual safety. Until we truly grasp this and allow our gaze to shift to a wider horizon, we will continue to be a part of the problem and the impetus for women to birth outside the system.

The only real legacy of the Barrett case has been the increased surveillance and control of pregnant women in Australia and, with it, deep divisions and distrust among women and midwives. Meanwhile, women continue to go underground as they seek to avoid mainstream care. After watching two days of online vitriolic and often polarised discourse on the court's decision in the Barrett case, I (Hannah) posted this message on social media:

> I have been pondering the Lisa Barrett case a lot in the past couple of days. I have watched the polarised discourse unfold and received messages from those who want me to condemn her and from others who want me to sanctify her. I will do neither – not because I don't think her standard of care fell far below what is acceptable; not because I easily dismiss this as not a midwifery issue because she was de-registered and hence not a midwife at the time (how do you ever stop being a midwife?); not because I am unaware of the horror of losing a baby/s when we are failed (I know that intimately). This case goes beyond the individuals involved to a wider system problem we have where traumatised women are driven to impossible choices and lack of options and recognition of women's right to choose and access midwifery care is deliberately obstructed, despite the overwhelming evidence of benefit. We can all make judgments about this one case and we would be missing the point – we have a system problem where women are choosing to birth outside the system because it is so sick. We have a system problem where private midwives are being hunted out of existence for vexatious reasons and we have some de-registering themselves and other unregulated birthworkers filling the gap. We have a polarised response from some midwives and birthworkers who in rejection of the obscene birth intervention rates leave their common sense and duty of care at the door and do harm to women and babies, and we have a system that takes no responsibility for the damage it is causing women and chooses to throw stones while being fully culpable for the crimes they accuse others of. And so my response is this: Let's fix the system and we will have less cause to debate the symptoms of that broken system. While I dismiss none of the gravity of this case, which I have been public about previously, and I feel the distress of those parents failed in this case, let's work together to make the system accountable. A manslaughter charge would not have been the answer here, but I think it was made clear the care was well below any acceptable standard. We need to stop being divided over this issue and become united in focusing on the real problem and join our energies together so we can make sure every woman has the respect and choice she is due. #ENOUGH.
>
> (Hannah Dahlen, Facebook, 6 June 2019)

We made clear, at the start of this book and throughout, that this is not a manifesto on freebirth or high-risk homebirth, and it is not an idealisation of unregulated birthworkers, inadequately trained health providers, or both. It is clear the harm resulting from all these scenarios can be significant and lifelong. When you are the 1:1000 or 1:100 who is harmed, and in some cases failed, then you see this whole subject differently. Our intention was to always ask why women are making this choice in the first place, how the system has failed them and how we can re-engage them into kind and competent maternity care.

We know that for women with low-risk pregnancies, attended by competent registered midwives who are well networked into a responsive system, homebirth is physically safe for women and babies (Scarf et al., 2018; Hutton, Reitsman, Simioni, Brunton, & Kaufman, 2019). However, as you have seen in this book, many women are also seeking care that is more than just physically safe. As I (Hannah) have written recently in a commentary, 'Perhaps we need to ask: is hospital birth safe or sustainable for low-risk women in developed and developing nations? To go down this path, we need to change the embedded narrative, to embrace a definition of safety that women instinctively understand and strive for, including physical, psychological, social, cultural and spiritual safety. It is time we recognized the need for all the professional and maternity consumer groups to unite and agree on the central principles needed to ensure women have safe options when they choose their place of birth, whatever that choice may be' (Dahlen, 2019).

A rigid, evidence-based approach, however, is not necessarily a human rights approach. This book has shown that many of the women seeking to birth outside the system did not access gold-standard care. Our aim in this book is to finally hold the system to account for failing to provide women with the care they are seeking and for bullying and harassing women who make 'off-menu' choices. The question we ask in this book is why do we get the mandate to condemn birth outside the system while we ignore our part in driving women way? It's time for all of us to work together to make birth safe (physically, psychologically, socially, culturally and spiritually).

This book is squarely aimed at the way in which maternity healthcare is being developed and structured across globe into rigid, hierarchical structures that pursue dehumanised, process-driven healthcare services that are hostile and disrespectful to women. Where generations of healthy women and babies are being forced, for convenience or financial, political and stakeholder reasons, to attend childbirth facilities structured to offer substandard care with impunity, conceal mistakes, shirk responsibility and shield careproviders who engage in horrific, abusive and coercive treatment.

There is work to be done, and it begins with learning, understanding and developing agreement over the way forward. We need to put aside our personal preferences and beliefs, and ask ourselves: what kind of system do we need to create that protects and supports the families we are bringing into this world?

The canary is still highly regarded … by some

While at the 2019 Normal Labour and Birth Conference in the UK, I (Hannah) met Maltese obstetrician Jean Calleja-Agius, who shared my enthusiasm for the concept behind the canary in the coal mine. She told me that, to this day in the small village squares in Malta, men are seen socialising on Sundays or after work with canaries in cages tucked closely and affectionately under their arms. It is not known if the men are descendants of miners. Coal mining never took place in Malta, which was known for its limestone quarries, the stone used for building in Malta. Malta was, however, a British colony for almost 200 years. Many of the British expats, especially the Welsh, may have passed on the stories of forefathers who were coal miners and who trusted their lives to their canary. These big burly Maltese men with hairy chests and masculine traits tend to the birds like pets (see Figure 21.2), bringing their canaries to cafés or bars, tenderly placing the cage on the table beside them before they start drinking one glass after another of homemade wine. When the evening ends, they tuck the canary cage under their arm and head off to their home, making sure to stay in the shade so as not to make the canary uncomfortable. These little songbirds are so revered they have become part of the community's social activities today. In 2006, Malta issued a postage stamp with a picture of the canary. The canary matters!

Conclusion

The writing of this book, and the research in it, has been a journey for us and for many of our authors. We made a decision to include these journeys, to deepen our collective understanding that the mainstream maternity system affects all of us: women and their families, health professionals, lawyers, coroners, government bodies, researchers, educators, regulators, professional bodies and policy-makers. When the canary falls silent in the coal mine, we all need to respond, with and for that canary.

So we leave you with these questions. What do we think of the canaries (the women we care for) in our coal mines (maternity care)? Do we heed their warnings? Do we listen responsively for their joy and their silence or do we ignore them and keep mining away, releasing more and more poisonous gasses and toxic fumes to destroy us all in the process? If we think ignoring the canary will lead to the demise of the canary only, we need to think again. We are all in this together. What is toxic for women will inevitably be, if it is not already, toxic for us, the maternity service providers. Being responsive and respectful to women in our care is about all our survival. The toxic maternity care environments women increasingly experience today are leading to more women choosing to birth outside the system. They are our canary in the coal mine and we need to listen now, for all our sakes.

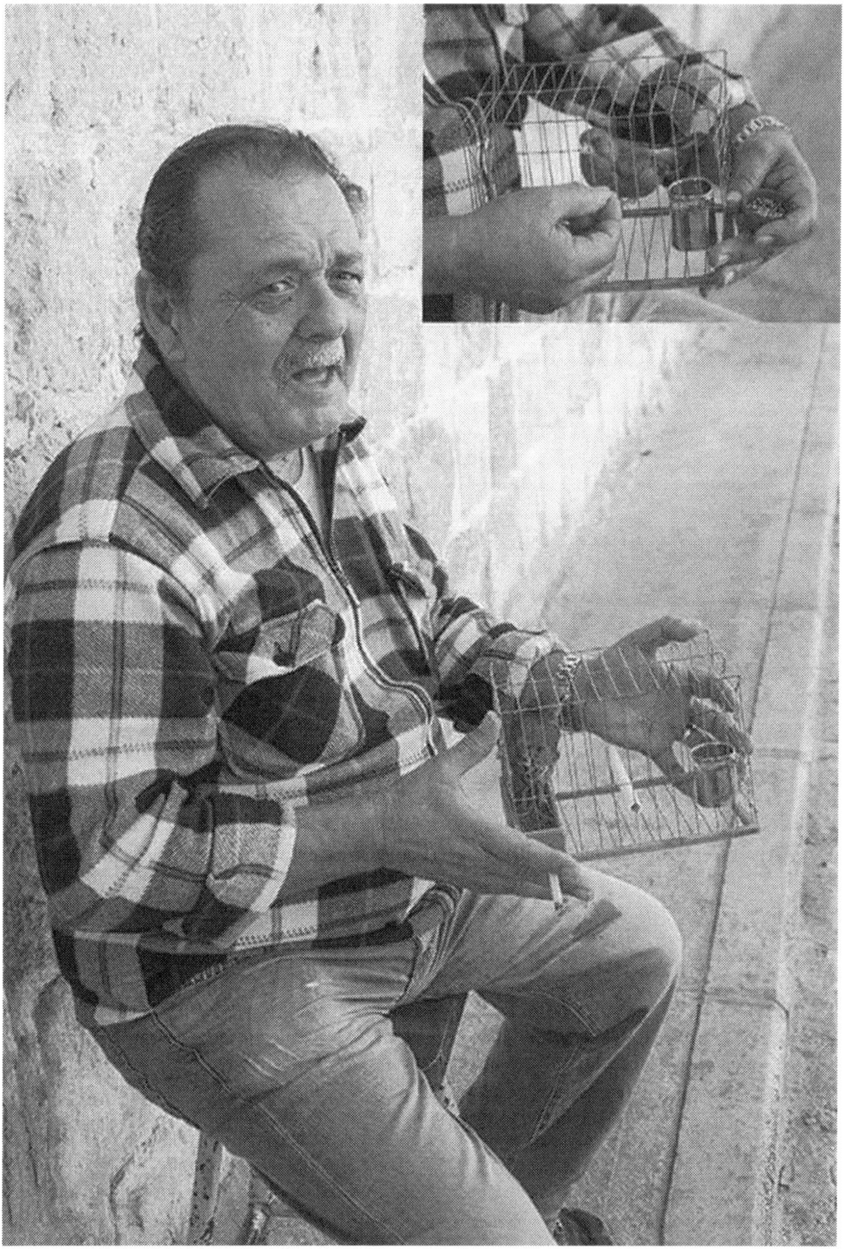

Figure 21.2 Maltese man with his canary
Source: Photo taken by obstetrician Jean Calleja Agius.

St Augustine said 'Give me other mothers and I will give you another world', but this should be phrased differently: 'Give me another world and I will give you other mothers'. We cannot expect our mothers to mother with strength and spirit if we crush that strength and spirit with our care during childbirth. Join us today to put a stop to the abuse and let's work together to give all childbearing women in the future 'another world' to mother in. Only then will women, their children, families and communities be able to give us the world we know is possible.

References

Allen, A. (2005). *Feminism and motherhood in Western Europe, 1890–1970: The maternal dilemma.* New York, NY: Palgrave MacMillan.

Bohren, M. A., Vogel, J. P., Hunter, E. C., Lutsiv, O., Makh, S. K., Souza, J. P., ... Tunçalp, Ö. (2015). The mistreatment of women during childbirth in health facilities globally: A mixed-methods systematic review. *PLoS Medicine, 12*(6), e1001847.

Dahlen, H. G. (2019). Is it time to ask whether facility based birth is safe for low risk women and their babies? *EClinical Medicine, 14*, 9–10. doi:10.1016/j.eclinm.2019.08.003.

Fixmer-Oraiz, N. (2019). Securing motherhood on the home front. In *Homeland maternity: US security culture and the new reproductive regime* (pp. 31–58). Urbana, IL: University of Illinois Press. Retrieved from: www.jstor.org.ezproxy1.library.usyd.edu.au/stable/10.5406/j.ctvfrxq2m.6.

Friedan, F. (1963). *Feminine mystique.* London: Penguin.

Goodwin, S. & Huppatz, K. (2010). *The good mother: Contemporary motherhoods in Australia.* Sydney: Sydney University Press.

Hallstein, D. L. O. (2010). Public choices, private control: How mediated mom labels work rhetorically to dismantle the politics of choice and white second wave feminist successes. In S. Hayden & D. L. O'Brien Hallstein (Eds.), *Contemplating maternity in an era of choice: Explorations into discourses of reproduction* (p. 7). Lanham, MD: Lexington Books.

Human Rights in Childbirth. (2019). Human Rights in Childbirth (HRiC) website. Retrieved from: https://humanrightsinchildbirth.org/.

Hutton, E., Reitsman, A., Simioni, J., Brunton, G., & Kaufman, K. (2019). Perinatal or neonatal mortality among women who intend at the onset of labour to give birth at home compared to women of low obstetrical risk who intend to give birth in hospital: A systematic review and meta-analyses. *EClinicalMedicine (Lancet), 14*, 59–70.

Miller, S., Abalos, E., Chamillard, M., Ciapponi, A., Colaci, D., Comandé, D., ... Langer, A. (2016). Beyond too little, too late and too much, too soon: A pathway towards evidence-based, respectful maternity care worldwide. *The Lancet, 388*, 2176–2192.

OVOItalia. (2017) First data on obstetric violence in Italy. *Osservatorio sulla Violenza Ostetrica Italia (OVOItalia).* Retrieved from: https://ovoitalia.wordpress.com/2017/11/04/first-data-on-obstetric-violence-in-italy/.

Piepmeier, A. (2013). The inadequacy of 'choice': Disability and what's wrong with feminist framings of reproduction. *Feminist Studies, 39*, 159–186.

Renfrew, M. J., Homer, C. S. E., Downe, S., McFadden, A., Muir, N., Prentice, T., & Ten Hoope-Bender, P. (2014). The *Lancet's* series on midwifery executive summary. *Lancet,* June 2014, 1–8.

Roberts, D. (2009). Race, gender, and genetic technologies: A new reproductive dystopia? *Signs: Journal of Women in Culture and Society*, *34*, 783–804.

Rose, N. S. (2007). *The politics of life itself: Biomedicine, power, and subjectivity in the twenty-first century*. Princeton, NJ: Princeton University Press.

Ross, L. J. (2006). Understanding reproductive justice: Transforming the pro-choice movement. *Off Our Backs*, *36*(4), 14–19.

Safe Motherhood For All Inc. (2017). Women's experiences of birth care in Australia: The Birth Dignity Survey 2017. Safe Motherhood for All Inc. Retrieved from: www.safemotherhoodforall.org.au/wp-content/uploads/2017/05/Dignity-Survey-Safe-Motherhood-for-All-Circulated.pdf.

Safe Motherhood For All. (2019) Respectful maternity care: The universal rights of childbearing women. Retrieved from www.whiteribbonalliance.org/index.cfm/act-now/respectful-maternity-care/.

Scarf, V. L., Rossiter, C., Vedam, S., Dahlen, H. G., Ellwood, D., Forster, D., … Homer, C. S. E. (2018). Maternal and perinatal outcomes by planned place of birth among women with low-risk pregnancies in high-income countries: A systematic review and meta-analysis. *Midwifery, 62*, 240–255.

Schmied, V., Kearney, E., & The Maternal Anxiety White Paper Group. (2018). Tackling maternal anxiety in the perinatal period: Reconceptualising mothering narratives. Health and Well-being White Paper Series, Western Sydney University. Retrieved from: www.westernsydney.edu.au/__data/assets/pdf_file/0010/1483885/Maternal_Anxiety_White_Papers_FINAL.pdf.

Snitow, A. (1992). Feminism and motherhood: An American reading. *Feminist Review, 40*, 32–51.

Solinger, R. (2005). *Pregnancy and power: A short history of reproductive politics in America*. New York, NY: New York University Press.

The White Ribbon Alliance For Safer Motherhood. (2011). *Respectful maternity care: The universal rights of childbearing women*. Washington, DC: White Ribbon Alliance.

Vedam, S., Stoll, K., Rubashkin, N., Martina, K., Miller-Vedam, Z., Hayes-Kleine, H., … The CCinBC Steering Council. (2017). The Mothers on Respect (MOR) index: Measuring quality, safety, and human rights in childbirth. *SSM – Population Health, 3*, 201–210.

Waggoner, M. (2017). *The zero trimester: Pre-pregnancy care and the politics of reproductive risk*. Berkeley, CA: University of California Press.

Wolf, J. (2011). *Is breast best? Taking on the breastfeeding experts and the new high stakes of motherhood* (p. 76). New York, NY: New York University Press.

World Health Organisation. (2014). Prevention and elimination of disrespect and abuse during childbirth. World Health Organisation – Sexual and Reproductive Health. Retrieved from: www.who.int/reproductivehealth/topics/maternal_perinatal/statement-childbirth/en/.

World Health Organisation. (2016). *Midwives voices midwives realities: Findings from a global consultation on providing quality midwifery care*. Geneva: WHO.

World Health Organisation. (2018). *WHO recommendations: Intrapartum care for a positive childbirth experience*. Geneva: WHO.

World Health Organisation. (2019). *Strengthening quality midwifery education for Universal Health Coverage 2030: Framework for action*. Geneva: WHO.

Glossary of terms

Aunty A term of respect and recognition given to a female elder in the Aboriginal community.

Australian College of Midwives (ACM) The peak national organisation and professional body for midwives in Australia (www.midwives.org.au/).

Australian Health Practitioners Regulation Agency (AHPRA) The national regulatory body for health professionals, including midwives, in Australia (www.ahpra.gov.au/).

Bait-and-switch A common but unlawful business practice of advertising or making representations that are fraudulent to entice consumers to purchase a good or service. It is especially prevalent in industries where consumers are not able to assess the quality of the good or service they are acquiring prior to consumption, such as the provision of maternity healthcare services. The 'bait' is the promise or representation that a particular service (such as skin-to-skin or waterbirth) will be offered. The 'switch' occurs when the woman arrives in hospital only to discover that the advertised services are either not offered or not available, and she is pressured to consider unwanted or unacceptable alternatives.

Birth centre Midwifery-led units providing home-like birth environments. They may be located within a hospital, alongside a hospital or standalone.

Borning Used to refer to a much wider and more symbolic process for Aboriginal people. Where one is 'found' refers to the rebirth of a 'spirit child' from the Dreamtime ancestors who belong to a particular area of Country which may be the grandmother's or grandfather's Country. The child has strong traditional affiliations to the Country where he or she was found and will later assume rights and responsibilities for Law, the land and its people. Women with particular familial and traditional affiliations, usually the grandmothers and aunts, are in attendance during birthing in an *alukura apmere alaltyeke* (a single women's camp in the country).

Breech presentation When a baby is lying bottom down or feet down in the uterus instead of the more common head down position.

Cholestasis of pregnancy Where women experience very severe itching in late pregnancy when hormones are at their peak and this goes away a few days after birth.

Community midwifery/birth Care provided in the community and most often used to refer to midwifery care and homebirth in the USA.

Country Sacred to Aboriginal and Torres Strait Islander people and denotes the traditional cultural land that 'owns' a group of people.

Dehumanisation, dehumanising The process of treating someone under your control as less human or as 'sub-human' through direct actions (commission) or lack of action (omission).

Doula A doula provides non-medical pregnancy, birth and/or postnatal support to women. This may include providing information, emotional support or physical support in labour such as massage (www.dona.org/what-is-a-doula/).

Dreaming Explains how things came to be for Aboriginal people and how the ancestral spirits made the earth and people.

Entonox A gas with 50% oxygen and 50% Nitrous which women can breathe through a mouthpiece during labour to help with pain relief. Also known as gas and air.

Episiotomy A surgical cut made at the opening of the vagina during childbirth.

Failsafe Failsafe is not intended to imply infallibility. Rather, it means a system that is intended to counteract the effect of an anticipated possible source of failure.

Freebirth A planned unassisted homebirth, whereby there is no midwife or medically trained birth professional in attendance.

Freebirther A woman who freebirths.

Freebirthing The act of having a freebirth.

Iatrogenesis Inadvertent harm introduced by medical care or treatment.

Janani Suraksha Yojana (JSY) Scheme Scheme introduced by the Government of India to increase institutional birth through the use of incentive payment schemes and pregnancy surveillance.

Kristeller manoeuvre Application of fundal pressure (pressure on the uterus) during the second stage of labour.

Lay-midwife Also sometimes called a traditional birth attendant, an unregistered birthworker who provides homebirth support services to women.

Legal or juridicial personhood The judicial act of recognising the legal rights and identity of a person. Legal personhood automatically attaches to anyone born alive. Debates about legal personhood usually arise in the context of a claim for foetal rights or the rights of a foetus before a live birth.

Medicare A publicly funded universal healthcare scheme in Australia. Medicare provides free or subsidised access to healthcare services for Australian citizens and permanent residents in public hospitals and from a range of care professionals such as medical practitioners, nurses and midwives who have been provided with a Medicare number (www.humanservices.gov.au/customer/subjects/medicare-services).

Medicare Benefits Schedule (MBS) A listing of the Medicare services subsidised by the Australian government.

Medicare Provider Number (MPN) A number used for Medicare claims processing. It is used to identify the practitioner and their practice location when processing claims.

Mob A term identifying a group of Aboriginal people associated with a particular place or Country. It is a term that is extremely important to Aboriginal people because it is used to identify who they are and where they are from.

National Maternity Services Review (MSR) A review conducted in 2009 that sought submissions from the public and interest groups on maternity services in Australia. The aim was to identify gaps and changes need and inform priorities for national action.

National Registration and Accreditation Scheme (NRAS) A registration and accreditation scheme for health practitioners that commenced on 1 July 2010 and was established by state and territory governments in Australia through the introduction of consistent legislation in all jurisdictions.

Nursing and Midwifery Board of Australia (NMBA) The regulatory board for Nurses and Midwives in Australia.

Pethidine A fast-acting opioid analgesic drug used commonly during labour for pain relief.

Pharmaceutical Benefits Schedule (PBS) The PBS provides timely, reliable and affordable access to necessary medicines for Australians. The PBS is part of the Australian Government's broader National Medicines Policy.

Postpartum haemorrhage (PPH) The traditional definition of primary PPH is the loss of 500 ml or more of blood from the genital tract within 24 hours of the birth of a baby. PPH can be minor (500–1000 ml) or major (more than 1000 ml). Major could be divided to moderate (1000–2000 ml) or severe (more than 2000 ml).

Post-traumatic stress disorder (PTSD) A type of anxiety disorder. Some people develop PTSD after experiencing a traumatic event. People affected may feel anxious and highly vigilant and have intrusive thoughts and memories of the trauma.

Privately practising midwives (PPM) Midwives who are self-employed or work within a group of PPMs; they are not employed by a health service. Most PPMs provide continuity of care across the full scope of midwifery practice and provide homebirth services. The women employ them directly.

Professional Indemnity Insurance (PII) Arrangements that secure, for the practitioner's professional practice, insurance from civil liability incurred by, or loss arising from, a claim that is made as a result of a negligent act, error or omission in the conduct of the practitioner.

Publicly funded homebirth programmes A midwifery model of care provided through the public hospital system and caters to women who are at low obstetric and medical risk. Midwives working within this model are employed by the public hospital and the midwives' hospital employer provides their professional indemnity insurance. Women's ability to access this model is limited and assessed against strict medical selection criteria and women must remain low-risk throughout their childbirth experience.

Shroud waving The practice of focusing in an unbalanced way on the potentially negative effects of a health implication to coerce a patient to take up the treatment or intervention you prefer.

Stretch and sweep A technique sometimes used to try to initiate labour. It involves the clinician inserting their index finger into the woman's cervix and sweeping around to separate the amniotic membrane from the cervix.

The exemption An exemption to the requirement of insurance provided under section 284 of the National Law from PII for PPMs providing intrapartum care in the home in Australia.

Trauma-informed care Care that assumes a person is likely to have a history of trauma (sexual, emotional, or physical). Providers try not to re-traumatise the person they are caring for, whether intentionally or unintentionally. The Five Guiding Principles are safety, choice, collaboration, trustworthiness and empowerment.

Twilight Sleep A morphine–scopolamine cocktail that used to be widely used as an anaesthetic/amnesiac during labour. It caused women to be unable to consciously remember labours in which they became highly agitated and were in tremendous pain yet were unable to actively communicate or participate. Twilight Sleep typically necessitated large episiotomies and forceps deliveries followed by resuscitation of morphine-drugged babies. Twilight Sleep was promoted as feminist progress, a release from the pains of labour. For about a year in 1914–1915, upper-class white women led a campaign for access to Twilight Sleep. Although it quickly became apparent that it was in fact bad for mothers and babies, it took decades to end the practice.

Unassisted birth *see* Freebirth

Unregulated birth worker (UBW) A person who attends women planning a homebirth but who is not a registered midwife or doctor. They may have experience or knowledge of childbirth and may be a doula, childbirth educator, lay-midwife or ex-registered midwife.

Vaginal birth after caesarean (VBAC) When a baby is born vaginally after the mother has had at least one previous caesarean section.

Vaginal examination (VE) A digital examination attended by a midwife or doctor to determine cervical dilatation and descent of the presenting part of a foetus.

Index

Made in the USA
Monee, IL
12 November 2026

0c110482-065d-4589-90d7-e5861d8edc5cR01